Physical Diagnosis

D1518652

CONCISE TEXTBOOK SERIES

- **Physical Diagnosis,** Siegfried J. Kra, M.D., editor
- **Dermatology,** James W. Patterson, M.D., and W. Kenneth Blaylock, M.D.
- **Obstetrics,** Ralph W. Hale, M.D., and John A. Krieger, M.D., editors
- **Anesthesiology,** Thomas J. DeKornfeld, M.D., editor
- **Essential Neurology, Third Edition,** William Pryse-Phillips, M.D., and T.J. Murray, M.D.
- **Psychiatry, Fifth Edition,** Merrill T. Eaton, Jr., M.D., Margaret H. Peterson, M.D., and James A. Davis, M.D.
- **Acute Internal Medicine,** Laurence B. Gardner, M.D., editor
- **Gynecology,** Ralph W. Hale, M.D., and John A. Krieger, M.D., editors
- **Endocrinology, Third Edition,** Ernest L. Mazzaferri, M.D., editor
- **Pediatric Allergy, Third Edition,** Michael R. Sly, M.D.
- **Rheumatology,** Robert A. Turner, M.D., and Christopher M. Wise, M.D., editors
- **Infectious Diseases,** Robert H. Waldman, M.D., and Ronica M. Kluge, M.D., editors
- **Clinical Nuclear Medicine Imaging, Third Edition,** Philip Matin, M.D., editor

IN PREPARATION:

- **Gastroenterology,** Frank L. Iber, M.D., and Richard Baum, M.D.

A CONCISE TEXTBOOK

Physical Diagnosis

Edited by

Siegfried J. Kra, M.D.
Associate Clinical Professor of Medicine
Yale University School of Medicine
New Haven, Connecticut

Medical Examination Publishing Company

NOTICE

The authors and publisher of this book have made every effort to ensure
that all therapeutic modalities that are recommended are in accordance with
accepted standards at the time of publication.

The drugs specified within this book may not have specific approval by the
Food and Drug Administration in regard to the indications and dosages that
are recommended by the authors. The manufacturer's package insert is the
best source of current prescribing information.

Medical Examination Publishing Company
A Division of Elsevier Science Publishing Co., Inc.
52 Vanderbilt Avenue, New York, New York 10017

© 1987 by Elsevier Science Publishing Co., Inc.

This book has been registered with the Copyright Clearance Center, Inc.
For futher information, please contact the Copyright Clearance Center, Inc.,
Salem, Massachusetts.

Library of Congress Cataloging in Publication Data

Physical diagnosis.

    (Concise textbook series)
    Includes bibliographies and index.
    1. Physical diagnosis.   I. Kra, Siegfried J.
[DNLM: 1. Diagnosis. 2. Physical Examination.
WB 200 P578]
RC76.P49   1987   616.07'54   87-7905

ISBN 0-444-01044-0

Current printing (last digit):
10 9 8 7 6 5 4 3 2 1

Manufactured in the United States of America

This book is dedicated to our students
who have endured our teaching for all these years,
and hopefully will continue to do so in the future.

Contents

Foreword

As modern medicine becomes increasingly oriented toward technologic approaches, the distinctively human features of patients have become increasingly neglected. Doctors often order technologic tests rather than talk, and may examine blood, specimens, films, and tracings rather than patients themselves. Nevertheless, anyone who cares for patients knows that the prime information to be considered for most medical decisions consists of the patient's symptoms, signs, functional capacity, emotional state, and other attributes that can be noted only from direct examination.

In this book, Dr. Kra and his colleagues have tried not only to describe the examination process, but also to improve the state of the art. The authors have produced a valuable distillation of their extensive experience in patient care. The book is dedicated to medical students and intended for them, but physicians of all ages can find many historical vignettes, clinical "pearls," and pragmatic recommendations that are entertaining and enlightening. The comments may not evoke universal agreement, but they have the advantage—rare in many books today—of being lively and forthright, and reflecting personal styles, adventures, and beliefs.

Although worthwhile for its instruction to contemporary medical students, this book will also be of interest to medical historians in the future. The text contains a thoughtful account of the way in which physicians practicing near the end of the twentieth century tried to arrive at an effective compromise between exploiting the majestic achievements of modern technology while avoiding its dehumanizing distractions from clinical art.

Alvan R. Feinstein, M.D., F.A.C.P.
Professor of Medicine and Epidemiology
Director, Robert Wood Johnson
  Clinical Scholars Program
Yale University School of Medicine
New Haven, Connecticut

ix

Preface

In the past 25 years, the practice of medicine has changed more drastically than it has in the past hundred years. Practicing medicine has become extraordinarily more complex and difficult each year. It would be ludicrous and presumptuous to have one or two authors claim themselves experts on all the areas of the body. Instead, each expert in his field tells us the best and most expedient manner of how to conduct a physical examination of his area.

Each section can stand by itself as a subspecialty. Naturally, the style will differ according to each contributor. The common thread that connects all the chapters is the method of physical diagnosis.

This textbook will prepare students to conduct a thorough physical examination and enable them to readily master the subspecialty clinics. A general outline of the anatomy and pathophysiology is included in many of the chapters so the student can better understand the physical findings.

I particularly wish to thank the students, Jeffrey Barkin, Charles Brackett, Martin Chenevert, and Autry Parker, for their excellent critique and help in making this textbook possible. I also wish to thank Dr. Lawrence S. Cohen and Dr. Donald Dock for his suggestions on the cardiopulmonary section, and my able assistant and typist, Madelyn Bartone.

Introduction

Physical diagnosis is the last bastion of the clinical practice of medicine. The art of diagnosis may soon become antiquated unless there is a revival of this ancient technique of using our own basic tools of the trade: *our senses*.

Can you picture one day in the life of a resident without blood gases, CAT scan, multigated nuclear scanning, and sonar of the abdomen and the heart? If all at once we had an electrical power failure and we no longer had the thallium stress test, the digital arteriogram, the nuclear magnetic resonance, the positron tomography, mammography, brain scan, and so forth, what chaos! Are there any more Osler's in our midst?

This book not only explains physical diagnosis, it also explains how to retain our identity as clinicians: our ability to diagnose an ailment without expensive cumbersome test—tests which should be used to verify the diagnosis, not to make it. Our trained brains must remain in command and not allow the technicians to become the warlords of our medical practices. The brilliance of our medical forefathers with their ingenious intuition and Sherlock Holmes' sense of detection must be carried on—propagated and retold in a precise clear fashion.

Physical diagnosis can be fun and rewarding, but doing it well requires training, retraining, and practicing—which is why our profession is called the *practice* of medicine.

Imagine, thousands of years of medical practice have passed and we still use the observations of Hippocrates (the father of bedside diagnosis!), Sydenham, Heberdon, Charcot, Laennec, Leopold Auenbrugger, Battista Morgagni, and Osler—these names will resound throughout this book, for it is they who taught us the art of physical diagnosis.

It is the principle of Hippocrates that will be followed in this book on physical diagnosis. "A great part, I believe, of the art is to be able to observe. Leave nothing to chance. Overlook nothing. Combine contradictory observations and allow yourself enough time.''

Listen to Hippocrates first description of the clubbing of fingers, a sign of pulmonary disease. ''Water accumulates, the patient has fever and cough, the respirations are fast, the feet become edematous and swollen, the nails appear curved, and the patient suffers as if he had pus inside, only less severe and more protected. One can recognize that it is not pus, but water. If you put your ear against the chest, you can hear a seethe inside like sour wine.''

''Study the patient rather than the disease,'' Hippocrates said. ''The patient's makeup, his surroundings, and his way of life are all important in evaluating his state of illness and likelihood of recovery. Observe the nature of each country diet, customs, the age of the patient, speech, manners, fashion, even his silence, his thoughts. If he sleeps, or is suffering from lack of sleep, learn the content and origin of his dreams. One has to study all these signs to analyze what they portend. Evaluate honestly.''

Hippocrates taught us that ''life is short and the art long.'' It is necessary for the physician ''to diagnose and treat.''

Physical diagnosis began when Hippocrates placed his ear directly on the patient's chest. ''In hydrops of the lungs, if applying your ear against the chest, you listen for some time, it boils within like vinegar, and again when the lung falls against the breast, the patient has a cough, he feels pains in his chest, a sound like that of leather is heard'' (this undoubtedly was the friction rub).

Leopold Auenbrugger published a book in Austria in 1780 that became the talk of Europe. The book was about his new invention, ''percussion.'' Auenbrugger made the simple observation that when you tap your fingers over a hollow log, it makes a different sound than a solid log. He applied the same principle to tapping his fingers over a lung filled with air which sounded like a drum, while a lung that is filled with fluid, as in pneumonia, made a different sound—a dull sound. An innkeeper's son, Auenbrugger observed his father slap the sides of the kegs of beer to determine at what level the fermentation had reached. The vibrations told his father whether it was liquid or solid in the casks.

Auenbrugger stated in his book, ''These volumes of sound depend on the cause which can diminish or increase the volume of air commonly in the thoracic cavity. Such a cause, whether it be in the solid or liquid mass, produces what we observe, for example, in casks, which, when they are empty, resound at all points, but, when filled, lose just so much of this resonance as the volume of air which they contained has been diminished.''

It took a French physician, Jean Nicolas Corvisart (1755–1821), to put the new invention into clinical use. He percussed lungs, recorded his observations, and verified his hypotheses and findings at the ''final court of appeal,'' the autopsy. Corvisart had a young man in his tutelage by the name of Rene Theophile Hyacinthe Laennec, born in February 1781, in Rouxeau, France.

Prior to the great French physician, Laennec, listening to the heart and chest was a rudimentary technique. The custom had been to apply the ear directly to the chest wall and sounds would be heard that the physician tried to interpret. It was quite a scene. The doctor would uncover the chest, and, if it was a female patient, place a napkin across her bosom and slyly remove it, and place his ear over the patient's breast. The patient would generally be sitting in a chair, and the good doctor, garbed in black, would contort his body and listen to the movement of the heart and lungs.

Laennec worked in the Hospital Necker in Paris, and felt great disgust with this manner of listening to the heart. As this was a charity hospital, most of the patients had lice and he had his share of these nasty creatures. Each night, returning to his apartment, he scrubbed his body with lye, usually to no avail. Furthermore, placing his ear on a young woman's breast distracted him so that "blood would rush to his head and cause a confusion of sounds."

Laennec was particularly chagrined with an obese girl who was suffering from a heart condition. Listening to her heart was useless, for only faint and distant sounds could be heard. Walking through the gardens of the Louvre one day, Laennec came upon a pile of litter where a group of children were playing with a hollow wooden beam. Two groups were at each end of the beam. While one group scratched and tapped at one end, the second group, their ears pressed to the other end, listened in childish amazement to the sound.

Laennec observed the scene and swiftly set out for the Necker Hospital in an excited state. Reaching the room of his patient, he seized a magazine, rolled it into a tight cylinder, and, to the amazement of the other doctors, placed one end of the crude instrument against the patient's heart and applied his ear to the other end. He could hear the heart sounds and also those of the lung. Emotions usually carefully suppressed by him were now stirred, "for the possibilities of the discovery were instantly seen."

To improve the instrument, he used a *corne de papier* on the famous Madame de Stael, who developed fluid in her lungs that Laennec discovered by means of his instrument.

Tiring of rolling up paper cylinders and tying them with string, Laennec learned to use a lathe and made solid batons, each about a foot long. He could hear the heart sounds better. He devised cylinders made of skin inflated with air. In the end, Laennec found that a light wood, preferably beech or linden, was the most satisfactory.

The instrument, at first, went under many names. He called it a cylinder himself. Others called it a baton; others a solo meter or a *cornet medicale*. It was Laennec who finally changed the name to stethoscope. Revolutionary as it was, Laennec became the laughing stock of the medical profession. The local Paris newspapers carried cartoons and caricatures of the new instrument.

A charming picture of Laennec and a general attitude towards the discovery is found in Kipling's story of the "un Arkele witches." Oliver Wendell Holmes, in his "stethoscope song," wrote amusingly of the "listening tube for sounding the heart":

> There was a young man in Bostontown
> He bought him a stethoscope nice and new
> All mounted and finished and polished down
> With an ivory cap and a stopper too.
>
> It happened a spider within it did crawl
> And spinned him a web of ample size
> Whereon there chanced one day to fall
> A couple of very imprudent flies.

The doctors being very sore
A stethoscope did they devise
They had a rammer to clear the bore
With a knob at the end to kill the flies.

Now use your ears all you who can
But don't forget to mind your eyes
Or you may be cheated like this young man
By a couple of silly abnormal flies.

Laennec, who suffered from asthma all his life, studied respiratory sounds by percussion and auscultation. He described, with an uncanny accuracy, emphysema, pneumothorax, and divided rales into moist rales or crepitations, mucous rales or gurgling, dry sonorous rales or snoring, and dry sibilant rales or whistling. He described the percussion signs of pneumonia. In spite of his efforts, any physician using a stethoscope in the 1800s was considered a charlatan.

Laennec not only auscultated the lungs, but also the heart. He described blowing murmurs, although he incorrectly thought they were physiological, and, for a number of years, a blowing murmur was not considered important. It was Laennec who heard sounds that nobody had ever heard with his wooden stethoscope, and coined such words as bronchophony, pectoriloquy, and egophony.

Men like Corvisart and Laennec thought they were able to differentiate for the first time between cavitary tuberculosis, pneumonia, and bronchiectasis. Perhaps the reader, the student, will also find a sound heretofore undiscovered.

Paris remained the medical center of the world, until 1830, when a gentleman by the name of Josef Skoda, a portly looking man, balding, who wore Benjamin Franklin glasses, became the leading clinician of the new Vienna school—the first medical teacher to lecture in German. It was this physician who classified the different sounds in the chest according to their pitch, their tone, going from hollow, dull, tympanic, muffled, high to deep. Skoda was a bachelor, a whimsical gentleman, dressed in bizarre clothing. Unfortunately, he had little concern for his patients; they were objects of his investigations. He had no interest in treatment and cared little for the humane side of medical practice. He was more interested in confirming his diagnoses by postmortem examination. He published a book that described the methodology of physical diagnosis which remained the guide for physicians for decades. He outlined its limitations and is quoted as saying that "diseases which are entirely different may show the same findings on percussion and auscultation, and vice versa, the same disease may show the right variety of findings when we percuss or auscultate because sounds depend not upon the chemical but upon the anatomical state of the organs."

What was next to follow in improving the technology of diagnosis were the laryngoscope, the bronchoscope, the ophthalmoscope, the signoidoscope, and so forth, up to the present day of incredible technology that should be used to confirm what is suspect as wrong.

Contributors

Caleb Gonzalez, M.D.
Professor of Ophthalmology, Yale University School of Medicine, New Haven, Connecticut

Peter Grannum, M.D.
Assistant Professor of Obstetrics and Gynecology, Yale University School of Medicine, New Haven, Connecticut

Siegfried J. Kra, M.D.
Associate Clinical Professor of Medicine, Yale University School of Medicine, New Haven, Connecticut

Keat-Jin Lee, M.D.
Assistant Clinical Professor of Surgery, Yale University School of Medicine, New Haven, Connecticut

Ronald D. Lee, M.D.
Assistant Professor of Urology, Yale University School of Medicine, New Haven, Connecticut

Sherwin B. Nuland, M.D.
Associate Clinical Professor of Surgery, Yale University School of Medicine, New Haven, Connecticut

Ethan D. Nydorf, M.D.
Assistant Professor of Dermatology, Yale University School of Medicine, New Haven, Connecticut

Arthur M. Seigel, M.D.
Assistant Clinical Professor of Pediatrics and Neurology, Yale University School of Medicine, New Haven, Connecticut

John Shine, M.D.
Clinical Instructor of Surgery (Orthopedics), Yale University School of Medicine, New Haven, Connecticut.

Alan Sholomskas, M.D.
Assistant Clinical Professor of Psychiatry, Yale University School of Medicine, New Haven, Connecticut

Thomas Vris, M.D.
Clinical Instructor, Section of Otolaryngology, Yale University School of Medicine, New Haven, Connecticut

Physical Diagnosis

1
The Art of History Taking

Siegfried J. Kra, M.D.

SOME GENERAL COMMENTS

History taking is an art. It requires much experience and a certain amount of intuitiveness to zero in precisely on the patient's problem. There is no area of medicine that requires a keener medical sense than taking a productive history. Preferably, it should be performed under comfortable, ideal conditions, with as much privacy as possible.

A good history can make the difference between a correct and an incorrect diagnosis. The patient must be encouraged to tell his/her tale of woe. Failing to ask the right questions can lead the clinician down the dismal path of failure, and the patient can suffer irreparable harm. I always say to my students, "Listen to the patients and they may give you the correct diagnosis." The more medical knowledge you have, the better you are able to take a history. It is the art of flushing out bits of relevant information that not even the patient realized existed.

Learning to listen is not easy. The mind must not be allowed to wander to the Miami Dolphins or that perfect person you just met. The patient can quickly detect if you are not fully concerned with his tale. So often, the patient complains about a physician: "He is a nice man, but he never listens. He does all the talking and is in too much of a hurry."

Take your time. Ask your questions, but wait for the answers, and do not rush to the next question before the patient has a chance to answer the previous one. This is not only discourteous, but harmful to the most precious commodity in medicine, the doctor–patient relationship. The doctor–patient relationship is sacred. It is during the history taking that it has its inception. Just as you have to make the preliminary assessment of the person who seeks your help, that person also makes his or her own quick judgments regarding your sincerity, your competence, your concern, your affability, and "Are you going to be able to help me?"

A question phrased indiscreetly with lack of sensitivity, or poorly timed, can not only impair the doctor–patient relationship but also close off any information that might have been reaped. The history taking should lead directly to the problem.

The tone of the interview should be sympathetic, firm, never autocratic, never condescending, but always understanding. The patient should at no time feel as a subaltern to you.

Your general appearance is not to be neglected. There should be dignity in conduct and in dress. Wearing a grease-spotted, tattered sweater and unclean clothing was fashionable for Albert Einstein, who was once heard saying at Princeton, "I am a scientist and not a tailor." It took quite a while for the students at Princeton to accept this foreigner with his unhealthy appearance before they recognized his genius. The patient does judge your appearance: your nails, your hair, your general tidiness. I once heard a patient say regarding a superb physician, "I know he's a great doctor, but his beard smells so, I can't go near him."

The physician of bygone days had a distinct appearance. During medieval days, physicians wore an unmistakable long black frock and a pointed mask while strutting through the plagued streets. Even today, some doctors of fashionable Harley Street still wear black striped pants, white shirts, and dark jackets. Happily, in our more relaxed society, we do not have to advertise our competence to the patients by our dress.

When the physician first meets his patient, the person should be addressed by his or her last name unless the patient is a child or a contemporary. It is disrespectful to begin an interview with a mature person with, "Well, Marge, what's troubling you?" Later on, when the doctor-patient relationship is better established, you can become more informal.

It is important to get an overall impression of the person at that first meeting. Is there a language difficulty? "Know your customer," one famous Yale professor once told me. The language you use has to be flexible and easily understandable. Not everyone knows the meaning of such phrases as exacerbation symptoms, in remission, angina, asymptomatic, spasmodic pains, preprandial or post-prandial pains, respiratory distress, impotent, febrile, episodes of syncope or vertigo, urinary frequency, and palpitations, to name a few examples from interviews between interns and patients.

The examiner should take into account the general intellect of the person interviewed, and be tactful enough to rephrase the questions so that the patient does not feel that he is an imbecile. Sometimes a good technique is to have a member of the family present, especially if the patient is older. The male patient has a tendency to play down the severity of his symptoms, especially pain. For this type of patient, it is inadmissible and unmanly to be sick, even in the 1980s. An example of this "macho" sort of man came to my office accompanied by his wife. The questioning went like this:

"Do you have any trouble with your bowels?"
"Not at all. I go regularly."
The wife quickly interrupts, "It isn't so. Why don't you tell him that you haven't been able to go to the bathroom for two weeks."
"Do you have any blood in your stools?"
"I never saw any."
The wife interrupts quickly. "He is embarrassed to tell you, Doctor. He's had blood in his stools every single day."

It has never been more important than now that a good doctor-patient relationship be established. The entire nonmedical world is pounding on our doors. We are being criticized for being insensitive, unattentive, careless, and overpriced, and there is always the spectre of malpractice. If, early on in your career, you learn to care and be caring, to listen, and retain the basic tools of the practice of medicine, you will probably eliminate many of the malpractice suits that might be directed against you.

Sir Jonathan Hutchinson, the famous 19th century surgeon, gave the following advice to his first-year medical students: 1) have a sense of humor, as there are so many unpleasant things that surround you; 2) have a sense of beauty because of the ugliness that you might face; and 3) work hard, especially if you're an average student, which you can make up with diligence. I would add, be humble and digni- fied; do not for an instant be supercilious or God-like. Don't be afraid to admit that you don't know. Treat the patient as a person and not a case! How I abhor the comment, "He is an interesting case!"

Take into consideration that elderly patients may have memory problems, hear- ing problems, and vision difficulties. You will meet some patients who are overly aggressive and may resent certain questions, such as those pertaining to sexual matters. Others are too shy or too sensitive, and the wording has to be carefully altered so as not to insult them.

Notice how the patient sits in the chair. Are the hands tightly clasped? Are the facial expressions filled with terror? (What is the doctor going to discover?) Many times the real reasons why the patient comes to see you are not obvious. The back pain may be a pretext of an altogether different problem, such as depression, impotence, or an unhappy marriage.

Listen carefully for the most important sentence that people use in the English language: "Oh, by the way . . ." This may come toward the end of the interview: "Oh, by the way, I meant to tell you, I have this nagging feeling in my chest." "Oh, by the way, I noticed some blood in my stools."

The patient has to do the talking. Use a sentence or two to stimulate the pa- tient to talk and to use his own words to describe, because the description of pain and other symptoms is so personal and subjective, yet it can be so very character- istic.

THE FIRST ENCOUNTER WITH THE PATIENT

If the patient does not know you by name, then introduce yourself: "I'm Dr. Jones." Always address the patient by the full name, as Mr. or Mrs. if it is an adult. Some patients resent being called by their first name at the first meeting, and doing so does not add to the dignity of the interview. However, when interviewing a child or a teenager it is appropriate to use a first name. Avoid such patronizing terms, as "dear," "sweetie," "darling," "mother/father," ("Sit down, mother, I want to talk to you."). People have names and are proud of their names and want to be called by them, regardless of social status or ethnic backgrounds. Do not start a con- versation with a patient who digs ditches by using his first name. You would not do so if he was president of a major corporation.

Somewhere along the line in the initial portion of the conversation, I find it useful to tell the patient when discussing sensitive topics that this is purely con- fidential and to remind them that a part of the doctor-patient relationship is that such information is private and cannot be revealed without their permission. Some husbands prefer that their wives not know everything, and vice versa. A wife that calls an hour later inquiring about the health of the husband should be very dis- creetly handled unless you have permission from the spouse to give all the informa- tion that you have received. Alas, human beings have a morbid curiosity about finding out details about another person. Friends, former spouses, and employers will often call inquiring, "How is John doing?" In essence, the patient is entitled to privacy and has the right to have medical information kept secret.

It is likely that your first experience in meeting the patient will be at the bedside, and the privacy that is needed will not be possible in a four-bed room.

A low tone would then be essential. Closing the curtains while conversing with the patient can at least create an atmosphere of privacy. When you enter the room, introduce yourself, and, if there are family members present, wait until they have said their proper goodbyes. In any case, it is best to begin the interview with a light greeting. Ask the patient's name, take a comfortable chair at his/her bedside, and be certain that the patient is comfortably placed. Even adjust the pillows, if necessary.

The chief complaint is a time-honored tradition in starting a history, and this still holds quite well, but it is unhelpful to say, "What's your major complaint?" The patient will quickly answer, "I have no complaints. I'm just sick." If you ask "What brings you here?", some may say "I don't know," or, in response to "What is troubling you?", "Nothing is troubling me, I'm just sick."

If the patient is in the hospital setting or in an office, it is a good idea to begin by telling "I would like to find out the reasons why you are here and about your illness, or the symptoms you have been suffering from, and, if you can tell me in your own words, just what is the trouble."

At this point, if the patient states, "I have severe headaches," that should be written down in your notes in the exact words that the patient has given you.

"And is there anything else?"

"I also have this terrible chest pain."

Allow the patient to give to you the list of complaints. The patient may state, "This may take a long time"; respond with, "I'm a good listener and I have plenty of time. I'm here to help you." Do not interrupt their thoughts by asking another question too soon, or by suggesting the answer.

In recording an oral history of the patient, begin with the history of the present illness. I usually begin my questions by asking when was the last time the patient felt well. When they will give you a fairly specific time, then begin with the major symptoms. For example, if the complaint is chest pain, where is it located on the chest? Ask the patient to point to the location. What sort of pain is it? Let the patient tell you the type of pain rather than you supplying the words. Is the pain mild, moderate, or severe? When did it start, what was the relation of the time, and what were they doing? Ask the patient to describe the chest pain. Let the patient tell you whether it increased in severity, whether it changed, and, finally, why they decided to consult a physician at that particular time. Did the character of the pain change (increase? decrease?), or did something else appear? To develop the story further, you might try to create a setting that the patient was in. This should be like a stage setting: get the entire scenery, the location, the surroundings, the temperature. Was it at their place of work? What was the time of day? Who else was present? Make an effort to get the entire scene in your mind. What was the patient doing? What were the other events occurring in their life?

"I just had a terrible fight with my boss, and it was very hot.
I went to the bathroom and then began to feel the chest pain."

The triggering of an event is essential in history taking. After you have the general setting, more specific questions regarding the complaint can be asked. How long it has been present? Where it is felt maximally? Is it localized? Does it radiate? Is it associated with other symptoms? Is the pain sharp? Severe? Mild? Did the patient ever have this sort of pain before, or do they know any person who has had this kind of discomfort? Is there anything the patient can do to improve the pain? Lie down? Run in place? Go to the bathroom? Apply a hot towel? For example, pain at night that originates from regurgitation of acid is often relieved by sitting up or worsened by bending down. Do not hesitate to have the patient explain what they mean. Sometimes patients will have difficulty communicating and will use words they have heard in a magazine.

> "I'm suffering from an arrhythmia."
> "What do you mean by an arrhythmia? What is actually
happening to your heart?"

If the patient is embarrassed by the symptom and seems to hesitate, it is a good technique to repeat the last statement that they made: "I have the pain only when I have intercourse." Silence may follow, and, at this point, you might repeat, "Only during intercourse?" The patient then will go on to describe it further, as a rule, or they might say, "I'm too embarrassed to discuss this." The patient must then be reassured that, as a scientist and a physician you can understand the embarrassment, and that perhaps they would like to return to it at a later time.

The social history should follow. Ask about the type of work that the patient does, looking for environmental insults—coal mining, factory work, working in chemical plants, and so forth. Personal matters should be left to another time for some people, but you can easily inquire about some of their habits, for example, if they smoke and how much, whether cigars, cigarettes, or pipes. You should inquire about the use of alcohol, but this has to be done in a very discreet way. Alcoholics very rarely admit to the fact that they are drinking too much. A subtle question is, "Do you drink any alcohol?" If the patient says "yes," ask "Can you give me an idea about how much? A couple of shots a day, or something in that order?"

You can get a very good sense of the patient's actual alcohol intake on the basis of the way the patient answers that question. Most nonalcoholics and non-serious drinkers will say, "Oh, I only drink once a month or so, if that much." Others who are more serious drinkers will say, "Well, I usually have a drink every night when I come home." Others will say, "I only drink on weekends."

"And what do you have to drink?"

"Well, I don't drink alcohol. I just drink beer." (Some patients do not regard beer as an alcoholic beverage.)

Inquire about whether the patient is taking any medications on their own. People who take over-the-counter prescriptions often do not consider them to be medications. Check on the use of aspirins, antihistamines, vitamins, and diet pills. Some patients may have been carrying prescriptions for years, such as tranquilizers. It is good practice to inquire about the use of cathartics, because their chronic use can raise havoc with the bowel. So often, the patient comes in with a gastro-intestinal bleed and is never asked if they are taking any aspirin or compounds containing aspirin. Today, in our antiplatelet prophylaxis, aspirin is so commonly used, and on a daily basis, that patients often forget that they are taking one or two aspirins every morning.

Inquire about whether the patient drinks coffee or tea, and if it is decaffeinated, and if they consume an unusual amount of antacids.

Ask the patient if he had any military service, how he lives, about marital status and any previous marriages, the number of children and their ages, and his family of origin, including if the parents are still alive and their ages, and the brothers and sisters.

Family History

It is not enough to ask if there is any illness in the patient's family; you must ask specifically if there is any tuberculosis in the family, for example, or brain disorders, such as Alzheimer's. Some patients are embarrassed to say there is mental illness in the family. That question has to be worded carefully. Hereditary diseases should be noted, especially chronic anemias, such as thalassemia, sickle cell, and hemophilia. I always inquire if there are any allergies in the family, although the patient may not have any as yet. For example, hay fever in a family could signal asthma at a later time. Is there a history of heart disease, diabetes, strokes, hypertension, seizures, or alcoholism?

Past Medical History

Ask the patient if they have had any illnesses in the past, if they have been immunized, if they have had any allergic reactions to medications, if there have been any operations, accidents, or hospital admissions that they can remember, and if their general health has been good. It is useful to obtain previous medical records from doctors the patient has seen before you. Always ask for the hospital records. Not only will this allow you to compare such things as electrocardiograms and radiograms, but you may also learn of illnesses and adverse reactions to medication that the patient may have forgotten.

Review of Systems

Some clinicians believe that the review of systems should be done at the time of the examination of each organ. I prefer to do a review of systems prior to the physical examination, because during the review of systems it will help to concentrate on certain areas, and the systems can again be reviewed during the time that the physical examination is performed.

Physical Systems

Skin: Has there been any itching of the skin or rash? Any moles changing in appearance? Any cancer of the skin ever in the past? Sudden flushing of the face?

Head and Neck: Are there any hearing problems, infection, ringing in the ears, vertigo? Have there been any enlargements noted in the neck, or any swelling? Has the patient felt any lumps in the neck?

Nose: Has there been excessive bleeding, dryness, obstruction, or constant postnasal drip?

Eyes: Has there been any loss of vision, or double vision? Does the patient wear glasses? Any need for change of glasses? Any infection, dryness or itching, or discharge in the morning?

Mouth: Have there been any painful ulcers? Any hoarseness or dryness? Do the gums bleed easily? Does the patient have his own teeth? Are there any sores on the tongue or gums? Are there lesions on the lips, or recurrent sore throats?

Breasts: Has the patient felt any lumps in her breasts? Any bleeding, discharge, infection, pain, or fullness? Any color changes of nipples, or retraction of nipples?

Respiratory System: Does the patient have a cough, or coughing up of blood, or has he been exposed to tuberculosis? Has he recently had pneumonia, or shortness of breath? Does he get frequent colds or recurrent pulmonary infections?

Cardiovascular Examination: Is there any shortness of breath, or swelling of the ankles? Has the patient ever had a heart murmur or rheumatic fever? Has there been any chest pain? Has he ever noticed palpitations, fast heartbeats, fainting spells, or dizzy spells, any weakness, lightheadedness, fatigue, awakening at night with difficulty breathing, excessive sweating, or wheezing? If you suspect coronary artery disease, ask regarding remote pains, such as pain in jaws, arms, or elbows. Each symptom, if the patient states yes, then has to be fully detailed with regard to when it appeared, description, duration, radiation, what makes it better, what makes it worse, and if the patient was concerned about the symptom.

Vascular System: Does the patient suffer from varicose veins? Are their feet cold, or do they get numb? Is there pain on walking? Do they get recurrent phlebitis or ulcerations, dizziness, or numbing of the face or body?

Gastrointestinal System: Is the patient's appetite good? Have they had any loss of appetite or weight loss, any intolerance to certain foods, swallowing difficulties, nausea, vomiting, belching, bloating, burping, blood, abdominal pain, diarrhea, or constipation? Has there been a recent change in bowel habits? Do they use excessive laxatives or antacids? Have they ever had any liver trouble or found the urine to be dark or yellow, or the skin yellow? If there is diarrhea, ask if there is blood; if there is mucous, is it green? Has there been any traveling? If the patient complains of belching, bloating, and burping, think of the gallbladder, for example, and again ask if there is any history of gallbladder trouble in the family.
Always get a complete description and follow-up on any positive answers.

Renal and Urinary Tract: Does the patient have blood in the urine, burning on urination, difficulty urinating, or frequent need to urinate at night? Is there a history of stones or kidney infection?

Hematologic System: Does the patient bleed easily? Is there anemia present in the family? Have they received transfusions? Are petechiae present?

Endocrine System: Is there polyuria, polydypsia, temperature changes, changes in appetite, libido, menstrual disorders, weaknesses, weight changes, presence of diabetes? Has the patient had voice changes, hair loss, increased or decreased weight, or heat intolerance? Does his/her face flush easily?

Nervous System: Does the patient have dizziness or numbness? Have they ever had tremors, incoordination, pain, motor problems, loss of memory, seizures, syncope, or sudden shaking spells? Have they ever had ataxia, or visual disorders? Also check for orientation to time and place.

Musculoskeletal System: Is there any pain, stiffness in the morning, backache, swelling of any joints, repeated traumas, fractures, or abnormal walking tendencies? Each symptom to which the patient says yes must then be carefully followed and outlined. If he/she complains of back pain, it should be noted if the pain is worse on walking, on lying down, on standing, and/or on bending. Ask if it radiates down one or both legs, when was its origin, did it occur after an injury, and so forth.

Gynecologic History: When was the last time the patient had a Pap smear? What was her age at menopause? Is there menorrhagia, metrorrhagia, spotting, discharge, or itching? Does she use contraceptives? Ask about the number of pregnancies, births, and abortions.

Always elaborate on any symptoms; no symptom should be disregarded.

Male Genitalia: Does the patient have any pain, tenderness, or discharge? Has he ever had an infection? This might be a good time to casually ask if there is any problem with having an erection. Bear in mind that some men do not know what the word "erection" means. It might be more simple to say, "Do you have any trouble with your sex life?" This could be further elaborated during the neuro-psychiatric questioning.

Neuropsychiatric Systems

This is an essential part of the examination and should be done if you feel comfortable with the patient and are now able to ask some specific questions. Ask if the patient has had any trouble sleeping. If the answer is "yes," ask him to describe the specific sleep pattern, if there is difficulty initiating sleep or the sleep is interrupted, and if they waken early in the morning, if they are totally exhausted, and if the sleep problem persists throughout the day. Ask about mood variations. Do they tend to get blue?

A sexual inquiry would be useful at this time; by now, it is hoped that a doctor-patient relationship has been established, and there is confidence in your role as a physician and that you are not just being nosy. A simple question in a light manner might be, "How are things at home with your spouse?" The patient might, at that point, start crying, or answer glibly that everything is wonderful: "We have a great marriage." If the patient says things are not so great, ask them to further elaborate.

"What do you mean, not so great? How is your personal life with your spouse?" The patient might then answer, "We have a very good sex life," or may say, "It's been just fine," indicating that he/she does not want to discuss it further. On the other hand, the patient might state, "There is no sex life." If you repeat, "No sex life?", it might come out that the wife has pain on intercourse, or that the husband is impotent.

A lack of sexual desire can signal many illnesses besides psychiatric background. Chronic illnesses, such as cancer, diabetes, and heart disease, often are accompanied with a loss of libido, especially as a result of medications that the patient may be taking, including tranquilizers, β-blockers, and hypertension medications. Depending on the patient, it might be perfectly proper to inquire about the use of marijuana or cocaine, because this is rampant in our society. If it appears that the patient may have an alternate sexual preference, that should be discussed in view of the possibility of AIDS. This has to be done very discreetly, and often-times the patient may not want to volunteer this information. If the patient is single, an inquiry about whether the patient lives alone may lead you into the subject. Inquiring about whether there is any desire to get married, the patient might openly say, "No, I don't plan to be married. I am a lesbian (or a homosexual)." If you find that there is great discomfort and unease, then it is best to leave that question alone for the time being.

Summary

After the review of systems has been completed, a summary of all the patient's symptoms might then be gone over in the following way: "It seems, Mrs. Jones, that your major problems are constipation, bloating, and chest pain. Did we leave

anything out?" Then comes that famous, "Oh, by the way. . ." as the patient reveals that she has been coughing up blood for a month, which she failed to tell you
during the review of systems.

At that point, there should be a fair idea of what the patient's illness might be.
The patient might even inquire and say, "Well, doctor, what do you think?" They
are asking for reassurance with that question, and it would be safe to say, "I will
have to do my examination on you first, and then we'll discuss your findings and
I'll be able to tell you more."

STUMBLING BLOCKS IN THE HISTORY TAKING

The Anxious Patient

If you are presented with the patient who continually wrings his hands, pours with
sweat, fidgets, or moves around with his eyes glaring, be wary of wording your
questions carefully, and encourage the patient to discuss his fears. These patients
are afraid to use words such as "cancer," "syphilis," or "asthma." You might proceed with asking them, "What is your major worry or fear?" If they refuse to
answer, the topic might be probed further with, "Are you afraid of dying?", "Are
you afraid of cancer?", and so forth. Throughout the interview with anxious patients, reassurance is essential: "I'm here to help you, and everything is going to
be fine."

The Garrulous Patient

Some patients talk on and on and get off the track of questioning. They will relate stories totally inappropriate to the conversation. The way to handle the patient
who goes on and on is to gently interrupt them and say, "Well, I would just like to
ask you again how long you have had the chest pain." The patient will usually
say, "Oh, I'm sorry, I am rambling." Above all, do not become exasperated or im-
patient, but inject a sense of humor and say, "I would like to talk to you all day.
I find you so interesting, but I do want to get at your problem." Always show
interest.

The Quiet Patient

Other patients sit quietly and do not want to talk at all. In these situations, you
might attempt to discover what are some of the things they like to do most. This
will give an entrance to their silence. The quiet patient may be depressed or suffering from a mental illness, or may just be shy or terrified of the entire interview.

The "Yes" Patient

There is the patient who will answer yes to every question. "Do you have chest
pain?" "Yes." "Do you have diarrhea?" "Yes." A positive review of all systems
may reflect an emotionally disturbed person. In this situation, it is best to say,
"Well, which one of these symptoms bother you the most?" If the patient insists
that every symptom bothers him equally, you have no other alternative but to explore each one. I know this is time-consuming, but, unfortunately, in this salad of
symptoms there may be a serious organic cause.

The Crying Patient

When the patient is crying, it is best to talk softly or offer them a tissue and wait
for the crying to cease. The patient may then volunteer information: "I'm not
really depressed, it's just whenever I talk about my father, I start crying."

The Dangerous Patient

There will be a time in your career when a patient will be confronting you who may be frankly psychotic. These patients can be dangerous, especially if they are psychopathic. It is best not to look them directly in the eyes, because that may anger them. If you feel the presence of danger, it is best to gently interrupt the interview and find another person to be present when it continues. Above all, do not attempt to comfort them by touching them, because some will take this as an aggressive act and strike out.

The Angry or Litigious Patient

Some patients are just plain angry, especially if they have been carrying an illness or a symptom for a long time and have not received any relief. They will make deprecating remarks to you about the last physician they saw ("He's a butcher" or "He's a barber). It is best to let the patient talk and let them tell you the story. In the initial part of this confrontation, it is best not to defend or make any judgments about your colleague. The patient will often say, "I know you can't say anything, that's your professional ethics, but I can't move my arm since she injected my nerve. Don't you think, Doctor, that was a terrible thing to do?" It is best to say, "I certainly feel that you have a lot of problems and we have to discover their cause, and I will do everything I can to help you." Do not become a partner in the patient's doctor conspiracy by saying, "That was terrible, what she did," even though the patient may be correct in their assessment of having been treated shabbily by the last physician. It will not endear you to the patient to agree with them because you may be next on the list of terrible doctors, or, later on, they may say, "Dr. Jones agreed with me."

This does not mean you should in any way cover up bad medical care. Instead, keep accurate records and do everything to correct the situation. There is nothing worse than to hear through the grapevine that the patient is complaining, "Dr. Jones gave me the wrong pills."

"How do you know he did?"

"Well, Dr. Smith told me that I got the wrong pills and that he could have helped me if he had seen me earlier."

Patients sometimes like to use physicians for their own selfish causes and needs. Alas, some patients will go from doctor to doctor in the hope of finding a litigious cause so they can reap handsome profits on their mishaps. If you maintain a professional tone, then you will not get roped into pointing an accusing finger at your colleague. As a matter of fact, most medical malpractice cases come to bear because another physician points out the malpractice. This is not to say that you should in any way hide the truth, because it is your duty and obligation to police your own profession. However, without having all the facts and the other doctor's records available, in no way should you take a stand. "If you came to me first, I would have helped you," is a degrading and dangerous manner in which to establish a doctor-patient relationship. Eventually, the patient will accuse you.

ON SEXUAL MATTERS

Undoubtedly, for both sexes, there will be a natural attraction to some patients. These feelings should not fill you with despair as long as you maintain a doctor-patient relationship. Patients, at times, tend to be seductive and make sexual advances and promises, especially in the presence of a young physician. This must be handled carefully, since the patient might turn your professionalism into a rejection. A certain light sense of humor helps, along with flattery and reaffirmation that you are the doctor and that you can only be helpful to this patient if you maintain a doctor-patient relationship.

2
Summary of the Patient Examination

Siegfried J. Kra, M.D.

HISTORY TAKING

The following basic information should be obtained initially for each patient:

Name

Age

Address

Marital status

Chief complaint

Present illness

Subsequently, more detailed information should be obtained regarding past, personal, and family history, and a review of systems should be performed.

Past History

Determine if the patient has ever had any of the following conditions: rheumatic fever, diabetes, high blood pressure, infections, scarlet fever, tuberculosis, arthritis, kidney trouble, heart trouble, murmurs, diphtheria, mumps, polio, tetanus, or rubella. Review old charts or other records, if possible. Also inquire as to:

Operations: date and where performed.

Accidents: any residual effects.

Medications used: over-the-counter, vitamins, laxatives, aspirin, or analgesics.

Allergies: medications, food, contact, asthma.

Personal History

Inquire about the patient's birthplace, recent travel, marital status, occupation, habits, use of alcohol and tobacco, sleep, exercise.

Family History

Determine if anyone in the patient's family of origin now has or has had diabetes, tuberculosis, cancer, hypertension, kidney disease, gout, arthritis, heart, mental, allergies, or anemia.

Review of Systems

General: weakness, fatigue, weight change, appetite, chills, fever, night sweats.

Skin: color changes, pruritus, infections.

Eyes: visual trouble.

Ears: hearing trouble.

Nose, Throat, and Sinus: discharge sinus, hoarseness.

Dental: history of caries, dentures, peridontal disease.

Breasts: discharge, masses, history of breast cancer.

Respiratory: shortness of breath, cough, sputum, wheezing, hemoptysis, last chest x-ray and where taken, use of cigarettes, cigars, pipe, marijuana.

Cardiovascular: chest pain, shortness of breath, paroxysmal nocturnal dyspnea, peripheral edema, murmurs, palpitations, Raynaud's disease, syncope, dizzy spells.

Vascular: cold feet, numbness, Raynaud's disease, blue toes, intermittent claudication, color change of extremities (paleness).

Gastrointestinal: nausea, vomiting, diarrhea, constipation, blood in the stools, change in bowel habits, difficult swallowing, belching, bloating, burping, pain, jaundice, use of antacids, heartburn.

Hematologic: Easy bruising, bleeding, anemia.

Urinary/Renal: dysuria, hematuria, frequency, urgency, hesitancy, renal stones, infections. *Males:* penile discharge, renal disease, testicular masses, pain, impotence, libido. *Females:* gynecologic history, age at first menstrual period, menopause, postmenopausal bleeding, abnormal menses, amount of bleeding, instrumental bleeding, postcoital bleeding, pruritus, history of venereal disease, last Paps, obstetric histories, full-term deliveries, pregnancies, abortions, living children, complications of pregnancies, infertility, libido, contraception.

Musculoskeletal: joint pain, swelling, redness, stiffness, deformity, muscle weakness, atrophy, gait.

Endocrine: heat/cold intolerance, increased appetite with no weight gain, weight gain, hair loss, hair increase, numbness, polyuria, polydipsia, polyphagia, redness of the face.

Central Nervous System: headaches, syncope, seizures, vertigo, double vision, paralysis, weakness, tremor, ataxia.

Psychiatric: nervousness, depression, insomnia (obtain a sleep history).

PHYSICAL EXAMINATION

Obtain the following information: vital signs, blood pressure, pulse, respirations, height, weight, and temperature. Note the patient's general appearance, and any voice abnormalities, cyanosis, paleness, or jaundice. Check the patient's skin for distribution of hair, surgical scars, rashes, pigmentations, and purpura, and note any nail changes.

Lymph Nodes: enlargements, mobility, tenderness, location, size. Check anterior, posterior, cervical, supraclavicular, axillary, epitrochlear, and inguinal.

Head: size, shape, tenderness over sinuses.

Eyes: conjunctiva, sclera, pupillary size reaction, protrusion, ptosis, arcus, gross visual acuity, gross visual fields, ophthalmologic examination.

Ears: tophi, discharge, hearing, description of drum.

Nose: septal deviation, color of septum.

Mouth and Throat: lips, tongue, gums, condition of teeth, dentures, palate, uvula, tonsils, posterior pharynx.

Neck: extension, flexion, pulsation, scars, masses, thyroid gland, position of trachea, carotid pulses.

Back: lordosis, kyphosis, mobility, thorax configuration.

Lungs: tactile fremitus, percussion, excursion of diaphragm, breath sounds, voice sounds, rales, wheezes, rubs.

Breasts: masses, discharge, size, consistency.

Heart: inspection, abnormal pulsation, bulging, apical pulse, parasternal heaves, thrills, auscultation: heart sounds, murmurs, ejection sounds, systolic clicks. Listen to aortic area, pulmonic area, mitral area, and left sternal border with patient lying down, sitting forward.

Abdomen: palpate liver, spleen. Pulsations, scars, tenderness, masses. Palpate each quadrant—right upper, right lower, umbilical area, left upper.

Musculoskeletal: lower extremity tenderness, swelling, redness, deformity, temperature. See if there is hair on the toes.

Extremities: flexion/extension of all joints, temperature, skin changes, calf tenderness, weakness, tenderness, atrophy.

Vascular System: check carotid brachial, radial, femoral, popliteal, pedial, posterior tibial pulses.

Neurologic: Is patient oriented to time, place, and day? Check cranial nerves 2-12. Sensory—pain, temperature, light, touch, vibratory. Motor reflexes—biceps, triceps, brachial, knee jerk, Achilles tendon, abdominal, and Babinski—Romberg's sign, and gait.

Male Genitalia: penis, scrotum. Check for inguinal hernia.

Female Genitalia: External—introitus, urethra, labia, clitoris, perineum. Internal—vagina, cervix, cul-de-sac, ovaries, Pap test, rectal, rectal sphincter tone, hemorrhoids, masses.

Prostate: smooth.

ADDITIONAL CONSIDERATIONS

Finally, the patient examination should include:

Patient summary.

General impression of the patient.

Laboratory examination: significant laboratory results or x-rays, electrocardiogram.

List of problems.

3
The Psychiatric History and Mental Status Examination

Alan J. Sholomskas, M.D.

I deliberately included a large section on the psychiatric history and mental status examination in a textbook of physical diagnosis, because psychiatry is intimately related to the practice of medicine. The physician must know how to do a thorough psychiatric history, since this is one of the most difficult parts in arriving at a proper diagnosis. It is easy enough to diagnose angina from a thorough history, but when physical complaints become intermingled with psychiatric complaints, and when no organic basis is found for a physical complaint, too often the physician will presume it is a psychosomatic manifestation. The well-rounded physician is also a good psychiatrist.

The psychiatric history provides a way to diagnose, or at least suspect, the presence of major psychiatric disorders. Such disorders must be recognized, because they have their own specific treatment.

I have included this as the first chapter on physical diagnosis, since the information presented here will assist the physician in performing all other aspects of patient examination.

INTRODUCTION

The psychiatric history and mental status examination (MSE) share equal importance with the neurologic examination in the neuropsychiatric assessment of the patient. The neuropsychiatric examination is more complex than examination of some of the other organ systems because it involves assessment of the brain at both physical and mental levels of functioning.

The psychiatric history and the MSE can be done quickly and are easily integrated into the overall history and physical examination. When positive findings are suspected or elicited, one can probe further in a systematic fashion.

PSYCHIATRIC HISTORY

The psychiatric history bears the same relationship to the MSE as does the general history to the physical examination. The psychiatric history prepares the physician for conducting the MSE and suggests areas for more detailed examination. It is important to remember when performing the psychiatric history and MSE that conclusions about diagnosis are fraught with pitfalls. First, each sign and symptom is part of a larger syndrome and is never pathognomonic. Each symptom may occur in a variety of psychiatric syndromes both primary (no known physiologic cause) and secondary (related to an underlying disease). Hence, diagnosing a patient as psychotic merely on the basis of reported hallucinations is an error, unless other symptoms of the psychotic syndrome are found to be present. Another error is to assume that if the patient is psychotic he is probably schizophrenic because that is the most common psychotic disorder in a young person. Psychiatric diagnostic labels can be applied too casually, and without a proper work-up a final opinion should not be rendered.

A second point is that many syndromes are undiagnosable in the acute stage. Although the history and MSE are necessary to delineate the specific signs and symptoms of an illness, further diagnosis must await completion of the work-up. Just as the signs of congestive heart failure on physical examination are insufficient to explain the cause or the reason for its acute occurrence at a particular time, so too do signs of a psychiatric disorder define only a broad area of disturbance. Schizophrenia, for example, requires ruling out physical disorders and obtaining a longitudinal history, including premorbid levels of functioning, family history, and variables such as response to previous treatment. If it is a first psychotic episode, the final diagnosis often will remain uncertain until the patient has been followed for a time. Just as no sign or symptom is pathognomonic for a specific syndrome, neither is any syndrome pathognomonic for a specific disorder.

Third, there are differential aspects to *behaviors* just as there are to signs and symptoms. A patient who is seemingly unconcerned about his headaches should not be assumed to show the "la belle indifference" of a hysterical conversion reaction. Alternative explanations may include the patient's being depressed or anxious, or that he is stoic by virtue of cultural and familial background. Or, the patient may be reluctant to reveal how painful the headache is lest the doctor order more tests and keep him in the hospital longer. There may be a variety of reasons, then, why the patient is seemingly unconcerned about his plight. Yet the underlying disorder can range from a conversion reaction to a brain tumor.

The specific aspects of the psychiatric history can be performed separately or be incorporated into the general history. An outline follows below, portions of which will be described in greater detail later.

Outline for the Psychiatric History

Demographic Data: name, address, sex, age, race, religion, marital status, occupation, language if other than English.

Referral Data: reason, source, process, timing of referral.

Chief Complaint: in patient's own words.

History of the Present Illness or Presenting Problem: chronologic account of patient's symptoms (including past episodes of same or related conditions); include mental and physical symptoms, psychologic and social-environmental stressors; patient's attitudes, reactions, and behaviors, including attempts to cope; quote from patient's own words.

Past Psychiatric History: premorbid personality traits or description (high-strung, moody, serious, carefree); past psychiatric episodes, treated or untreated symptoms or problems, stressors and precipitants; past psychiatric hospitalizations, treatment type (include drugs, dosage, duration, number of electroshock treatments), outcome, follow-up care.

Past Medical History: same as for general medical history with special attention to illnesses that may interact with psyche and vice versa (e.g., hyperthyroidism in patient with anxiety); medications and relevant laboratory values; all abnormal values; alcohol, illicit drug use, over-the-counter drugs, caffeine, tobacco, nutritional habits.

Review of Systems: in addition to routine review, include symptoms relevant to psychiatric status (e.g., palpitations, headaches, diaphoresis, gastrointestinal distress in patient with anxiety attacks); include all positives in other less relevant organ systems; central nervous system symptoms (seizures, headaches, focal signs, syncope, weakness, head trauma); sexual history and functioning.

Social and Developmental History: Childhood: labor and delivery, Apgar score, milestones, childhood experiences and behaviors, fears, school performance, peer relationships, play; physical or emotional problems, handicaps; sleep and appetite patterns; temperament.
Adolescence: age of puberty, dating, hobbies, activities, bodily concerns or deficits; relations with school, society, peers, parents; sexual history; antisocial behavior, truancy, petty crime, drug or alcohol use.
Adulthood: education, occupation, marital history, social and military history; sexuality; hobbies and use of leisure time; personality style, values, goals; current social situation including family constellation, socioeconomic status.

Family History: role of parents, siblings, extended family; family functioning including history of divorce, separation, unusual living arrangements; abuse; incest; family's social, cultural, religious values; history of alcoholism, psychiatric illness, chronic illness, genetic disease, suicide, unusual or erratic behavior; deaths, divorce; family "skeletons."

Chief Complaint

The physician should inquire about any psychiatric symptoms likely to be associated with the complaint(s) in question. For instance, if the patient complains of abdominal pain, the physician should make inquiries about symptoms of depression, anxiety, and other disorders that might be related. Or, if drug-seeking is suspected, an inquiry into the use of drugs and alcohol should be included. The possibilities are numerous but can be shaped by the areas in question.

Past Psychiatric History and Past Medical History

In this portion of the interview, the physician should inquire about previous "counseling," "trouble with nerves" or emotions, and times when the patient has not functioned normally. Any psychiatric hospitalizations or other professional contacts should be tactfully sought after. If relevant, previous suicide attempts or accidents might be questioned. ("Did you ever try to hurt yourself in any way? What happened? Were you treated for this? Did you talk to anyone about it?"). The physician should never be reluctant to ask about suicidal feelings or acts if there is any suspicion at all. It is your prerogative as a professional and your duty as a physician. Rarely will a patient hide a previous suicide attempt once you convey genuine interest and helpfulness.

If the patient has a previous psychiatric history, your awareness of possible physical disturbances is especially important. Not only the physician but often the patient himself will rationalize his symptoms as, "Well, it's probably just my nerves." Maybe the patient is correct, but the physician has the obligation to explore the complaint(s) fully. Anxiety is only one of the differential possibilities.

A psychiatric patient should always be asked the name and nature of his illness and what treatment he was or is receiving.

> A 22-year-old man presented to the emergency room (ER) with what appeared to be an acute oculogyric crisis. Although the ER resident had never seen such a reaction, his suspicion of it was prompted by the knowledge that this mute patient, unable to speak because his throat muscles were in spasm, was in psychiatric treatment. Specific questions to the man's wife revealed that the patient had taken his first dose of haloperidol earlier that day. An intravenous injection of diphenhydramine rapidly enabled the grateful patient to talk again and confirm the sequence of events.

It is also important to know the psychiatric history of a patient in order to suspect conditions seen more frequently in certain patients: water intoxication in a schizophrenic patient, anorexia in a depressed individual, inappropriate antidiuretic hormone syndrome in a patient taking tricyclic antidepressants, toxic megacolon in a patient on high doses of phenothiazines, or anticholinergic delirium in a patient taking an antidepressant and thioridazine are a few examples.

The medical history should inquire of all patients about drug-taking and drinking behavior—in any age group. A serious omission is to see an apparently demented elderly patient and not ask about alcohol or drug intake. The use of over-the-counter medications should also not be forgotten. Bromides, cough and cold medicines, analgesics, sleeping medications, sympathomimetic diet aids, antihistamines, and many others can cause illness.

If the patient has been ill before, such as with chest pain, inquire how he handled it before. What were his perceptions of the problem then and now? What are his expectations now? Does he have any ideas about why this happened and what should be done about it? Answers to these questions can be of great help in learning about the patient's interaction with the disease process and can thus enrich the physician's understanding of how to maximize the patient's treatment.

> A 48-year-old man who suffered an anterolateral myocardial infarction 2 years before, in response to the questions above, described guiltily how he had abstained from all sex after his infarction. However, on this night he had drunk excessively at a party, become amorous, and enjoyed a vigorous sexual extravaganza with his wife until severe chest pain set in. Initially too embarrassed to tell the intern, he confided this to a perceptive resident, who then not only learned the reason for the patient's ER visit but also identified an important area for rehabilitation once the patient was treated and discharged.

Review of Systems

The system review should always inquire about symptoms relevant to the patient's complaint and also specifically about psychiatric functioning: changes in mood, sleep, appetite, and sexual functioning; anxiety or tension; worries and fears; unusual sensory experiences; and changes in personality or behavior.

To illustrate some of the principles involved in history taking, the sexual history, which is often difficult for the inexperienced clinician, will be taken as an example. First, the examiner should recognize that, although sexuality may be a sensitive topic for both patient and examiner, it is an important area of assessment because both physical and psychologic conditions can cause sexual problems.

The physician should begin with general questions: Have you had any difficulty in your sexual life? Has your spouse noticed anything about your sex life that concerns him/her? Have you had any problems with interest in sex? Your ability to perform sex? Reaching an orgasm? Having an erection/lubricating during intercourse? When was the last time you had a sexual experience? Can you tell me something about it?

In clinically relevant situations it may be necessary to determine whether and what kind of sexual contact the patient has had. The physician has an obligation to inquire into these areas but should do so tactfully and with sensitivity. A physician had the following conversation with a young man with a penile discharge:

DOCTOR: Before this symptom began, when did you last have a sexual experience?
PATIENT: Oh, about a month ago.
MD: Can you tell me about it?
PT: It was just someone I met at a bar.
MD: Do you know anything about this person?
PT: Just that they weren't a virgin.
MD: Was this a male or a female?
PT: It was a guy.
MD: What kind of sexual experience was it?
PT: Well, there was oral and, uh, anal intercourse.
MD: And were you the active partner or the passive one or both?
PT: Well, we each did it.
MD: Did what? Penetrated the other?
PT: Uh, yeah, that's what we did.

In this questioning important clinical information concerning homosexual anal intercourse was elicited that provided the basis for further clinical evaluations appropriate to the circumstances.

Another sensitive area may involve asking a married person about extramarital affairs. One might ask simply, "Considering this rash you have, have you had sexual contact with anyone besides your husband/wife?"

It cannot be emphasized too strongly that the clinician must utilize his role as a physician to gather the information required on the basis of clinical necessity but that it can and should be done with tact, diplomacy, and consideration in an objective and nonjudgmental manner. Avoid flippant remarks ("How's your sex life?"), moral judgments ("You should try to do something about your homosexuality"), misinformation ("Only men masturbate") or gratuitous comments ("Your wife must be sexually deprived with you sick for so long"). It may almost appear unnecessary to mention these points to the reader, but in fact it is possible for even well-meaning clinicians to become uncomfortable about sexual issues.

Social and Developmental History

When the physician inquires into the patient's developmental history, psychological development should also be included. High fevers of childhood, bedwetting or sleepwalking beyond early childhood, fearfulness at going to school, nervous habits, learning difficulties in school, and problems with peers or parents suggest but a few examples of childhood problems that may have an impact years later (febrile seizures can predispose to later seizure disorders; school phobia sometimes is a precursor of adult anxiety disorder). The nature of the patient's current problem may suggest what developmental areas to investigate.

> A 23-year-old man with a history of impulsive behavior and a bad temper was seen after falling from a ladder while frenetically painting his house. After minor treatment, he was referred to a psychiatrist, who learned, among other things, that the patient had a history of learning disabilities and disciplinary problems as a child, that he had been accident prone, and that he still displayed a short attention span and low frustration tolerance. When he was treated with tricyclic antidepressants, in conjunction with other psychiatric treatment, his attention deficit disorder (formerly called minimal brain dysfunction) and his impulsivity improved considerably. The developmental history in this case was crucial to making the adult diagnosis.

Family History

In psychiatry, just as in general medicine, it has become increasingly important to know a patient's family history. Schizophrenia, manic-depressive illness, alcoholism, unipolar depression, certain anxiety disorders, and some dementias all show a genetic background. Suicide, too, although not clearly an inheritable behavior, tends to run in families and constitutes a risk factor for patients with such a family history. Attention deficit disorder (formerly called hyperkinetic syndrome or minimal brain dysfunction) and many learning disabilities likewise occur with greater frequency in families of patients with these disorders. In a patient presenting with an atypical psychosis, for example, who has a family history positive for manic-depressive illness, this diagnosis must be suspected despite a confusing presentation. Therefore, the physician must always gather family data whenever possible.

Because patients do not always know of psychiatric disorders in their families, the physician should be prepared to ask other family members as well. Questions should try to gather descriptive data in addition to specifics such as "Has anyone in your family suffered from depression?" One may need to ask a series of questions in order to obtain a family history. Note the following questioning of a patient with a depressive episode. The patient denied any history of manic-depressive illness in the family.

PHYSICIAN: Well, then, you said your father's brother was hospitalized for depression. Do you know what caused his depression?
PATIENT: I don't know. He had several depressions but only was in the hospital once.
MD: How long was he hospitalized?
PT: I think at least a couple of months. They gave him shock treatments.
MD: And did he continue in treatment after discharge? Did he take any medication?

PT: I think he saw a doctor for awhile but I don't know about medication.

MD: Did he ever have episodes where he acted differently, like the opposite of depressed? Sort of speedy or super-energetic, not needing much sleep, and being busier and more active than usual?

PT: I remember once my father said he would have times when he would be particularly obnoxious.

MD: What did he do, for instance?

PT: Well, he would call all the relatives in the middle of the night trying to borrow money for some business he was starting. And I remember when I once talked to him he was talking a mile a minute. Also, he would write all kinds of crazy letters to the newspapers about all sorts of things, although I don't think any ever got published.

Further questioning by the physician brought out clearly an episode of changed behavior in the uncle characterized by sleeplessness, hyperactivity, pressured speech, grandiosity, reckless driving, and excessive spending, which lasted for several weeks and subsided gradually. On this basis, a manic episode was suspected in the uncle, which contributed an important new perspective to the patient's depression.

Finally, a family medication history is often useful. In the above example, the nephew may not have known of his uncle's manic episode but he might have reported that his uncle was taking lithium carbonate. Also, because a drug that is effective for an individual may often be effective in biologic relatives, knowing, for example, that a close relative responded to imipramine but not to amitriptyline could help in deciding which drug to use for the patient.

THE MENTAL STATUS EXAMINATION

The mental status examination is part of the general physical examination and is most useful only in the context of a complete evaluation of the patient. A point that sometimes causes clinicians confusion is where the psychiatric history ends and the MSE begins. The MSE properly includes only observations made of the patient's behavior and his subjective experiences during the interview process. It does not include information acquired from the history. If a patient describes recent beliefs that someone is trying to harm him, that information belongs in the psychiatric history. However, if at the time of the interview that belief is still current, then this possible delusion is included in the MSE.

A patient may have recently experienced visual hallucinations but, if he denies them during the interview and the examiner has not detected any instances of the patient's appearing to hallucinate, then the MSE is negative for hallucinations. The importance of this is obvious. A patient may have hallucinated 2 days before but is not hallucinating now. This could mean that the condition is subsiding or that the patient is responding to medication. Mental status examinations may be done serially during evaluation and treatment, and it is important to document the presence or absence of specific findings at each examination. A demented patient, for example, may show changes that could indicate worsening, improvement, or fluctuation. Without specifically delineating the findings over time, the patient's course can be unclear.

It is equally important to record only objective findings in the MSE, not opinions or conclusions. Furthermore, specific details should generally be noted in writing up the examination. For example, the statement that "the patient was manic" is not acceptable. This is a diagnostic description, not a mental status finding. Although it is somewhat more acceptable to say, "the patient had paranoid delusions," it is much more useful to describe the actual delusion. This conveys greater information, which may prove useful if the delusions improve or change in content, for example, or may even help to resolve unclarity about whether the finding is actually a delusion.

> An elderly lady recently admitted to a nursing home told the examining physician that her son was out to kill her and she feared for her life. The physician wrote on the examination that she was "delusional." He discovered later, however, that the woman's son was a paranoid schizophrenic who had indeed attempted to kill her while in a psychotic state. Because he lived with her, admission to the nursing home was in part a response to the impossibility of the living situation.

The MSE is both structured and unstructured. It is necessary to allow the patient to talk spontaneously without immediately limiting his verbal productions. Otherwise, valuable clues to his thinking and affect may be lost. However, there are portions of the MSE in which the physician must obtain data by specific questioning. Part of the skill of doing an MSE is being able to strike a balance between these styles of interviewing.

Part of the MSE can be derived in the process of taking the patient's history. Questions about orientation and memory are less necessary when the patient is able to render a careful, chronologic history and is able to manipulate times and places in the current situation. Ideas about the patient's verbal productivity and thought patterns can also be inferred to varying degrees from the overall interview.

The examiner should have an outline in mind. It is often useful to carry a 3x5 card with the points to be covered in the MSE. A mental outline can be reviewed before and during the exam to make sure all areas are assessed. In general there are four main areas of the MSE: general appearance, behavior, and attitude; speech and thinking, including content and process; emotional state; and sensorium, or intellectual functioning. Each area can be subdivided into several categories, but if the physician remembers to summarize just these four areas, he will have laid down the cornerstones of the examination.

The variety of information obtainable in each of the four areas can be almost limitless, reflecting the protean possibilities of individual human beings. An outline of the MSE follows, to be fleshed out in detail afterward. Examples will be given in each section and several common syndromes will be described at the end to exemplify composite mental status examinations.

Outline for the Mental Status Examination

General Appearance and Behavior: age, race, sex, body type, nutritional status, hygiene, dress, gait, posture, use of specific descriptive adjectives; motor activity (agitation, retardation, tension, hyperactive, hypoactive) and abnormal movements (tics, tremors, posturing, stereotypies); relation to interviewer (cooperative, candid, indifferent, defensive, suspicious, hostile, guarded, seductive, teasing, collaborative, compliant, helpful, suppliant); characteristics of speech (halting, dysarthric, stuttering, slurring, aphasic, mumbling, foreign accent).

Flow of Speech: speech patterns (dysarthric, hesitating, scanning, slurring, stuttering); rate and rhythm (pressured, spontaneity, poverty, loquaciousness, laconic; circumstantiality, tangentiality, perseveration, verbigeration, palilalia, echolalia); use of words (neologisms, word salad, paraphasias, word approximations); associations (looseness, thought blocking, derailment, rambling, clanging, non sequiturs).

Content of Speech: obsessions, compulsions, ruminations, phobias, derealization, depersonalization, somatic anxiety complaints, delusions (grandiose, erotic, somatic, paranoid), hallucinations (auditory, command, visual, olfactory, gustatory, tactile, hypnagogic, hypnopompic).

Emotional State: objective versus subjective; contagiousness; affect (amplitude, range, stability, quality, appropriateness, relatedness); mood (irritable, angry, annoyed, cheerful, happy, euphoric, pleased, apathetic, subdued, depressed, anxious, fearful, terrified).

Sensorium: orientation (time, place, person); attention and concentration (Serial Sevens Test, Digit Span); calculations; memory (immediate, short-term, long-term; amnesias [retrograde and anterograde]; pseudomemories, confabulation; deja vu, jamais vu; verbal and visual memory); intelligence (information, vocabulary); abstraction (proverbs, similarities); judgment; insight; perception and coordination (complex tasks, reading, writing, drawing, copying).

General Appearance and Behavior

In interviewing a patient the physician must remember to introduce himself to the patient, make the patient comfortable, explain the purpose of the interaction, and be aware of the patient's feelings about the process. Here the clinician observes the patient as a person and must try to derive a description of the patient that paints a picture for someone reading the description. Age, sex, race, body type, and nutritional status, as well as items of dress, hygiene, hair and eye color, gait, posture, and mannerisms are all noted. Levels of alertness and attention are noted, too, in order to detect, for example, organic mental disorders.

The following is an example of such a description:

> This 42-year-old white man, grossly overweight with his stomach
> protruding through a torn sport shirt, breathed heavily as he sat
> in the chair wiping his perspiring face with a soiled handkerchief.
> Black-rimmed eyeglasses kept slipping down his nose and his eyes
> stared intensely at the examiner as he anxiously told the examiner
> he was being followed.

The physician should describe the degree and type of the patient's motoric activity: restless, bradykinesic, pacing, squirming in the chair, wringing his hands, sighing, eyes darting, avoiding looking at the examiner, or jiggling his foot throughout the interview, for example.

Increased motor behavior is called *agitation* and increased frequency of goal-directed behaviors is called *hyperactivity.* Lack of body motion or stiffness suggests *bradykinesia* or *hypoactivity.* Furrowed brow, downturned mouth, and watery eyes suggest depression. Extreme hypoactivity or hyperactivity suggests catatonia, which will be described later. Perspiration, rapid breathing, increased palpebral fissures, and tremulousness suggest anxiousness.

Abnormal motor movements such as *tremors, chorea, tics,* and *dystonia* can indicate neurologic dysfunction. Other abnormal movements can be seen in psychiatric disorders. *Posturing,* the assumption of odd postures by a patient, can be seen in psychoses. *Catalepsy,* maintaining the same position or an odd posture for an extended time, is seen in catatonia. *Echopraxia,* the patient's copying of the examiner's motor behavior, can also be seen in catatonia. *Stereotypies,* non-goal-directed, automatic, repetitive motor behaviors (such as shaking one's head constantly) are seen in psychotic disorders.

The patient's way of relating to the examiner should be noted: cooperativeness, friendliness, candor, indifference, haughtiness, fearfulness, irritability, suspiciousness, needing constant reassurance, and the like. This may change as the interview progresses and even in subsequent interviews, reminding the examiner of the need for caution in forming first impressions.

Flow of Speech

Mental activity can be divided into process and content. The process of thinking (as indicated by speaking), also known as the flow of speech or productivity, can be increased as in the pressured speech associated with anxiety, agitation, mania, or anger, or can be decreased as in paranoia, depression, anxiety, dementia, aphasia, or psychosis. The degree of spontaneity, the fluency, the tone, and any other qualities of the speech pattern should be noted. Speech may be halting, slurred, inaudible, boisterous, loud, scanning, stuttering, vague, evasive, firm, hoarse, interrupted by crying, or mumbled. Speech patterns can give clues to mood, neurologic disorders, psychotic disorders, or personality disturbances, and analysis of speech patterns is crucial for diagnosing the various types of aphasias.

Disorders of thinking are reflected in what the patient says, but his speech is usually normal. Patterns of speech as reflected by articulation, quantity, and quality are distinct from patterns of thinking, but it should be noted that patterns of thinking and patterns of speech are used more or less interchangeably. To quote Taylor (14), "thought process is characterized by its rate, pressure, rhythm, idiosyncrasy of word usage, tightness of associational linkage and forms of associational linkage." For the nonpsychiatrist exploration of these concepts in detail is unnecessary, but the more common varieties of thought processes will be reviewed.

Circumstantial Speech

Speech that is excessively filled with detail but eventually reaches the communication goal is called circumstantial speech. "Beating around the bush" is a colloquial description of circumstantiality that is found in anxious and/or obsessional patients who take a long time "to come to the point." It can also be seen in some neurological patients, in some psychotic individuals, and can be seen in chronic epileptics, alcoholics, borderline mentally retarded, and some passive-aggressive persons.

Tangential Speech

Speech that never reaches the goal but moves from one related idea to another in tangents is called tangential speech. It can be seen in anxious states, early stages of mania, psychosis, organic mental disorders, and intoxications.

Perseverative Speech

Perseveration is a pattern in which thoughts are repeated several times with the patient being unable to shift to a new idea. For example, each time a patient was asked a different question, he kept repeating his age. This is most often seen in organic states but sometimes in psychosis as well. (It should be noted here that patients may perseverate behaviors as well as speech.) *Palilalia* is a type of perseveration in which phrases are repeated, particularly those occurring at the end of sentences: "I'll be there, there, there." *Verbigeration* consists of a spontaneous repetition of meaningless words or phrases and is quite rare, being found mainly in chronic, regressed schizophrenics.

Idiosyncratic Speech

Idiosyncratic speech is often seen in mental disturbances. *Neologisms* are unique words coined by the patient that may represent one or several real words or concepts condensed into a single word. For example, one patient referred to her neighbor, an old crone who spied on her through her window blinds, as a "witch-watch." Occasionally, patients with organic mental disorders will create them. Speech replete with many neologisms is called *word salad.*

Paraphasias

Paraphasias are words that substitute for the correct words; they can be seen in either psychoses or organic mental disorders. Neologisms and *word approximations* (similar words such as "clock" for "watch") are examples of paraphasias.

Association

After evaluating a patient's rate, rhythm, and use of words, the associational aspects of thinking should be analyzed. Terms like "incoherent," "illogical," and "irrelevant" are rough examples, but these terms are imprecise. Instead, the psychiatrist refers to the *tightness* or *looseness of associations* when evaluating the form of speech. Loose associations can be described as paragraph looseness, in which the patient changes topics after a few sentences; sentence looseness, in which one sentence has no apparent connection to another; or word looseness (or word salad), in which not even a coherent sentence is verbalized.

Mild looseness can be seen in anxiety and agitated states such as mania. More severe degrees are often seen in psychotic states. An acutely psychotic patient might say to the examiner: "Is this the hospital where I am brother Paul? My father told me never to say never to nobody and if that were the case, then tell me, where are the business suits? The man was worried and I came along, probably at lunchtime in the open rain. Where did that girl go?"

Thought Blocking

Thought blocking refers to the sudden cessation of speaking and thinking. The patient stops in the middle of a sentence or interview and momentarily seems unresponsive. This can occur in a petit mal patient with "absence" attacks, in an anxious individual who loses his train of thought, and in psychotics who may report having experienced either no mental activity at all or else the intrusion of a hallucination which interrupted their thinking.

Derailment

Derailment refers to the interruption of one thought with subsequent continuation on a parallel but different line of thought. Usually the derailment is punctuated with blocking or a pause: "My head has been hurting for a week now. [*pause*] I read where you shouldn't give aspirin to kids with the flu." It is seen in schizophrenia and in chronic brain disease.

Rambling

Rambling occurs when the patient's speech is not goal directed and associations are not tight. It is seen in acute organic states, such as in an alcoholic in the emergency room. Parts of speech may make sense but the conversation seems to wander and the goal is never reached: "I'm an old baseball player, did you know that? My first wife knew that. Could hit a ball a mile. Never struck out. You don't look like a ballplayer to me. Never could make any money at it. Had to work in a factory. Forty years in that pit, never missed a day. And now it's closed. Man can't find a job if his life depended on it."

Clang Associations

Clang associations are important because, although uncommon, they are most often seen in mania and occasionally in organic brain disorders. These are associations connected on the basis of sound and overlap with the rhyming and punning of words sometimes seen in manics: "I wanted to drive my car. You know, drive it far. Far, far away. Away, away. I'll find a way. I know the way. Way to go, way to go."

Non Sequiturs

Non sequiturs are words or phrases unrelated to the previous word or phrase or to the examiner's previous comment: "Where do you live?" "Well, yes that can happen at times." These are also found in schizophrenia and organic brain disease.

In listening for these patterns, the examiner must utilize the patient's spontaneous speech as well as that given in response to specific questions. It takes practice to listen carefully and detect such abnormalities because our minds often fill in the blanks or correct errors to allow the patient to make sense. We can thus impose our own estimate of what we think the patient means, which is fine, so long as we also observe where the patient has problems in communication.

Content of Speech

Thought content, of course, is imbedded in the patient's thought processes and may contain specific signs and symptoms. Content can include general themes as well as specific types of thoughts, emotions, behaviors, perceptions, and other miscellaneous experiences. Again it is important to note that many of these signs and symptoms will have been more properly included in the psychiatric history rather than the MSE.

Obsessions

Obsessions are repetitive thoughts that intrude into the patient's mind against his/her control. They concern most commonly thoughts about doing forbidden things involving sex, cleanliness, or aggression.

Compulsions

Compulsions are behaviors of a repetitive nature that the patient feels compelled to carry out, which are not pleasurable and which he attempts to resist. These involve commonly touching, checking, counting, and washing.

Ruminations

Ruminations are repetitive thoughts that are less discrete and less resisted than obsessions. They usually involve appropriate issues but in an excessive manner, such as constantly worrying about money when one's finances are adequate.

Phobias

Phobias are irrational, unreasonable fears. *Simple phobias* are common and involve concrete objects such as snakes, insects, or dogs or common situations such as high places or water. *Social phobias* involve social situations such as public speaking, eating in restaurants, and crowds. *Agoraphobia* is a complex of phobias involving fears of traveling, crowded places, or being trapped in places where immediate exit is impeded (such as the first pew of a church).

Depersonalization/Derealization

Depersonalization is the feeling that one's body and self are in a daze or dream, or are unreal. In *derealization* the person feels that the environment is altered as if it is unreal or changed, or as if he/she is in a dream.

Somatic Anxiety

Somatic anxiety involves physical symptoms that occur secondary to tension and anxiousness, most commonly heart palpitations, tension headaches, knot in the stomach, perspiring, lightheadedness, diarrhea, and muscle aches. Note that any of these symptoms can be due to organic disease and are only considered somatic anxiety symptoms in the context of a diagnosed anxiety disorder. Thus, one should consider them somatic complaints until the etiology becomes known. They will appear either in the history or review of systems and only appear in the MSE if the patient experiences them during the interview.

Delusions

Delusions are more complex phenomena of major importance. Also referred to as apophany, they are defined simply as fixed false beliefs not in keeping with one's cultural environment or not validated consensually. In other words, they do not reflect an accurate perception of one's environment.

It is sometimes debatable whether an idea is actually a delusion. The more bizarre or unlikely sounding it is, the greater the likelihood it is a false belief. Sometimes the clinician cannot tell without outside verification. For example, a wife may complain that her husband accuses her of having an affair, which she insists is not true. One might be hard pressed to learn the truth in this situation: Is he delusional or is she concealing the facts? If she then reported that he searched the house in a bizarre and frenetic manner each and every time he returned home and that he purchased electronic equipment to detect occult sounds, the possibility of a delusion then becomes more believable. In evaluating a delusion that could be realistic, it is particularly important to be neutral about it until further data are gathered. Elderly people, for example, may make legitimate complaints that can sound like delusions.

There are four basic types of delusions: somatic, paranoid, erotic, and grandiose.

Erotic delusions are uncommon and involve the belief that a specific person or persons is/are in love with one despite evidence to the contrary.

Grandiose delusions, frequently seen in mania but seen in other psychotic states as well, center around beliefs involving special powers or capabilities. They are thus often accompanied by a grandiose or expansive mood, as will be described later. Believing that one is Jesus Christ is a common, if cliched, grandiose delusion.

Somatic delusions are commonly found in psychoses and in some depressions, particularly in the elderly. They are also present in organic brain disorders. They can involve any organ system and can be quite bizarre, like that of a depressed 80-year-old woman who was convinced her insides had rotted away.

Paranoid delusions are the most common variety and involve infliction of intended harm to the patient by known or unknown others. It is important to recognize that paranoid feelings occur on a spectrum of intensity. At the milder end is *suspiciousness,* which is not always present but is often out of proportion to reality when it occurs. An example is a machinist who is suspicious that his co-workers talk about him but is not absolutely sure. *Ideas of reference* are further developed notions in which the patient's suspiciousness borders on delusional but is elicited only by a stimulus from the suspected person. Hearing his co-workers laugh, the machinist mentioned above assumes they are laughing about him. Finally, there are *clear-cut delusions* in which the belief is always present; for example, the machinist is convinced that his co-workers are planning to harm him by short-circuiting his machine. Delusions may be limited or circumscribed (only the machinist's co-workers are against him), or generalized in varying degrees (many others, including maybe even you, the examiner, are after him). They can range from the almost believable to the bizarre, such as a patient reporting that animal urine is pumped through his vents at night to vaporize and asphyxiate him. A specific type of delusion, called a *delusional percept,* is sometimes described in which the patient has a delusion that only occurs referentially: oncoming flashing headlights mean his life is in danger from the FBI agents in the car. If the car does not flash its headlights, the delusion is not activated.

It can be very difficult at times to elicit delusions, but they are very important. Patients who seek medical care for obscure complaints are sometimes delusional. So too may be an occasional person requesting plastic surgery. Of course, delusions can be a part of an obvious psychiatric syndrome such as schizophrenia. Delusions can also be the presenting sign of a medical illness: the patient on steroids who accuses the nurses of poisoning his juice, the hypothyroid patient who claims her bedridden husband is having an affair with neighborhood girls, or the postoperative patient who is convinced the Mafia have restrained him in the hospital in order to kill him.

Illusions

Illusions are relatively uncommon except in delerious, highly anxious, or histrionic patients, and in some psychotics. These are misinterpretations of sensory data—noises, smells, shadows, bodily sensations—to which the patient assigns incorrect meanings. They can be harmless, like mistaking the phone for the doorbell, or more upsetting, like mistaking a shadow for a rapist.

Hallucinations

Hallucinations are subjective sensory experiences without corresponding external stimuli that can occur in any sensory modality and may occur in more than one sensory modality within the same individual.

Auditory hallucinations are the most common type and may involve hearing voices, noises, or ineffable sounds. Voices are the most common type and can range from mumbled whispers that cannot be discerned as true words to complex sentences maintaining a running commentary on the patient's activities. Auditory hallucinations are common in a wide variety of syndromes: schizophrenia, affective psychosis, alcoholism, and some bereavements and hysteria. Thus, a patient need not be psychotic to suffer a hallucination.

A special type of auditory hallucination, known as a **command** hallucination, is of importance because it is widely believed that patients who experience them may act upon the voice's command and hurt themselves or others.

Visual hallucinations are also common in many states but especially so in both dementias and delirium of whatever cause. They can also be seen occasionally in bereavement and hysteria.

Olfactory hallucinations involve detecting smells or odors that do not exist. Occasionally occurring in psychotic states, they must always raise a suspicion of temporal lobe involvement such as by a brain tumor or temporal lobe seizures. In such cases, a pungent or burning smell is sometimes described.

Gustatory hallucinations involving tastes (usually strange or unpleasant) also occur in psychosis, depression, and organic states.

Tactile hallucinations, or sensations of touching such as bugs crawling on the skin (formication) occur in schizophrenia, alcoholism, affective illness, and amphetamine intoxication. They must be distinguished from real but bizarre-sounding sensations such as those that may occur in patients who have injected themselves with heroin diluted with quinine.

Hypnagogic hallucinations, those occurring during the transition from wakefulness to sleep, and **hypnopompic** hallucinations, occurring in the transition to wakefulness, can occur in organic and alcoholic states but are also seen in narcolepsy and as a side effect of certain drugs, such as tricyclic antidepressants.

In probing hallucinatory experiences, it is important to determine the time, place, content, frequency, patient's attitude toward them, and previous history of hallucinations in order to make a differential diagnosis. Although the content of hallucinations and delusions may be intrinsically interesting to the examiner, they have no correlation with diagnosis. They do relate to the patient's background, life experience, and culture, but the specific content cannot be used to formulate etiology.

Emotional State

In assessing emotional state, it is important for the examiner to note not only the patient's expressed (or objective) emotional state and the reported (or subjective) emotional state but the examiner's emotional response as well. The latter is important because the examiner's interaction with the patient may influence the patient's emotions, just as the patient's emotions may influence the examiner. Thus patients who are euphoric, anxious, depressed, or irritable may induce similar feelings in the examiner. In such cases, the examiner's response can be a clue to the patient's emotional tone.

> One resident, after interviewing a young, seemingly calm woman, felt tense and anxious after the interview, sighing, his shirt damp, and was relieved that the interview was over. The supervisor, who had sat in upon the examination, reflected to the resident that the patient had indeed been quite tense despite her superficially calm manner: she, too, had sighed, rarely smiled, held her body stiffly in the chair, crossed her legs tightly throughout the interview, and clenched her fists several times. The resident realized then that his own feeling of anxiousness was disproportionate to the actual stress of the interview and had been "caught" from the patient.

The examiner's behavior and affect can influence the patient's affect as well.

> A frenetic young woman arrived 30 minutes late for her intake interview with the resident, who was doing his last evaluation before his vacation. Already feeling irritable, he challenged the lady's lateness when she came in the room. The woman was irritable and withholding during the interview, in which she discussed the terrible situation she was in (divorcing her husband). The resident noted in his report that the woman was angry, sullen, and uncooperative with the interview, which surprised the social worker who had referred her to the resident for treatment. Only after another visit did the resident learn that the woman was in fact very cooperative, compliant, and even dependent, and had behaved somewhat atypically because the resident's behavior had both threatened and irritated her.

Affect is the term used to refer to the patient's overall emotional capacity and expression. It can be described by depth or amplitude, range or variability, stability, quality, appropriateness, and relatedness. **Mood,** on the other hand, is a transient manifestation of affect, and includes the observable mood as well as what the patient experiences. Usually, both will be similar or congruent: an anxious patient will acknowledge his anxiety. However, a patient's presentation sometimes can be misleading, and one must be aware that the patient's internal experience may be belied by his exterior demeanor. This is common, for example, for patients in pain, particularly if the pain is chronic. More than one chronic pain patient has been labeled as "indifferent" or not really "in pain" because he did not grimace, cry, whine, writhe, and moan.

The expression of a mood depends on many things: duration, previous experiences with physicians, and cultural and intellectual background, for example. Thus it is important to ask what the patient is feeling and to acknowledge this, even if the observable mood differs. Moods can be described in a variety of ways familiar to us all: angry, irritable, annoyed; happy, cheerful, ecstatic, euphoric, elated; apathetic, subdued, depressed; anxious, fearful, terrified.

The more global concept of affect, however, is defined by several parameters. **Amplitude** or depth of affect might be described as the intensity or the quantity of mood; it also suggests a degree of believability. A very angry patient will show intense anger by his physical and facial expressions (and probably verbally as well) and the examiner will be likely to take it as real. Someone who pretends unsuccessfully to be angry will not convey the depth of emotion shown by the really angry person unless he is a particularly good actor.

Variability, or range of affect, refers to the capacity to display different depths of affect. If the angry person displays only a monotone of feeling, whatever the intensity, his range of affect is said to be constricted. In contrast, a full range of affect allows for grading and modulation in the levels of emotion expressed, whatever emotion it may be. Thus, sadness may grow intense or subside in response to changes in the interview. Constriction also applies to the patient who displays basically one mood, despite fluctuations in the interview situation. Thus, a patient who remains angry even when discussing neutral or pleasant topics shows constricted affect.

The **stability** of an affect is reflected by the ability to shift from one mood quality (anger, fear, cheerfulness) to another and to shift in intensity. Normally, such shifts occur gradually. Rapid or unexpected shifts in mood and intensity are called unstable mood or lability. Such phenomena are seen in mania, organic mental disorders, and various personality disorders, such as histrionic personality. In organically impaired patients, a patient may shift from sorrow to laughter, or from laughter to rage, in a matter of seconds, often without any external cue. Neurologists sometimes call this "emotional incontinence" as though certain emotions were unexpectedly leaking out. Labile is probably more descriptively accurate, however.

Appropriateness refers to the degree to which the patient's mood matches the content of his speech or thinking as adjudged by the examiner. A patient who laughs when describing his mother's death would be judged to have inappropriate "affect" (this technically should be called inappropriate mood, but the more general term is in common usage despite its imprecise nature). A paranoid patient, convinced that her boss is trying to have her fired, would have an appropriate mood if she were angry or fearful. Even though her thinking is pathologic, her emotions parallel the thought content and therefore are appropriate. Inappropriate affect is not pathognomonic; although it may occur in organic or psychotic states, it can also be expressed by someone who is simply anxious.

Relatedness refers to the ability of the (it is hoped) normal examiner to experience warmth, rapport, or emotional connectedness with the patient—the ability to empathize with the patient. Talking to someone's answering machine instead of to them would provide an experience similar to a lack of emotional relatedness. People who are psychotic, especially schizophrenics, may convey a feeling of aloofness, coldness, emotional distance, or lack of rapport. The words may be there but the feelings are absent. Such patients are sometimes described as having *blunted* or *flat* affect.

Such flatness is a combination of constrictedness, or restricted range, and low intensity or depth, and is reflected in minimal facial expression, staring, poor eye contact, monotonous voice, and unexpressive bodily movements. Again, such lack of relatedness is not pathognomonic for any particular disorder, occurring in psychosis, organic states, depression, personality disorders, and physical illness.

Sensorium

The sensorium refers to the cognitive or intellectual functioning of the patient and most commonly includes orientation, memory, abstractive ability, attention-concentration, information and vocabulary, judgment, and sometimes insight. It was organized in its formal methodology by Adolph Meyer in 1902, but systematic research to establish its value it has been surprisingly neglected. It is the part of the MSE often done by neurologists in conjunction with the neurologic examination, and indeed tests of higher cortical functioning may overlap with this part of the MSE.

In appropriate cases, this part of the exam may be minimized, because many of the data can be obtained via the interview. In cases where the examiner has reason to suspect a deficit, or where a formal examination is required for purposes of comparison with previous tests, a more "in-depth" examination is performed in which all of the areas are tested. For the inexperienced clinician, it is advisable to perform formal exams on patients of all ages, backgrounds, and conditions in order to acquire experience with the range of normal responses.

Orientation

Orientation refers to the patient's ability to discern his location in space and time, and his identity. **Time sense** is the most vulnerable to disturbance, and this can happen to anyone. Who has not had the experience of forgetting which day it was during a long vacation away from home? One might even forget the month, if the vacation overlaps two months. However, in a stable environment, loss of time sense can indicate pathology. The more severe the disturbance of time sense, the more severe the underlying problem. Thus, not knowing the time of day or exact date may be a minor deviation; losing track of the month and year is more significant; and not knowing the season or whether it is day or night can reflect the most profound disorientation in time. It is important not to take this for granted in a suspected patient.

An elderly man was casually asked by an attorney to give the date. He replied that it was Sunday, which it was, and the attorney assumed the man was oriented. However, the physician asked the date (which the patient avoided), the month (which was off by a month), and the year (which was off by 50 years). The man had seen a calendar in his room indicating the day, and his true deficit became apparent only on specific probing.

Orientation to place is lost usually only after time sense and may require probing in certain cases. If the patient has driven to the clinic by himself, it is likely he knows where he is; conversely, if a patient knows he is in New York but doesn't recall the exact address, this may be normal (for example, in an elderly person being brought by his child).

The answers people give under abnormal circumstances can be quite interesting. A stroke victim was convinced he was in a bed in a department store (which had gone out of business years before, reflecting memory loss as well!). A woman knew she was in a university hospital but thought it was in California, not New York. A man knew he was at Jones Rest Home, but claimed it was a restaurant where his wife worked.

Orientation to person is the last to be impaired and is rarely seen except in severe cases of organicity. Occasionally, acutely psychotic individuals will also show loss of identity, although they may also be delusional and believe they are someone else. Nevertheless, they still will have some identity, whereas an organically impaired individual may not offer any identity at all, or may remember only his or her first name. A young woman eventually diagnosed as having an ependymoma was disoriented with regard to time, place, and person. She did not know her own name, and when asked by the examiner: "Is it Linda or Mary?", she replied, "I don't know. Do you know?" This symptom as well as the lack of previous psychiatric history was one of the red flags raising the suspicion of an organic process, despite the lack of focal neurologic signs. In fact, it could be considered a focal finding of the MSE.

Attention and Concentration

Attention reflects the ability to attend to a specific stimulus without distraction by extraneous environmental stimuli. It is distinct from alertness, which involves a more basic process of arousal or wakefulness allowing a patient to respond to any stimulus in the environment. An attentive patient must be alert, but an alert patient need not be attentive.

Impairment can range from mild inattention, which can occur normally in boredom or preoccupation, to gross impairment, which can occur in delirium. A wide variety of syndromes can affect these functions. *Distractibility* can be seen in anxious states, mania, psychosis, and organic syndromes, and impaired concentration can be seen in depression and in dementias, for example. In altered levels of consciousness deviating from normal alertness, impairment can be seen progressively in drowsy states, stupor, and finally coma, where no attention at all is present.

Concentration or vigilance, the capacity to maintain attention over an extended period of time, such as by focusing voluntarily on a specific task or object, can be inferred from the course of the interview and examination or can be tested formally. The *Subtraction of Serial Sevens* test, originated by Emil Kraepelin in the early part of this century (having the patient start with 100, or 101 if tested before, and subtract 7 until no number remains), is a traditional way to assess this function. If the patient has difficulty, it will be reflected in slowness, hesitancy, losing track of the previous number, or giving up. Serial 5s and 3s can be used if patients cannot subtract by 7s, and counting backward from 20 to 0 can be utilized in patients already known to be impaired. In the latter case, inattention can be sometimes seen in the failure to go beyond 10 or 12 in the countdown. Finally, if patients refuse numbers, it can be useful to request that "world" be spelled both forward and backward.

Slight changes in attention, such as those produced by delirium, can be detected with some sensitivity with this task. Increased anxiety, perseveration, starting over, slowness, depreciating the test or examiner, or refusing the task are different ways in which difficulties can be manifest.

Other tasks such as digits forward and backward are also used. *Digit Span* is performed by asking the patient to repeat a series of digits given by the examiner. The examiner should begin with three digits read at the rate of one per second, without pauses or inflections. If the patient fails on the first trial, a second trial of the same number of digits should be given. The test is stopped after two failures at a given series length. The length of the series should start with three digits, then four, and so on until the patient is unable to do them. Then, series should be given for the patient to repeat in reverse, starting with two digits at a time. The usual response is to do five to eight digits forward and four to six backward. A discrepancy of more than three digits between forward and backward span is also abnormal. Experience with normal patients will enable the examiner to evaluate this test more ably. Deficiencies reflect impaired concentration, which in conjunction with other findings may suggest a cognitive problem, a psychiatric problem, or both; by itself the test is nonspecific.

Calculation

Calculation tests require the patient to do arithmetic problems mentally and therefore test attention, concentration, and intelligence. Patients can be asked to perform subtractions or additions of two- or three-digit numbers or to "make change" from a hypothetical transaction ("How much change would you get from a $5 bill if you spent $3.75?"). Although this is a common test, steeped in tradition, it is rarely of practical value, as will be discussed later.

Memory

Memory is a complex function, involving a number of different subfunctions. For purposes of examination, memory can be classified into *long-term* (or *remote*) *memory* of months to years, *recent memory* of hours to weeks, *short-term memory* of minutes to hours, and *immediate recall* of seconds to about a minute. Short-term and recent memory are sometimes lumped together.

Immediate recall is rarely if ever affected, even in Korsakoff's syndrome (a disorder of memory due to damage to memory structures, most commonly from thiamine deficiency). Only in altered states of consciousness and severe bilateral damage to the hippocampi is immediate recall affected.

Short-term memory can be affected in intoxications, acute brain disease, and states of psychomotor epilepsy, whereas recent memory is more often disturbed in chronic brain disease. **Recent memory** can be affected by bilateral hippocampal infarctions, herpes simplex encephalitis, and Korsakoff's syndrome, as well as by dementias such as Alzheimer's disease.

Long-term memory is often the last to be affected, but it is a myth that it remains intact in dementia. In such illnesses long-term memory will often be impaired irregularly (so-called spotty memory), but it is almost always found to be impaired if the examiner probes carefully. In Korsakoff's syndrome, however, long-term memory remains intact.

Adequate concentration and attention are necessary to assess memory accurately. Decreased concentration will therefore go hand-in-hand with impaired memory because the former interferes with the latter.

Immediate recall can be tested by Digit Span, or by repeating any series of words or numbers (but not backward, because this is a different mental function). It can also be tested by presenting four unrelated items (such as dog, pencil, the color red, and loyalty; note the different categories of abstraction) and ask the patient to immediately repeat them. Then, the patient can be asked again 5 to 10 minutes later to test short-term memory. Recent memory can be tested by asking what the patient had for breakfast that morning or dinner the night before (assuming you have a way of verifying this).

Long-term or remote memory is the most stable form of memory and can be assessed via the history. It may be "spotty," which can fool the unwary examiner. Overlearned material may be preserved, so that the patient can tell you all about the history of a leg injury 20 years before but recall little about other past events. Asking the patient to name several presidents is a frequently used test; if asked to recall them in backward order it becomes a test of concentration also. Frequently patients will complain, "I don't follow current events" or "I'm not interested in politics." Major recent events, like a big news story or tragedy, can be inquired about, but some patients will have been isolated from newspapers and television, so caution is necessary.

Questions can be asked concerning the dates of the major wars, Kennedy's assassination, and Watergate, which most people know something about. Personal events are better preserved, so questions like "When were you married? How old are your children? When did you graduate high school? Do you remember the names of any of your teachers? What was your first job? How old are your parents?" can be asked.

It is useful to note that patients are more likely to forget neutral or non-personal data, such as the dates of World War II or the last six presidents in order, than personal items such as dates of their birth, graduation, marriage, and the like. Impairment on these latter items is therefore of greater significance. It is not uncommon, for example, to find demented patients who cannot recall their birth dates or their ages.

Amnesia, or the inability to remember past events, can be due to brain disease or psychiatric disturbance. The television variety of amnesia, seen in dissociative states in people who "forget" for psychologic reasons, is rare. *Fugue states* are states in which individuals travel or move away for long periods of time and are unaware of their past identity and circumstances. In a *dissociative state* the individual will have varying periods of time during which he will have seemingly functioned normally yet later have no recall of what happened during those periods. In contrast to organic amnesias, such patients will be capable of new learning and will not be confused (i.e., disoriented to time and place).

Amnesia due to malingering, as in those with a pragmatic need to "forget," is also uncommon. The *Ganser syndrome,* or *syndrome of approximate answers,* involves the person's giving of slightly incorrect answers, such as saying it is Monday when it is actually Tuesday or May when it is June. When doing calculations, such an individual will answer as though deliberately trying to be slightly inaccurate (10 times 10 equals 101). This syndrome is seen after head trauma and in persons incarcerated in prison.

The most common types of amnesia are those induced by brain dysfunction. *Retrograde amnesia* is the inability to recall events prior to an injury or illness. *Anterograde amnesia,* conversely, is the inability to remember after the event. Head injuries, seizures, intoxicated states, and delirium can all produce amnesia. Electroconvulsive therapy also causes a transient amnesia, which tends to be anterograde rather than retrograde. Most cases of anterograde amnesia, however, tend to be permanent, whereas retrograde amnesia is usually transient except for the minute or two before the event.

Some psychiatric states, such as acute psychosis or mania, can lead to lack of recall of the acute stage in both anterograde and retrograde fashion. Whether this is a true amnesia or a psychologic mechanism of denial is uncertain. Clouded, dreamlike states occurring in psychosis are sometimes called *oneiroid states;* such patients appear dazed, confused, or perplexed.

Sometimes patients will appear to remember accurately but actually are recalling false memories. The memories can be the result of brain disease or psychosis and have been called **pseudomemories** and *retrospective falsification*. **Confabulation** is seen in mania and organic states but is usually associated with the latter. It involves a false reconstruction of memories that are not available to the patient. Such an individual, for example, may not recall what he did the previous day but will recount a plausible description of events that upon attempted verification turns out to be untrue. One can sometimes elicit this by suggesting a false statement to the patient, which the patient then agrees with and elaborates upon. For example, a 52-year-old alcoholic man was asked, "How was your visit with your wife yesterday?" The man replied, "Oh, it went very well. We had a good visit. She said she'll come again." In fact, the man was divorced and his ex-wife lived across the country.

Confabulation is classically associated with Korsakoff's encephalopathy. in which the patient is unable to "make" new memories. Thus, recent events are not registered and cannot be recalled. Confabulation occurs to fill in the gaps. However, confabulation can be seen in many organic disorders, as well as the fantastic varieties seen in delusional psychotic patients, manics, sociopaths, and even in normal children.

Two psychiatric symptoms that can also be subsumed under memory are **deja vu** (already seen) and **jamais vu** (never seen). The former is the phenomenon of experiencing an event as though it had happened previously, such as feeling that one has been in a particular place before, even though it is one's first visit. Jamais vu is the converse: feeling that a familiar experience is unfamiliar. These phenomena occur very infrequently in normal persons but with greater frequency in psychomotor epilepsy, toxic states, and sociopathy.

All that has been discussed so far involves verbal memory. Another memory capacity that can be tested but is usually omitted in the routine MSE is **visual memory.** This is the ability to recall items visually, and it can be tested by having the person "find" several objects placed in hiding, with the patient watching, after an interval of 10 minutes or more. Usually at least three of four objects will be recalled. Sometimes, geometric drawings are used: they are presented to the patient for a few seconds and withdrawn, and then the patient is requested to draw them from memory. Or a patient can be shown 10 or 20 pictures of common objects and then requested to name as many as possible from memory when the pictures are removed. Such tests can be found in standard texts if the reader is interested.

Fund of Information

It is useful to have some estimate of the patient's overall intelligence. In part this can be estimated from his/her performance on tests of information and vocabulary. However, educational background must be known in order to interpret the results of testing. A PhD in mathematics would be expected to perform at a different level than a maintenance man with an eighth-grade education. Given that information, one can partly estimate fund of knowledge or information as well as vocabulary from the interview and history.

The Wechsler Adult Intelligence Scale-Revised (WAIS-R) test asks many questions to measure information in its Information subtest. Most examiners in a clinical situation will not have the time or necessity to ask many information questions. If the patient can recall six presidents, this provides an estimate not only of memory but also of information as well. However, common questions that can be asked include: "Name four large cities in the United States. How many miles from New York to California? How many ounces in a pound? At what temperature does water boil? What is ice? Why do we have laws?"

Vocabulary is the best estimate of IQ and tends to be the most stable over time. It gives the best estimate of preexisting, or premorbid, intelligence even when the brain has been diseased. In severe disease states, the vocabulary will decline also but will generally be the last intellectual function to do so. The examiner can note the patient's use of complicated words or ability to understand the examiner's words (especially if the examiner lapses into medical jargon) or can ask the definitions of words.

One can create one's own list, but the words should be of increasing difficulty. A sample list might include airplane, donkey, diamond, nuisance, join, fur, bacon, tint, fable, stanza, plural, affliction. The patient must be able to give a reasonable definition or use the word correctly in a sentence. Standardized lists can be found in textbooks, with suggested scores for estimating above- and below-average IQ. However, for most clinical purposes, it is necessary only that the examiner make some estimate of intelligence, and this will become more accurate after the examiner has tested many patients. If there are questions, for example, as to whether the patient is mentally retarded, more formal testing can be ordered and past information on school performance can be obtained.

Abstraction

The ability to abstract—to mentally transcend the concrete and tangible and think at "higher" or theoretical levels—is quite vulnerable to both organic disturbances and psychotic processes. The ability to generalize, to use deductive and inductive reason, and to think symbolically are aspects of abstractive capacity.

Usually the interview will reveal examples of the patient's ability to conceptualize, manipulate symbols, and organize information in complex ways, but more formal testing may be required. Proverbs and similarities are two traditional ways in which this function can be tested.

A patient can be given a **proverb** to interpret, telling him: "A proverb is a saying. What do people generally mean when they say (*fill in proverb*)?" There are many common proverbs, with varying levels of difficulty. A few common ones are: don't count your chickens before they're hatched; don't cry over spilt milk; two heads are better than one; a stitch in time saves nine; a rolling stone gathers no moss; the squeaking wheel gets the grease; and empty barrels make the most noise.

The examiner should use the same set of proverbs over and over to develop experience in the range of responses and the difficulty involved. "Two heads are better than one," for example, is the simplest for most people to interpret. "Empty barrels" is often difficult if not heard before by people of average intelligence, although highly intelligent people do well. At least an eighth-grade education is required to be able to abstract proverbs, and it is by no means a pathognomonic test.

Psychotic patients may give idiosyncratic interpretations that bear little relationship to the proverb, or they may be personalized. A schizophrenic woman, for example, when asked about "a stitch in time," stated, "People are always trying to sew up time but it can't be done. God alone can do that, and the heathens had better learn that." A manic responded to "don't count your chickens" with clang associations: "Hatched? That's no match. Who's a match for a chicken? Chicken shit, is all!"

Individuals of low educational background or low IQ and organically impaired persons tend to give concrete responses: "Well of course two heads are better. Two of anything is better than one" (missing the abstract point of two people working together to intellectually solve problems). "Well, you shouldn't cry over spilled milk; just buy another quart."

Anxious people can also show concreteness, and people experiencing intense emotions can give somewhat inappropriate responses. A woman in the throes of divorce who was angry, hostile, and agitated but otherwise not afflicted with a psychiatric or organic disorder replied to "catching more flies with honey than with vinegar" by stating, "That's what happened to my husband. That sweet bitch seduced the SOB. Well, we'll see what tastes bitter after this when I get through." Although somewhat concrete, and certainly personalized and off the point, her response clearly is determined more by the intensity of feelings than by her desire to attend appropriately to the examiner's question, which may have seemed rather irrelevant to her concerns.

Similarities, which require the patient to identify an abstract quality common to different objects, is a frequently used test but has little value, except perhaps as a projective test in the same way as proverbs. (A projective test is one with ambiguous stimuli that allows the patient to interpret it in personal ways that may reveal aspects of personality and internal thoughts and feelings. The divorcing woman, for example, responded to the proverb with a "projection" of her own concerns onto the examiner's question.) If proverbs are concrete, similarities will usually be also. If the fund of information is equally impaired, the patient's concreteness is likely due to intellectual or educational impoverishment.

Common similarities may include identifying the similarity between items of fruit (what do an apple and orange have in common), common objects (airplane and bicycle, table and chairs, glove and shoe, guitar and trumpet) or more complex concepts (pound and yard, ice and steam, justice and equality, 47 and 83). Patients with low IQs or poor education may concretize them, as may brain-diseased patients. Psychotic patients may give strange or bizarre interpretations. Anxious people may concretize. Some demented patients may say, "They're different. They're two different things. They're not alike."

Judgment

The ability of an individual to understand and conform to the common modes of societal behavior and to understand the consequences of deviations from conventional values and mores can sometimes be impaired in disease states. A person who uses bad judgment chronically may be suffering from a personality disorder or a chronic illness, or may come from a background of poor or inadequate socialization.

A person who shows episodes of impaired judgment on a background of generally good judgment needs to have some assessment made as to the cause of the episodes, whether it be drug or alcohol abuse, a psychotic state, or what psychiatrists call "impulse disorders." The latter are disorders characterized by impulsive behaviors, either episodic or continual, that bring the patient in conflict with others and society, such as setting fires, outbursts of violence, gambling, or excessive speeding.

Any psychiatric disorder can create a substrate for errors in judgment; for example, psychoses frequently lead to inappropriate behaviors such as undressing in public, swearing abusively in a public place, quitting a job suddenly for minor reasons, buying two new cars when the patient has no appreciable income, or attempting to walk to California to get exercise. Such impairments in judgment can stem from delusional thinking, auditory command hallucinations, or excited states that press for some immediate activity. Persons in states of drug intoxication or withdrawal, panic or high anxiety, or relentless anger can perform activities that indicate poor judgment.

Patients with brain disease can show impaired judgment, which can sometimes be the first indication of the disorder.

A 60-year-old bank president began frequenting bars and going
out with promiscuous women over a period of several months.
He neglected his work and frequently left the phone off the hook.
He began wearing old clothes to work and was irritable and abusive
to his secretary. He walked around nude at home frequently, even
when guests were present. His change in behavior, all of which
reflected impaired judgment, prompted his wife to take him to the
family physician. After much difficulty, he agreed to see a neurologist and was diagnosed as having a frontal lobe meningioma.

Judgment can be estimated from the patient's overall behavior during the
examination and interview and can be tested in part by asking such questions as:
"What would you do with an unstamped letter you found on the street addressed
to someone in Montana?" "What would you do if you had a flat tire on the highway
but no spare?" More detailed questions appear on the WAIS-R, such as: "Why are
criminals put in prison?" "Why should a promise be kept?", and so forth. The patient
might also be asked what his plans are for the future, and what he would wish for
if given three wishes.

Insight
Patients may or may not understand what is wrong with them. The bank president had no insight that anything was wrong, insisting that his behavior was "being
my own person for a change." Similarly, a depressed patient might declare, "I'm
not depressed, I'm just sick from that antibiotic the doctor gave me." Insight is
of little diagnostic value but has been traditionally included in the MSE. Its main
importance is to help the examiner anticipate the kind of response the patient may
make to recommendations for treatment or evaluation. Knowing that the patient
has no insight into careless behavior, as with the bank president, enables one to
modify the approach to take. The family physician, for example, told that patient,
"You need to be in the best possible shape for all the changes you're making in your
life. I want you to see a special doctor for some tests to verify that you're all
right." Had the doctor confronted the patient too strongly with his behavior, the
patient likely would have protested and refused further help.

Perception and Coordination
Some authorities encourage at least a brief assessment of the patient's visual
and perceptual-motor systems. This is of limited value in "functional" psychiatric
disorders, although dysfunction may occur in the anxious patient who performs
poorly, or the depressed patient who performs slowly. For the patient with organic brain disease, defects can be discerned that may occasionally appear in brief
testing, but as a general rule the examiner is unlikely to uncover problems in most
patients that would not have been otherwise suspected.
Asking the patient to write their name and a grammatical sentence and to read
a sentence are easy and rapid tests for **dysgraphia** and **dyslexia**. Inability to write
or read precisely can indicate a problem to be further evaluated.
Constructional ability is the capacity to construct, draw, or copy a simple
figure and is mediated by the nondominant parietal lobe. The patient can be asked
to copy a geometric figure, such as a circle, a cross, a row of dots, or a three-
dimensional cube, or to draw from memory a clock with a specific time. Severe
distortions of the drawing, rotations, and perseveration (i.e., drawing too many
dots) usually point to some organic impairment. The examiner observes the patient's
ability to reproduce angles, corners, relationships of lines, and orientation in space.

Apraxia, a defect in the integration of motor skills from conception to performance, reflects brain dysfunction. *Ideomotor apraxia* refers to the inability of the patient to carry out motor acts as instructed by the examiner (stick out your tongue, close your eyes). Sometimes impaired patients can still perform the task if it is modeled by the examiner. Ideomotor apraxia can be seen in dysfunction of the dominant parietal lobe or from interruption of fibers between the dominant temporal-parietal area and the frontal lobe.

Ideational apraxia represents a still higher level of dysfunction and causes breakdowns in performance on complex tasks involving several steps. For example, a patient is told: "Fold a piece of paper twice and with your right hand put it in your pocket." Any error, such as folding it once or omitting putting it in the pocket, indicates an abnormality.

Other examples of cortical dysfunction include **right-left disorientation** (the inability to distinguish right from left on one's body and in the environment), **agnosia** (the inability to recognize and sometimes to name an object), **aphasia** (any of a number of defects in language processing that produce errors in choice of words and grammar), and **anomia** (a type of aphasia in which a patient cannot name an object presented to him although he can recognize it).

Reliability and Caveats for Use of MSE Tests

It is important to emphasize the fact that many of the standard MSE tests exist as much by tradition as by clinical utility and that the examiner needs to be aware of their limitations. In a recent study, Keller and Manschreck (7) reviewed the literature on the sensorium part of the MSE and offered a number of conclusions. They found *orientation* to be reliable and useful in distinguishing organic and nonorganic disorders. They found *memory* tests to be highly reliable (i.e., reproducible by other examiners or by the same examiner at different times) but not always valid (indicative of real dysfunction) because of factors such as intelligence, age, anxiety, and depression. They noted that the standard tests of *attention* and *concentration* measure an individual's capacity to sustain effort but do not test inattentiveness, increased attentiveness, or distractibility. With respect to *general information,* there is some evidence of its usefulness in distinguishing organic illness and it has high retest reliability for a given patient; its practical usefulness is limited, Keller and Manschreck claimed, because cutoff scores may be inapplicable to individual patients as opposed to statistical groups. *Calculation* is influenced by attention, concentration, and intelligence and has little practical use except in the rare syndrome of dyscalculia, or Gerstmann's syndrome, which involves the angular gyrus of the left parietal lobe (it consists of acalculia, right-left disorientation, finger agnosia, and dysgraphia). Finally, *insight* is of no proven aid in diagnosis of either psychiatric of neurologic disorders.

These tests are not designed to be used in isolation, but together with other information may produce a richer picture of the patient's overall mental functioning. Also, formal tests do not replace the more naturalistic observations every examiner must make with respect to the patient's behavior and communications during the overall interview and examination. As an example, an experienced clinician can detect the presence of distractibility in a patient from his behavior during the clinical interview. More formal tests of concentration, then, can be applied to support the clinical impression of distractible behavior. Conversely, it is very unlikely that the patient would appear distractible only on formal testing and not evidence this in the examination situation.

Similarly, memory testing needs to be formalized at times in order to detect and define disorders that might be missed in a cursory examination, although any clearly profound disturbance would be easily detected in the general examination without special testing. Bearing in mind that memory dysfunction can also occur in nonorganic states, it is important to delineate the type and degree of difficulty and monitor it at subsequent examinations. Therefore, although it may at times be difficult to distinguish a functional from an organic disorder (as in depression versus a dementia in an elderly patient), it is of great importance to delineate that there is memory dysfunction present.

CLINICAL EXAMPLES

It is difficult for the inexperienced clinician to learn signs and symptoms in isolation. Only when placed in a framework, as in a constellation of findings related to a disease entity or syndrome, do they become meaningful. Similarly, the signs and symptoms of the psychiatric history and MSE can be difficult to learn without a context in which to place them. It is the function of teaching in psychiatry in general and in psychopathology in particular to integrate the building blocks of examination into a cohesive understanding.

Although it is beyond the limits of this chapter to review these broad areas, illustrating how the data of this chapter can be synthesized may prove useful to the student. Several clinical vignettes will be presented to help convey a sense of relatedness of the data discussed here to clinical situations.

Mania

The manic syndrome, although most commonly associated with the primary disorder of manic-depressive illness (known as bipolar affective disorder to psychiatrists), can also be a syndrome secondary to a variety of physical illnesses and drugs. Central nervous system tumors and infections, seizure disorders, corticosteroids, isoniazid, procarbazine, L-dopa, and bromides are known causes of secondary mania. Thus, although one can diagnose the syndrome of mania from history and MSE, it is not possible to diagnose manic-depressive disorder without further evaluation.

George was a 29-year-old music school teacher who experienced a hectic schedule leading up to a Memorial Day series of concerts he was organizing. A week prior to his hospitalization he began not sleeping and felt his energy was increased so that he did not feel any need to sleep. He began to believe that he was ordained to do important things. On May 30, while in church, he felt that God was speaking to him through the minister. At this time he suddenly felt he had a special mission to become president of the United States at the next election and perhaps even become "President of the World."

George shared his ideas with his friends, who urged him to see a doctor. Because he was somewhat concerned about his blood pressure, he agreed to this. His friends told the doctor that George had become "progressively excited" in the prior month, but continued to handle his job excellently. If anything, he seemed to be much more productive than usual, although they were concerned he was working too hard. George described to the physician that for the past 2 weeks he had had no appetite and had lost 20 pounds; he felt there wasn't time to eat. He also felt increasingly interested sexually and had approached women numerous times in the month before. His physician was able to persuade George to be admitted to a psychiatric unit. On admission to the hospital, his MSE was as follows.

> He was a tall, mesomorphic, blond man, dressed inappropriately
> in tennis clothes. He was somewhat dishevelled, with uncombed
> hair, a heavy growth of beard, and the odor of sweat. He was
> cooperative and unusually cheerful and friendly. His mood was

euphoric, and his affect inappropriate to the seriousness of the situation. He behaved as though he were at a party rather than in a psychiatric unit. His speech was pressured and revealed flight of ideas. He showed clang associations, as revealed in his interpretation of proverbs. He denied feeling suicidal or homicidal but evidenced delusions in the form of believing that God was sending him messages to be president of the United States. He was oriented to time, place, and person. His recent and remote memory were adequate, but he could do only one digit forward and two back. He was unable to do serial 7s but did do serial 3s hesitantly with one error. He was easily distracted and thus had trouble attending to the examiner's questions. His fund of knowledge was fair but estimated to be below that expected for his education. His responses to proverbs and similarities were concrete and personalized: in response to "two heads," "I wish I had two heads, then I could get more done; so I just have to think twice as fast"; in response to "empty barrels," "We should roll out the barrels and just have a good time. Let's have a real old fashioned Fourth of July and show the people what we can do for this country"; in response to "What do an airplane and a boat have in common?", "Was it Paul Revere who said one if by land two if by air?" His social judgment was poor, as reflected by the comment that if he found an unstamped letter addressed to Montana he'd probably deliver it himself since he expected to go to all the states to carry his message. His insight was lacking, because he felt there was nothing wrong with him except perhaps high blood pressure.

George thus showed some of the symptoms of mania in his history and had an MSE consistent with an acute psychosis with manic elements. Although dementia or delirium might need to be ruled out, his memory dysfunction seemed due more to impaired concentration from his acute illness. A complete work-up showed that George was suffering from the first manic episode of a manic-depressive disorder.

Depression

Like mania, depression is also a syndrome that has to be further defined. In the elderly, it often takes the form of a depression with psychotic symptoms such as delusions and hallucinations.

Murray was a 70-year-old optometrist who was reluctant to retire. Since Labor Day, 1980, he had become obsessed with his health following a leg cramp sustained while swimming; he worried about permanent damage. In November, a sister died suddenly, and in December his 82-year-old brother, to whom he was very close, passed away after a brief hospitalization for cardiac disease. Following this last event, Murray began having difficulty falling asleep, would awaken several times during the night, and couldn't sleep past 4 AM. He noticed trouble concentrating and remembering things, and he cut back his practice. He ruminated about his brother but was unable to cry. He felt his worst in the morning and had to push himself to go to work. His appetite dwindled, he lost 15 pounds, and he began to hear a voice telling him he was not competent to practice and should retire before he killed someone. He also began to feel that his money was running out and he would soon be in the poorhouse. He gave up doing the family accounts, and let his wife do all the driving. When he began to talk of killing himself to "get it all over with," his wife brought him to the emergency room, from where he was admitted to the hospital. His MSE was as follows.

> The patient was a dapper, impeccably dressed man in a three-piece suit, appearing his stated age with a somewhat rigid, formal posture and trembling hands. He moaned softly at times throughout the interview. He was irritable with the examiner but answered all questions frankly. His speech was slow and halting with some tangentiality and circumstantiality. Several times during the interview he abruptly stood up and began pacing the floor in circles, moaning "I wish I was dead. I wish my brother was here," while wringing his hands. He performed serial 7s with many errors, as he did also with serial 3s, and he accomplished six digits forward but only three backward. Proverb responses were concrete ("Don't cry over spilt milk" was interpreted with the statement "I can't cry over anything"). He was unable to remember any of three objects after 5 minutes, but his recent and remote memory were excellent. He was hypervigilant and overly attentive to noises outside the room. He blocked at one point and stated that he thought he had heard someone speaking other than the examiner but he couldn't make out the words. He insisted he was impoverished and couldn't afford the hospital despite the examiner's statements that his insurance was in effect and would pay. He was worried that his leg had not recovered from the swimming episode and that it might be cancerous inside. He was able to name objects correctly and draw figures without distortion, and he could read and carry out complex commands adequately.

Murray thus gave evidence of an agitated depressive state with psychotic symptoms typically seen in depression (a voice criticizing him and delusions of poverty). He also expressed somatic delusions, which are commonly seen in depression, and his history of a variety of symptoms affecting his sleep, appetite, energy, interest, and so forth was entirely consistent with a depressive disorder.

Dementia

Antoinette was a 70-year-old woman who became gradually irritable, suspicious, and confused. Her husband, who was an alcoholic, noticed these changes only slowly and so she became considerably worse before he took her to their family physician. That physician referred her to a neurologist, who diagnosed probable primary degenerative dementia (Alzheimer's disease) on the basis of clinical history, mild cerebral atrophy on computed tomography scan, mild generalized slowing on electroencephalogram, and no positive physical findings to suggest any other cause for her dementia. She was then transferred to a nursing home, where she was seen by a psychiatric consultant who noted the following MSE.

> She was a pleasant women with wispy white hair, wearing a bathrobe and ambulating slowly in the company of her husband. Her gait was somewhat unsteady and she appeared restless. Her mood was labile—she became tearful at times and then quickly shifted to a pleasant or even cheerful mood. Her affect was inappropriate, puerile, and shallow. She was alert and animated

but very distractible, with a short attention span. She was garrulous in her speech, being tangential and often rambling nonsensically. She confabulated fluently when asked questions she didn't know ("How old are you?" "Well, I'm much older than I used to be. Probably around 60 or 70. I don't really keep track that much anymore."). She had some word-finding difficulties and could not recall her husband's name, calling him "honeybun" instead.

She was disoriented to time and place, believing it was November, 1999 (actually it was June, 1984) and couldn't identify the season. Her remote memory was impaired; she was unable to recall her year of birth, the ages of her children, or the year of her marriage. She could recall three items immediately after presentation but none after 2 minutes. She could not remember her lunch, although she confabulated an unlikely menu of pancakes and steak. She could recall no presidents except Roosevelt. She could not do serial 7s or 3s and could count backward from 20 only to 15. She copied several geometric figures poorly and could not draw a recognizable clock. She showed perseveration in both her writing and her speech. Her judgment was severely impaired, her proverbs were inappropriate or concrete, she could not do similarities, and her insight was nil.

Although not part of the MSE per se, a brief neurologic examination revealed abnormal snout, grasp, and sucking reflexes, which corroborated the impression of dementia. Thus, Antoinette showed signs and symptoms of dementia, and her MSE indicated changes in mood and affect, behavior, orientation, memory, and concentration and attention; impaired judgment; lack of insight; and specific cognitive deficits on formal testing.

Delirium

A 42-year-old man who fancied himself an Elvis Presley look-alike complained of symptoms consistent with depression and agitation since his boss threatened him with the loss of his job 2 weeks before. He became sleepless, lost his appetite, could not concentrate at work, and paced continually at home, ruminating about his future. He was irritable and several times nearly struck his wife. He began therapy with a psychiatrist, who placed him on thioridazine and amitriptyline to ease his agitation and treat his depression. Unknown to the psychiatrist, the patient was also taking several different antihistamines for a sinus condition. Five days after beginning the psychotropic medications, his wife called the doctor reporting her husband to be confused, seeing things, and acting strangely. He was then seen at the physician's office, where the following MSE was obtained.

The patient was a stocky, flushed gentleman, dressed in old clothes, perspiring profusely and breathing heavily. His eyes seemed to bulge out and he was restless. He appeared to be cooperative but seemed unable to attend to the doctor's questions. His speech was disjointed and tangential, rambling at times, and showing derailment and looseness of associations. He mumbled some of his words and showed some slurring of speech. His mood was anxious and fearful, with some lability in which he would become suddenly tearful or angry. His affect was intense and at times inappropriate. He described seeing monkeys outside his window and believed they were real, although he had some suspicion that they might not be. He complained that loud noises hurt his ears and that he felt strange sensations on his skin. He was disoriented as to day of the week, date, and month but knew the year. He knew he was at the doctor's office but could not state the address. He was aware of the city and state but had difficulty recalling them without prompting. He remembered his date of birth but not his marriage date. He remembered his two children but was unsure of their ages. He remembered none of three objects after 2 minutes, could not recall his last meal, and could not name any presidents in sequence.

He could not do serial 7s past 93, complaining that he "couldn't think well." He was unable to do calculations. He spelled "world" correctly forward but misspelled it backward. He was able to do only four digits forward and two backward. He showed both concreteness and idiosyncratic responses to proverbs (in response to "two heads," "Everybody should have two heads if they're smart"). On similarities he was concrete (dog-cat, "They both have tails and ears"). On questions of judgment he gave inappropriate responses (to the situation of a fire in a theater, he responded, "I'd get the hell out; every man for himself"). He had some sense that something was wrong with him and wanted help from the physician. He was unable to draw a clock without misplacing the numbers and forgetting the hands. His signature was barely legible due to tremulousness.

This patient showed signs of a delirium characterized by disturbances in behavior, thinking, and affect, and cognitive problems including disorientation, memory impairment, trouble concentrating, concreteness, impaired judgment, and poor visual-motor function. Further evaluation confirmed the tentative diagnosis of an anticholinergic delirium.

Catatonia

Emily, a 57-year-old woman with a history of lymphoma and leukemia, was referred for psychiatric consultation for her "depression." The consultant had little history except information relating to her hematologic disorders and a history of past treatment for depression with antidepressants. At the present time she was taking no medication. He obtained the following MSE.

The patient was awake and apparently alert, sitting in a chair in her room motionless. She did not react when the psychiatrist entered the room, and she did not respond when addressed. In attempting a physical examination, the patient was resistant and refused to cooperate, although she continued to remain mute. She showed facial grimacing, although her face was often blank and staring. She occasionally made strange movements of her body, including purposeless alterations of posture (posturing). When she held one of these postures for over 10 minutes, the examiner described her as having catalepsy. When the examiner attempted to move her arms out of her postures, she resisted (this is known as gegenhalten). A bit later he was able to move her arm above her head, where it remained, an example of waxy flexibility. Finally, she imitated his folding his arms, an example of echopraxia. Because the patient was mute, the examiner could not test her cognitive functions or her language. He described her mood as angry, alternating with indifference, and her affect as severely constricted, showing no range.

Thus, Emily exemplified many of the features of the catatonic syndrome, which can also include stereotypies, echolalia, verbigeration, and rigidity. Such patients can also appear excited and behave bizarrely, oblivious to their surroundings and the consequences of their actions. Some clinicians automatically associate catatonia with schizophrenia, especially catatonic schizophrenia, but as Gelenberg (4) demonstrated in a classic article, the catatonic syndrome has many causes, including affective disorder, hysterical and dissociative states, neurologic disorders (such as tumors), metabolic disturbances (such as diabetic ketoacidosis and porphyria), viral infections (such as encephalitis), toxic substances (such as mescaline and phencyclidine), and therapeutic drugs (such as the phenothiazines, which may themselves be used to treat catatonia). In Emily's case, central nervous system involvement from her hematologic disorders caused her catatonic syndrome; she died 10 days after the consultant saw her.

Paranoid State

Helen, a 42-year-old woman originally from Barbados, was brought by her sister to the outpatient psychiatry clinic. The patient had had an episode of psychosis 10 years previously, which had been treated successfully with antipsychotic medication. Years before that, the patient was described as being unusual in her behavior, maintaining that she had psychic powers. Two weeks before her visit to the clinic, she developed hallucinations of voices of both sexes commanding her to do such things as take off her shoes or steal a scarf from a store. She thought that people were talking about her and that she could help the President in freeing the Iranian hostages. She also felt that her psychic powers had returned. Over the past week her sleeping had become disturbed and she had quit her job as a domestic. A MSE revealed the following information.

The patient was an attractive black woman, looking her stated age, wearing a colorful scarf. She was guarded and reserved with the examiner and spoke reluctantly. Her mood was mildly depressed, her affect bland and constricted but not inappropriate. Her speech was coherent and goal directed but sparse. There was an evasive quality to her speech and she refused to elaborate when asked. She admitted to hearing voices during the interview telling her to leave and to be careful not to say too much lest she be hospitalized against her will. She thought the examiner might be one of the people who had been talking about her earlier that week. She was oriented "times three" (that is, to time, place, and person), recalled correctly three of three items with both immediate recall and 5 minutes later. She recalled personal dates accurately and had an adequate grasp of commonly known historic events. She did serial 7s rapidly and correctly but refused to continue after 65. Calculations were correct. Proverbs and similarities were resisted as unnecessary. In her opinion something was wrong but she was not sure whether it was her problem. She showed a paranoid flavor to her social judgment; when asked about an unstamped letter, she said it should be mailed but since someone might be watching, she would walk on by.

In sum, this woman gave evidence of a paranoid syndrome with hallucinations, delusions, ideas of reference, and no signs of organicity. There was no grandiosity or suggestion of mania in the MSE, but there was a hint of some depressed mood, not reflected in the kind of delusions she expressed (that is, they were mood-incongruent delusions as opposed to the mood-congruent type found mainly in depression) or in her sensorium (that is, the reduced concentration or memory often seen in depressives was not present). The history gave a suggestion of possible grandiose beliefs (talking to the President about the hostages) but this did not surface in the MSE.

Helen thus gave evidence of a paranoid disorder, which could be due to a psychiatric disorder (such as manic-depressive illness, schizophrenia, or a true paranoid state) or could be secondary to a neurologic disorder (tumors, degenerative diseases, temporal lobe epilepsy), a metabolic disorder (lupus erythematosus, Wilson's disease, pellagra, porphyria), an endocrine disorder (hypoadrenalism, hypoparathyroidism), an infection (syphilis, malaria, trypanosomiasis), alcohol or drug abuse, or toxic agents (amphetamines, steroids). Thus, her paranoid disorder required further diagnostic evaluation.

Personality Disorder

Frank, a 25-year-old man, presented to his general practitioner complaining of vague pains in his back and head. He denied any previous psychiatric history but stated he had suffered headaches for some years. He recently moved into town as a result of a job change and needed a new doctor. He asked for a tranquilizer or painkiller, saying it was necessary to keep him working. He said it would likely be only a temporary measure because he expected he would feel better once the stress of the job and the move subsided. He emphatically stated he had never been an abuser of drugs. He gave the name of an out-of-town physician but stated he could not remember the exact address or telephone number. The following MSE was obtained.

He was a handsome, neatly dressed man in a three-piece corduroy suit. His collar seemed too tight and he seemed tense. He had greeted the physician with a loud voice and a brisk handshake, and had sat down without being asked. He made good eye contact, and indeed was almost piercing in his glance, with a facial expression that often resembled a sneer. He seemed superficially cooperative but an evasive quality appeared that showed itself in changing the subject or bombarding the physician with constant chatter that distracted the examiner from his questions. His mood seemed somewhat irritable but pleasant; his affect had a shallow, insincere quality that was reinforced by gratuitous comments like, "I heard you have a superb reputation as a diagnostician, Dr. Jones." His manner was supercilious and condescending, and the physician's questions were met with glib and brief answers. He denied any psychiatric symptoms, explaining his head pain was diffuse and "excruciating" and that he had been "thoroughly evaluated and only Valium works." When the doctor suggested a small dosage to start, the patient countered almost sarcastically, "That wouldn't touch a fly." The patient appeared oriented with intact recent and remote memory except for discrepancies in his medical history that were inconsistent with his recall of all other events. He dutifully answered questions testing his concentration, abstraction, and judgment. To the question of finding an unstamped letter, he replied, "Of course I'd mail it; I'm not one of those dishonest people who would hold it up to the light to see if it contained any money."

Thus, Frank showed no evidence of any major psychiatric disorder, psychosis, or organic brain dysfunction within the available history and MSE, although suspicions were clearly raised as to the possibility of drug abuse. Possible problems were reflected in a style of relating that to an experienced clinician might suggest a personality disorder, such as an antisocial or narcissistic personality disorder.

However, personality disorders can rarely be diagnosed with certainty without a longitudinal history, which is unlikely to be obtained from the patient in a brief contact. This man could also be a genuine headache sufferer with some "obnoxious" personality traits, or an anxious individual who presents irritably in a strange situation. In such an interaction, the examiner would do well to remember also that, even if the primary problem is drug abuse, the patient still represents an individual in trouble. To become annoyed and hostile in return is not only unprofessional but might lead to further serious difficulties in both diagnosis and treatment.

Physicians see many people with a variety of personality disorders. The history or MSE in such people may be somewhat typical, as with a histrionic or paranoid personality disorder; or the individual may appear to have some kind of personality problem, although it may be difficult to specify; or the person may seem completely normal during limited contact with the physician. What appear to be specific personality problems may in fact be secondary to another, more important illness. For example, a manic-depressive in only a mild state of mania may appear to be annoyingly narcissistic. Thus personality disorder should not be diagnosed on the basis of a MSE, and often not even with a psychiatric history. Finally, any individual, no matter what his personality style, may have any other disorder, either psychiatric or medical. The patient's personality should not distract the physician from his task of evaluating and helping the patient to the fullest.

REFERENCES

1. American Psychiatric Association: *Diagnostic and Statistical Manual of Mental Disorders,* ed 3. Washington, DC, American Psychiatric Association, 1980.

2. Folstein MF, Folstein SW, McHugh PR: 'Mini-mental state.' A practical method of grading the cognitive state of patients for the clinician. *Psychiatr Res* 1975;12:189-198.

3. Kaplan HI, Sadock BJ (eds): *Comprehensive Textbook of Psychiatry IV.* Baltimore, Williams & Wilkins, 1985.

4. Gelenberg AJ: The catatonic syndrome. *Lancet* 1976;1:1339-1341.

5. Granacher RP Jr: The neurological examination in geriatric psychiatry. *Psychosomatics* 1981;22:485-499.

6. Jenkyn LR, Walsh B, Culver CM, Reeves AG: Clinical signs in diffuse cerebral dysfunction. *Neurol Neurosurg Psychiatry* 1977;40:956-966.

7.   Keller MB, Manschreck TC: The bedside mental status examination—reliability and validity. *Comprehensive Psychiatry* 1981;22:500-510.

8.   Krauthammer C, Klerman GL: Secondary mania: Manic syndrome associated with antecedent physical illness or drugs. *Arch Gen Psychiatry* 1978;35:1333-1339.

9.   Lezak MD: *Neuropsychological Assessment,* ed 2. New York, Oxford University Press, 1983.

10. Mesulam M-M (ed): *Principles of Behavioral Neurology.* Philadelphia, FA Davis Co, 1985.

11. Stasiek C, Zetin M: Organic manic disorders. *Psychosomatics* 1985;26:394-402.

12. Stoudemire A: The differential diagnosis of catatonic states. *Psychosomatics* 1982;23:245-252.

13. Strub RL, Black FW: *The Mental Status Examination in Neurology,* ed 2. Philadelphia, FA Davis Co, 1985.

14. Taylor MA: *The Neuropsychiatric Mental Status Examination.* New York, SP Medical & Scientific Books, 1981.

4
Examination of the Lungs

Siegfried J. Kra, M.D.

I once heard a younger colleague say that physical diagnosis of the lungs is a waste of time because a chest radiograph may show a lesion or infiltrate that you could never find on a physical diagnosis. It is true that small lesions and tumors and infiltrates often are not detected by the physical examination, but that does not depricate physical diagnosis; it points out its limitations. Once you are out in practice, a chest radiograph may not always be available, and you will have to rely on your learned skills to diagnose pneumonias, pleural effusions, and so forth.

Before discussing the actual physical diagnosis method of the lungs, a review of certain landmarks is necessary.

THE LANGUAGE OF EXAMINATION
OF THE CHEST AND THORAX

The *suprasternal notch* is located at the top of the manubrium. The *sternal angle* is that spot at which the manubrium and the body of the sternum join. It is a protrusion called the angle of Louis, and it is the point of attachment of the second rib. Location of this reference point will enable you to count the ribs for identification and reference points.

The *midclavicular line* is that line extending downward from the middle of each clavicle. The *anterior axial line* extends downward from the anterior axillary fold. The *intrascapular area* is that portion of the posterior thorax lying between the scapulae.

THE OUTLINE OF THE LUNG

The right lung has upper, middle, and lower lobes; the left lung is divided into an upper and lower lobe. The apex of each lung extends approximately 2-4 cm above the inner third of the clavicle. Looking at the back of the patient, the left upper lobe and right upper lobe complement each other, extending laterally toward the apex of the scapula. The left lower lobe and right lower lobe make up most of the portion of the back.

Looking at the right side of the patient while his arm is raised, the right upper lobe is in the lateral fold, a little triangle below is the right middle lobe, and the right lower lobe is posterior to both. With the patient's left arm raised, the left side of the body can be divided by an oblique line extending posteriorly and anteriorly to the sixth rib; above this is the left upper lobe and below it the left lower lobe.

Facing the patient directly in front, the right upper lobe and the left upper lobe are on the left and right sides of the patient, respectively. The right upper and middle lobes are divided by a horizontal fissure, and the right middle lobe extends below the nipple and covers part of the right upper quadrant of the abdomen. The right lower lobe is slightly to the left of the right middle lobe (facing the patient). The left upper lobe makes up most of the anterior portion of the chest, with the left lower lobe extending slightly into the axilla.

THE PULMONARY HISTORY

It is useful to obtain a complete smoking history on the number of cigarettes, pipes, and cigars smoked per day, and the number of years smoking has continued. Remember to include the occupational history, because some pulmonic disorders result from the type of work that a person does. Certain occupations, such as sandblasting, working in an iron foundry, and the mining of coal, lead, and zinc, are associated with silicosis.

Does the patient have a cough? Ask about duration, onset, relation to body posture, time of day or only at night, and whether it occurs when lying flat. Is the cough present only in the morning upon rising, as in smoker's lung? Is there early or more bronchitis? Shortness of breath at rest, or with effort? Decreased exercise tolerance, sudden onset of dyspnea wheezing, history of asthma, allergies, choking episodes? Effort coughing? Wheezing with exercise can mean asthma.

Although it may be distasteful to the physician to look at sputum, the quantity, the color, the viscosity, and the odor can yield a wealth of information. Yellow or green pus in globs is an important sign of an inflammation in the tracheobronchial tree. Lung abscesses have putrid sputum, and bronchiectasis produces a large amount of purulent sputum that separates into distinctive layers. Emphysematous patients tend to produce a grayish-whitish mucoid sputum. Streaks of blood may signal cancer of the lung, benign tumors, and bronchiectasis. There is a rusty-colored sputum in classic lobar pneumonia, as well as infarction of the lung resulting from pulmonary embolism. The characteristic foamy red sputum seen in pulmonary edema accompanying left ventricular failure is unforgettable. Patients with mitral stenosis may have recurrent coughing up of blood. Arteriovenous fistulas and telangiectasia of the lung should not be forgotten as a cause of hemoptysis.

PHYSICAL INSPECTION

The lung examination should be conducted with the patient sitting up with his chest exposed anteriorly and posteriorly. When the patient is lying down, the chest cannot expand symmetrically, and inaccurate percussion and auscultatory sounds may result.

The presence of cyanosis is as important a part of the lung examination as it is for the heart. Cyanosis is apparent when 5 g of unoxygenated hemoglobin is present in the capillaries. Anemic persons may not appear cyanotic, even if the

PO_2 is low, because there is not enough unoxygenated hemoglobin to produce cyanosis. Polycythemic patients have a dusty hue, even though the PO_2 level in their blood is normal.

Check the lips, tongue, earlobes, and nails for the presence of cyanosis. Clubbing of the fingers is a useful sign in pulmonary pathology. It is found in chronic pulmonary disease, such as interstitial fibrosis of the lung, and cystic fibrosis, and is sometimes associated with bronchiectasis and carcinoma of the lung. Formerly, when empyema ran rampant prior to the antibiotic era, clubbing was a common finding.

Make note of the chest configuration:

A *barrel chest* is associated with pulmonary emphysema but is not diagnostic.

In *funnel chest,* the lower sternum is moved posteriorly and can cause displacement of the heart and lungs to an abnormal location, causing difficulties in interpretations.

Chicken breast, in which the sternum is pushed forward, changes little the lung physiology.

Observe surgical scars and the pattern of blood flow on the chest: a large, dilated, visible vein could mean obstruction of the superior vena cava.

Is there retraction or bulging of the rib interspaces? Retraction on inspiration may indicate obstruction of flow of air into the respiratory tract. Bulging of the interspaces occurs in massive pleural effusion and tension pneumothorax, and is seen during forced inspiration in patients who have emphysema or asthma. Bulging of the chest also may be seen in tumors of the thoracic wall, aortic aneurysm, and children with marked cardiac enlargement.

Respiration

The normal respiratory rate in the adult is from 8 to 16 breaths per minute. Inspiration is generally longer than expiration in the normal individual.

Observe the type of breathing present. Dyspnea or shortness of breath may be obvious to the examiner, but the patient may not be aware of it. Dyspnea may be inspiratory or expiratory. *Inspiratory dyspnea* occurs when there is severe laryngitis, obstructions such as tumors or foreign bodies, or extrinsic compression of the trachea or bronchi. It is accompanied by an inspiratory retraction.

Expiratory dyspnea is associated with obstruction in the bronchioles and smaller bronchi, as in obstructive emphysema, bronchitis, and asthma. Expiration is prolonged and forced because of obstruction to the outflow of air.

Apnea is temporary cessation of breathing; *tachypnea* indicates increased respiratory rate; and *hyperpnea* is an increase in depth of respiration.

Hyperventilation is an increase in depth of respiration and rate. Causes include diabetic acidosis, emotional states, and excessive exercise.

Pleuritic breathing is the sudden cessation of inspiration because of pain due to pleuritis. This is, in essence, shallow breathing.

Periodic breathing is rapidly increasing rate and depth of inspiration followed by shallower breathing that finally ceases.

Stertorous respiration is the breathing found in some dying patients—rattling or gurgling produced by the passage of air through secretions that accumulate in the trachea and bronchi. It is also called rales or the death rattle.

Sighing respiration has to be differentiated from dyspnea. Some patients state, "I am very short of breath," when, in reality, they are only sighing. This is not a sign of organic disease.

Cheyne-Stokes respiration was described by Cheyne himself as follows: "His breathing was irregular; would entirely cease for a quarter of a minute, then it would become perceptible though very low, then by degrees it became heaving and quick, then it would gradually cease again. This revolution in the state of his breathing occupied about a minute during which time there are about 30 acts of respiration." This type of respiration is found in brain tumors, cardiac disease, chronic nephritis, meningitis, and pneumonia.

Palpation of the Chest

Palpation of the chest is a good way to determine respiratory excursions. Place both hands on the back of the chest, on the lateral portion of the rib cage, thumbs pointing toward the center parallel to the 10th ribs. Ask the patient to inhale deeply. This will allow you to feel the motion of the chest. Observe if there is decreased or increased motion of the chest (poor motion is seen in emphysema). Gentle tapping of the chest wall with the finger might elicit a tenderness of the pleura found between the ribs that is sometimes seen in pulmonary embolism. A similar maneuver should be done on the anterior portion of the chest, the thumbs pointing toward the center and the hands grasping laterally.

Palpation should include locating the position of the trachea. The spaces of the trachea on either side should be determined by placing your fingers in the suprasternal notch and moving them along to either side. Normally the space should be an equal distance on both sides. A trachea that is moved to one side can indicate a shift of the mediastinal structures produced by tumor, pleural effusions, or pneumothorax. In pneumothorax, there is a shift of the mediastinum toward the opposite side. Pleural effusions may push the mediastinal structures to the opposite side also. Atelectasis of the lung caused by a mucus plug, tumor, or foreign body will cause the mediastinal structures to shift toward the affected side.

TACTILE FREMITUS

The term "fremitus" means vibration. It is the perception by the hand of the vibratory sensations of the thoracic wall produced by speaking. Ask the patient to say "one, two, three" or to say "thirty-three" (or, if you wish to be international, say in French, "trent-trois," which is very effective). The sounds that arise in the larynx are transmitted through the tracheobronchial system and into the bronchi of each lung onto the smaller bronchiole and on to the alveoli, causing the thoracic wall to vibrate as a large resonator.

To examine for fremitus, place the palmar aspect of the fingers against the chest wall. Both hands are used in the corresponding areas, so that you can compare both sides. Others prefer to use the ulnar aspect of the hand with the fingers extended or sometimes with the fingers close to the palm. I prefer using one hand at a time and moving it to the corresponding place. I also find that the palmar surface of my hand is much more sensitive than the ulnar.

Normal vocal fremitus is most evident in the region where the large bronchi are closest to the thoracic wall over the upper thorax and the anterior and posterior side of the chest. Fremitus, obviously, is going to vary according to the thickness of the chest. In obese people fremitus will be diminished, and in thin people it will be increased. Small patches of pathology in the lung are not going to cause any change in vocal fremitus. This is a method of detecting large areas of abnormalities. It stands to reason that anything that will increase transmission of sound, such as lung consolidation, will increase fremitus. Fremitus, as a rule, is felt more clearly on the right.

Decreased fremitus will occur with any condition that interferes with the transmission of the sound waves from the lungs to the chest. For example, in fusions of fluid in the pleural sac, thickening of the pleura, or an infiltrating tumor will diminish or abolish fremitus. Atelectasis will cause fremitus to be diminished or absent.

PERCUSSION

Just as the stethoscope is the badge of the physician, so is percussion a distinguished sign of a practicing physician. Your hands are going to stimulate the chest wall and its contents to produce vibrations that will be felt by the fingers and perceived by the ear.

A pitiful medical chart I recently observed described an elderly woman who arrived with bilateral pleural effusions evident on chest radiograph. The intern examining the patient raced through the examination, briefly remarking in the chart that there were some rales present and the patient had a pleural effusion. Surely a more detailed description would have enabled the intern to make a better diagnosis and would be another step forward in the continuing saga of the fight for diagnostic clinical examination.

Percussion is an ancient technique that Leopold Auenbrugger (1722-1809) was credited for bringing into clinical practice:

> The signs of hydrops of the chest on one side of the thorax, besides the general signs which I have presented, the affected side (if it is not entirely filled with fluid) is weakened and is perceived to be less moveable on inspiration. Moreover, on percussion, there is no resonance in any part, but if it is half-filled with fluid, a greater resonance obtained in that part which is not filled with fluid.

Percussion has its limitations. Any lesion that is more than 5-8 cm away from the chest wall, or that is smaller than 3-4 cm in diameter, will not change the percussion sound. In the same fashion, fluid is the pleural cavity, if it does not exceed 350 mm, will not change the percussion sound. On the other hand, trust your fingers, because pleural effusions altering percussion and fremitus can be detected by the physical examination before the chest radiograph demonstrates the fluid.

Method of Percussion

Percussion is not easy to learn. I suggest you practice on yourself or a friend, or on a mattress, on a wall, and on a desk in order to appreciate different sounds. Extent your hand on the chest, placing it on the portion that you are going to examine; stretch out the middle finger, and place it firmly on the contact surface (Figure 4.1). Only your fingers should send out the message for the chest to vibrate. Gently arch the fingers of your other hand as if you are going to play a piano. Using only your fingers to percuss, tap the middle fingernail of the extended hand, keeping your wrist tucked slightly. Do not use your entire arm, banging away, but, instead, use the right middle finger if you are right-handed or vice versa if you are left-handed. It should be partially flexed and poised to strike the mark.

Notice the flat sound that you get when you strike a desk in contrast to the booming sound on your abdomen or a wall and the dull sound of the mattress.

Sounds elicited on percussion, termed "resonance," are noted in most patients unless they have thick muscular chests or are obese. A dull sound, like that

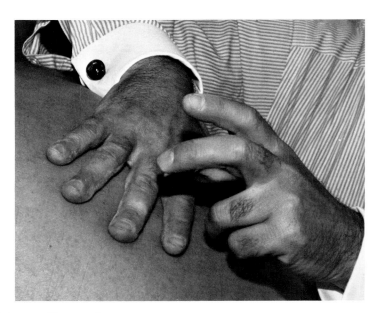

FIGURE 4.1   Percussion.

produced by tapping on a desk, indicates an absence in resonance, and the flat sound, as from tapping on a mattress, indicates a decrease of resonance. Tympanic resonance has a musical, drumlike quality with a particular pitch and a higher tone. Percuss your stomach and you will hear the tympanic sound.

As Auenbrugger noted, thin persons have a tone that is clear; this is less distinct in fleshy individuals. In obese individuals the sound is almost suppressed because of the massive fat. The anterior portion of the thorax is more resonant from the clavicle to the fourth true rub, "for there the breast and the pectoral muscles increase the mass and indistinct sounds result."

Percussion of the Anterior Chest

The patient should preferably be sitting up. Begin percussing down the right anterior portion of the chest and observe that the sound is resonant until the edge of the mass of liver in the fourth intercostal space is reached. At about the sixth intercostal space, the sound is flat because the lung does not overlap the liver. Then percuss the left side of the chest. The resonance will diminish and finally become flat as the chest cavity is interrupted by the mass of the heart. It is imperative that symmetrical points on the right and left sides of the chest are compared, one intercostal space with the other.

Percussion of the Posterior Chest

On the upper portion of the posterior aspect of the chest there is less resonance, and the interscapular area is much more resonant than over the scapula. Compare each side of the chest. Note that the shoulder muscles will be more developed on the extremity with the dominant hand, and there may be more dullness on percussion of that side.

Percuss the right and left clavicles and the supraclavicular area and compare the two, because a tumor lodged in the apices may cause decreased resonance.

It is traditional in the physical examination to outline the diaphragmatic excursions. Ask the patient to take a deep breath, inhaling as deeply as possible, and to hold it. Percuss downward until the resonance changes to a flat sound and make a mental note of this location. Then ask the patient to exhale and to again hold his/her breath, if possible. Again percuss downward, noting the level of the change in resonance of the lung. Normally this level is approximately 4 to 6 cm on both sides on inhalation and exhalation.

Interpretation of Abnormal Findings

Diaphragm
Evidence of an abnormally low diaphragm and decreased mobility suggests pulmonary emphysema. A higher than usual diaphragmatic excursion could result from increased intra-abdominal contents. Subdiaphragmatic abscess can cause decreased motion of the diaphragm on the affected side.

Hyperresonance
When there is more than the normal amount of air in the lung or chest cavity, percussion will yield a hyperresonant sound such as that found in pulmonary emphysema or pneumothorax. In emphysema this hyperresonance is usually bilateral, whereas in pneumothorax it is almost always unilateral. An increased percussion sound is sometimes found over lung cavities.

Dullness
Consolidation of the lung resulting from pneumonia yields a dull percussion sound, as do neoplasms and atelectasis. Any condition that interferes with transmission of the vibration from the chest wall can cause dullness—pulmonary fibrosis, empyema, and pleural effusions. However, Skoda noted that the area above a large pleural effusion may yield a tympanic sound (see below) called skodaic resonance.

Tympany
This sound results when percussing over cavities of at least 4 cm in diameter. In the past, when cavitary disease of the lung secondary to tuberculosis was much more frequent, tympany was a common finding.

Metallic Resonance
This is a high-pitched note, and it means that the cavity lies close to the chest wall and is surrounded by smooth muscle.

Bellmetal Resonance
Once a cavity is located, light percussion with a coin upon another larger coin laid over the cavity will produce a high-pitched, jingling sound.

Cracked-Pot Resonance
This is a soft muffled sound that one would hear on tapping a cracked pot. This sound is heard with the presence of large cavities that communicate by a narrow opening.

AUSCULTATION

A quiet room is essential for auscultation. The bell or the diaphragm of the stethoscope may be used. Every area of the lung should be auscultated—the anterior, posterior, and lateral portions. Listen for vesicular breathing, which is heard in most of the thorax; bronchial breathing, heard over the trachea; and bronchovesicular breathing, a combination of these two. It is essential that the patient be sitting up whenever possible. The patient should be encouraged to take deep breaths, full inspirations and expirations, in a rhythmic manner. Always ask the patient to cough first to rid the lungs of secretions because they can sound like adventitious sounds, or added lung sounds (see below).

All of the sounds discussed here are useful early in the diagnostic process. For example, a preliminary diagnosis of pulmonary consolidation from pneumonia may be made before obtaining a confirmatory radiograph.

Breath Sounds

Vesicular Breath Sounds

Vesicular breath sounds are produced by air rushing in and out of the alveoli. These sounds are loudest during inspiration. Vesicular breath sounds are normally heard over most of the thorax. They are moderately loud and deep and can be imitated by making an "ooh" sound and then slowly inhaling the air. Vesicular breath sounds are not high pitched, and they lack either a musical or a rasping quality; the character varies slightly with inspiration and expiration. The expiratory sound is softer, sometimes inaudible.

Bronchial Breathing

The vibration of air in the tracheobronchial system produces bronchial breathing, which can be traced from the mouth to the bronchi. Bronchial breathing is also known as tubular breathing, first described by Laennec. It is a distinct sound that can be imitated by uttering the German gutteral "ch" and then exhaling, and it has the same character in inspiration and expiration.

Over the vertebral prominences and in the interscapular area, bronchial breathing is heard quite distinctly in combination with vesicular breath sounds; this combination is referred to as bronchovesicular breathing. Pure bronchial breathing is normally heard only over the trachea and at the right apex where the primary bronchi are. When heard anywhere else in the chest, bronchial breathing is pathologic. For example, consolidation of the lung resulting from pneumonia causes bronchial breathing. The damping action of air surrounding the filled alveoli is diminished, allowing high-frequency bronchial sounds to be transmitted.

Abnormal Breath Sounds

Rales are added lung sounds arising from small bronchi or alveoli; there are discussed further below. Other kinds of abnormal breath sounds heard over cavities and in pneumothorax are primarily of historical interest, rarely heard today.

Cavernous Breathing. Cavernous breathing, heard over cavities surrounded by infiltrated pulmonary tissue, was first described by Austin Flint. It is nothing more than bronchial breathing, and is identical to the sounds heard over the trachea. The metallic breath sounds noted during percussion may also be heard with the stethoscope over a cavity.

Amphoric Breathing. Amphoric breathing is like the sound obtained by blowing over the opening of a hollow bottle. It is unusually low pitched and is found in open pneumothorax and large cavities.

Adventitious Sounds or Added Lung Sounds

Rales

The term "rales" (from the French râles, rattles) was used by Laennec to describe the "noisy" murmur in a dying person caused by air forcing its way with difficulty through the sputum that the lungs are no longer able to expel. They occur as air passes through secretions in a respiratory tract containing abnormal moisture. Rales are classified by site of origin as tracheal, bronchial, and so forth. Some clinicians have divided rales into three categories: fine, medium, and coarse. *Fine rales,* such as crepitant rales, have a crackling quality that has been described as the sound produced by holding a hair close to the ear and rubbing it between the thumb and finger. Fine rales heard at the end of inspiration, not cleared by coughing, often may be the first sign of congestive heart failure or pneumonia. *Medium rales,* resulting from air passing through the bronchioles, do not have a fine crackling quality. *Coarse rales,* such as gurgling rales, occur higher up in the respiratory tract in the trachea and bronchi. These are loud bubbling sounds produced by air going through the passages.

Rhonchi

Ronchi are continuous sounds resulting from air passing through the trachea, bronchi, and bronchioles. They are heard during both phases of respiration, although they are usually more prominent during expiration than inspiration. They can vary in pitch and in intensity. These continuous sounds are produced as the result of narrowing of the large air passages. *Sibilant rhonchi* are high pitched whistling sounds. *Sonorous rhonchi* are low pitched and snoring in character.

Wheezes

Wheezes are high-pitched whistling sounds resulting from air passing through a partial obstruction. This is generally a sound that is heard on the right and left sides of the lung. If it is heard on only one side, the physician should suspect a unilateral obstruction, as from a tumor. If wheezing results from asthma, it is heard predominantly in expiration. Wheezing that occurs during inspiration and expiration may result from a tracheal obstruction.

Pleural Friction Rubs

Friction rubs are frivolous sounds. They appear swiftly and may appear and then disappear. A pleural friction rub can be a creaking, soft, rubbing sound, and sometimes it is confused with a heart murmur. It was described by Hippocrates in pneumonia: "The lung is congealed to the ribs and squeaks like a leather strap." It is a sound heard during inspiration and expiration, or sometimes during expiration only. It may be the first sign of a pleuritis, and, as fluid forms in the pleural cavity, the sound disappears.

In any patient who complains of pain upon inspiration, a friction rub should be sought. Most friction rubs are heard at the inferior limit of the axillary line or at the base of the lung. This is where the movement of the viscera over the parietal pleura is greatest. These sounds are rarely heard in the apical portions of the lungs because there are often adhesions present and there is rarely any motion between the pulmonary and costal pleura.

Pleural friction rubs must be searched for carefully. Do not forget to auscultate in the midaxillary line at the base of the lung, where rubs are often heard in pleuritis. Sometimes asking the patient where the pleuritic pain is felt and placing the stethoscope on that spot enables the physician to locate a friction rub. The loudness of a friction rub is increased with the speed of motion of the pleural surface. Having the patient breathe rapidly and deeply, if possible, will aid in locating the rub. However, this may cause pain to the patient.

Crackling rales may sometimes sound like pleural friction rubs. Rales generally are limited to inspiration, whereas friction rubs are heard during both inspiration and expiration. Also, pleural friction rubs are not influenced by coughing, in contrast to rales, which may lighten or even disappear.

In the presence of pericarditis and pleuritis, pleural friction and pericardial rubs may be heard together. In order to distinguish a pericardial rub from a pleural friction rub, ask the patient to hold his/her breath. The pericardial rub will persist.

Voice Sounds

Auscultation of the voice is sometimes useful as part of the physical examination. Bronchial breathing and voice sounds are high overtones.

Bronchophony

The analog to bronchial breathing is called bronchophony. Before bronchial breathing occurs, bronchophony may be evident. It can be imitated by speaking, in a low or whispering voice, words with high vowels, such as "seen."

Egophony

The compressed lung border above a large pleural effusion causes egophony, which resembles bleats like those of a goat. Laennec coined the term from the Greek roots *aix,* meaning goat, and *phōnē,* voice. Egophony is commonly heard above pleural effusions of moderate size in the same area where skodaic resonance is present. The noise can be imitated by closing the nostrils with the fingers while counting aloud: "1, 2, 3."

Hamman's Sign

Patients who develop interstitial or mediastinal emphysema have a cracking, crunching sound that is synchronous with the heartbeat. This sound is heard best in the left lateral recumbent position.

Whispering Pectoriloquy

Whispering pectoriloquy refers to the transmission of the whispered voice through the pulmonary structures. Normally, the whispered voice is only faintly heard in areas where bronchovesicular breathings are normally heard. At the base of the lung the whispered sound disappears; if it can be heard, this indicates consolidation of the lung.

A SUMMARY OF PULMONARY FINDINGS

Diseases of the Bronchi

Acute Bronchitis
Signs are bilateral:

1.   Normal vocal fremitus
2.   Normal percussion sound
3.   Vesicular breath sounds
4.   Scattered rales, medium or small, occasionally sibilant

Emphysema

1.   Barrel-shaped chest
2.   Widened intercostal space
3.   Diminished respiratory excursions
4.   Diaphragm moves little
5.   Dull tympany or hyperresonance on percussion
6.   Breath sounds diminished in intensity
7.   Expiration prolonged
8.   Heart sounds distant

Asthma

1.   Expiratory dyspnea during the attack
2.   Dull tympany or hyperresonance on percussion
3.   Inspiration decreased in intensity
4.   Expiration prolonged and forced
5.   Sibilant and sonorous rales

Diseases of the Lung

Lobar Pneumonia
Early stages:

1.   Percussion sound normal to slightly tympanic
2.   Breath sounds normal or slightly diminished
3.   Inspiratory crepitant rales, sometimes a friction rub

These may be present before x-ray charge.
Stage of consolidation:

1.   Increased vocal fremitus
2.   Flatness on percussion
3.   Bronchial breathing, crepitant rales

Infarction of the Lung
There may be no physical signs unless the infarction is large.

1.   Increased vocal fremitus
2.   Dullness on percussion
3.   Bronchovesicular bronchial breathing, moist rales

Abscess of the Lung
There may be no physical signs if the lesions lie deep in the lung.

1.   Dullness on percussion over the lesion; may or may not be present
2.   Breath sounds diminished, vesicular bronchial breathing, moist rales

Pleural Effusion

1.   Vocal fremitus absent
2.   Flatness on percussion
3.   Breath sounds diminished
4.   It may be bronchial, if the lung is compressed beyond the effusion; rales may be present.

Pneumothorax

1. Vocal fremitus absent or diminished
2. Hyperresonance or tympany on percussion; bellmetal resonance may be present
3. Displacement of dullness over heart to unaffected side
4. Breath sounds absent or distally amphoric

Hydropneumothorax

1. Vocal fremitus absent or diminished
2. Flatness on percussion
3. Breath and voice sounds absent

Atelectasis

1. Vocal fremitus decreased or absent
2. Breath sounds decreased vesicular or absent
3. Dullness on percussion

Some Diagnostic Pearls

1. Wheezing on one side of the lung may be due to obstruction of a bronchus by a tumor.
2. Remember, all patients who wheeze are not asthmatic. Wheezing may be of cardiac origin.
3. Wheezing that occurs equally during inspiration and expiration may be the result of an obstruction above the bifurcation.

REFERENCES

1. Felson B: *Chest Roentgenology,* ed 2. Philadelphia, WB Saunders Co, 1973.

2. Snider GH, et al: *Simple bedside test of respiratory function. JAMA* 1959;170:1631.

3. Comroe JH, et al: *The Lung,* ed 2. Chicago, Year Book Medical Publishers, Inc, 1962.

4. Baum, GL: *Textbook of Pulmonary Diseases,* ed 2. Boston, Little, Brown, and Co, 1974.

5. Fraser RG, Pare JAP: *Diagnosis of Diseases of the Chest,* ed 2. Philadelphia, WB Saunders Co, 1977.

6. Braunwald E, West JB, Moser KM: Disorders of the respiratory system, in Petersdorf RG, Adams RD, Braunwald E, Isselbacher KJ, Martin JB, Wilson JD (eds): *Harrison's Principles of Internal Medicine,* ed 10. New York, McGraw-Hill Book Co, 1983, Sect 3, pp 1498-1508.

7. Delp MH, Manning RT: *Major's Physical Diagnosis: An Introduction to the Clinical Process,* ed 9. Philadelphia, WB Saunders Co, 1981.

8. Bates B: *A Guide to Physical Examination,* ed 3. Philadelphia, JB Lippincott Co, 1983.

9. Judge RD, Zuidema GD, Fitzgerald FT: *Clinical Diagnosis: A Physiologic Approach,* ed 4. Boston, Little, Brown, and Co, 1982.

5
Examination of the Cardiovascular System and the Lymphatic System

Siegfried J. Kra, M.D.

THIRTY-SECOND SUMMARY OF EVENTS IN THE CARDIAC CYCLE

Beginning with systole, the ventricle contracts, causing a sharp rise in the pressure and ejecting the blood from the left ventricle. As the ventricle relaxes (diastole), the pressure falls off almost to zero. During systole, the aortic valve opens and blood is ejected from the left ventricle into the aorta. At this time, the mitral valve is closed, preventing blood from flowing back into the left atrium. In diastole, the aortic valve is closed, preventing backflow of blood from the aorta into the left ventricle. The mitral valve is opened and blood flows from the left atrium into the relaxed left ventricle. As diastole occurs, the pressure of the left atrium exceeds that of the left ventricle and blood flows from the left atrium to the left ventricle as the mitral valve is opened. There is a slight rise in pressure in both chambers before the onset of ventricular systole, as a result of atrial contraction. As the ventricle begins to contract pressure rises, finally exceeding the pressure of the left atrium and closing the mitral valve. The first heart sound (S1) is produced as the result of closure of the mitral valve.

As the pressure of the left ventricle rises, it exceeds the diastolic pressure in the aorta, and the aortic valve is forced open. Ordinarily, the opening of the aortic valve is not heard except in pathologic conditions, but it may be accompanied by an ejection sound (ES). When the ventricle ejects the blood, the ventricular pressure begins to fall below the aortic pressure and the aortic valve shuts, producing the second heart sound (S2). As the left ventricle pressure drops during ventricular relaxation, the mitral valve opens when the pressure falls below that of the left atrium. The opening of the mitral valve is generally not heard except in pathologic conditions. An opening sound (OS) is heard in mitral stenosis. A period of rapid filling follows as blood flows early in diastole from the left atrium to the left ventricle, producing the third heart sound (S3). Atrial contraction late in diastole produces the fourth heart sound (S4).

Similar events occur on the right side of the heart, involving the right atrium, the right ventricle, the tricuspid valve, the pulmonic valve, and the pulmonary artery. Pressures of the right ventricle and pulmonary arterial pressures are lower than pressures on the left side of the heart, and the events on the right side usually occur later than those on the left. Two heart sounds are generally heard corresponding to these events: the first resulting from the left side valve closure, and the second resulting from the right side valves closing.

GENERAL COMMENTS

The examination of the cardiovascular system is one of the most challenging and rewarding experiences for the clinician. This is the time when your eyes, ears, sense of touch, and sometimes the sense of smell are coordinated in a precise manner in order to arrive at a clear diagnosis. Prior to the advent of modern technology, the diagnosis that was made on clinical grounds was not confirmed, except at the autopsy and in surgical specimens. I recall during my medical training that, when the professor of cardiology said that there was the presence of an S3 or S4 opening snap, I naturally accepted his diagnosis even though I was unable to hear it. Today, as never before, with the aid of phonocardiography, Doppler echocardiography, digital arteriography, cardiac catheterization, and positron emission tomography, we can confirm what we thought we heard.

The major noninvasive instruments that have made auscultation more meaningful than before are the echocardiograph and the phonocardiograph.

William Harvey was one of the first to record that the movements of the heart "can be heard in the chest," but doctors in Europe thought he was daft. Aemilius Pariss wrote in 1647, "nor we poor deafs, nor any other doctor in Venice can hear them, but happy is he who can hear them in London." The art of auscultation requires a stubborn, tenacious application of the ear until everything is heard that should be heard. Initially, auscultation is filled with frustration and an "I'll never hear it" attitude. Then comes that golden moment as the diastolic murmur is heard for the first time—the beginning of diagnostic skill in the practice of medicine.

THE CARDIOVASCULAR HISTORY

During general history taking, it may become evident that the focus of the patient's medical problem is cardiac. This section gives a brief review of some specific details to be asked for in a cardiac history.

The *family history* can be extraordinarily useful from an epidemiologic and practical point of view. Ask the patient if there is a history of myocardial infarction, congenital heart disease, or heart murmurs in the family. Had there been any sudden deaths in the family, especially in younger persons? The clue to idiopathic hypertrophic subaortic stenosis may lie just in that one question, since this illness runs in families. Is there hypertension in the family?

A past history of *rheumatic* or *scarlet fever* should be carefully noted. Ask if the patient was a blue baby.

Ask if a *heart murmur* is or ever has been present. If the patient answers, "Yes, I've had a heart murmur since I was a child," congenital heart disease may be present.

Fatigue is a major symptom of heart disease, reflecting low cardiac output, such as that found in valvular or coronary artery disease and early congestive heart failure. A recent onset of fatigue is particularly important, especially in an individual who has been vigorous and now has lost considerable stamina.

Has there been the presence of a *dry cough,* especially at night? This can be an early sign of heart failure.

Have there been any *dizzy* or *fainting spells*? Dizzy spells, or syncope, are a common symptom in severe aortic stenosis and other valvular or cardiac illnesses. Dizzy spells can also result from arrhythmias, orthostatic hypotension, transient ischemic attacks, or brain tumors. There are many other causes of syncope, which can be found in any standard textbook of medicine.

Inquire regarding *shortness of breath* (dyspnea). If present, is it of recent onset? Is it present only on effort or even when resting? Shortness of breath with effort can be the earliest sign of congestive heart failure. However, it is very common for people who have no heart failure to complain of shortness of breath when climbing stairs. Physical effort puts greater demand on the heart, increasing the wedge pressure (as in mitral stenosis), resulting in shortness of breath. An old-fashioned, useful manner of ascertaining dyspnea is to walk down a hall with the patient and observe whether he/she is short of breath. Ask if the shortness of breath occurs at night—does the patient suddenly awaken short of breath or wheezing? Wheezing can be a powerful indicator of congestive heart failure ("All patients who wheeze are not asthmatics").

Ask about *swelling of ankles,* which may reflect heart failure.

Ask about the presence of *palpitations*: "Do you ever hear your heart beat fast or irregular?" Many patients tell you that their heart races. Discover the time of onset: Is it with effort or at rest? After drinking coffee? With excitement? Does it occur with no reason? Sometimes tapping out different heartbeats helps the patient describe his/her palpitations better. For example, it would be easy enough to tap out sinus tachycardia, multiple premature ventricular contractions, sinus arrest, and atrial fibrillation. The patient may be able to correctly identify which condition he/she suffers from prior to examination and confirmation of findings with an electrocardiogram and Holter monitor.

One of the most important symptoms that the physician must look for is *chest pain,* or *heaviness* or *tightness* in the chest. It is essential to discover whether this chest pain is of cardiac, musculoskeletal, or gastrointestinal origin; a thorough history can help to differentiate the three. Included in the history should be the symptom of *heartburn,* which can be a very common sign of coronary artery disease, and also is a common sign of disease of the esophagus, regurgitation of acid, duodenal ulcer, or GB disease.

The classic symptom of angina will often be described by the patient clenching a fist on his/her chest, or using words like, "I feel like there is an elephant sitting on my chest." A severe, tight, constricting feeling causing an oppressive sensation, along with the fear of sudden death, are some of the other classic descriptions.

The physician should inquire regarding the duration of the chest pain or pressure, in terms of both the number of years it has been present and the length of time each occurrence lasts. Is it continuous? The type of pain should be characterized: squeezing, constriction, strangling, compression, burning, heaviness, pressure, or a sticking, gnawing, aching pain. The location of the pain should be also stated. Is it substernal (over the breastbone) or precordial (over the heart)? Is it found in the pit of the stomach? In the back? Does the pain radiate to the back? To the shoulder? To the arm? How frequent are the attacks: More than once a day? A few times a week? A few times a month? A few times a year?

Characterize the onset or the cause. Does it occur at rest, as might be found in spasm of the coronary arteries, or does it occur with walking, climbing, or tension? Is it related to meals, or does it occur after meals? Is it worsened by walking in the cold or walking against the wind? Is it brought on by fatigue or spontaneously? Does it occur while standing up, lying down, on intercourse, or

even with smoking? Some patients will state the pain in their chest will only occur after they smoke.

The relief of the pain needs to be noted. Is it relieved by nitroglycerine, by
itself, by whiskey, by rest, or by a warm drink or antacid?

After the pain has been characterized in such a manner, the physician can then
come to a conclusion as to whether the pain comes from the gastrointestinal tract
(pain relieved by antacids, or sometimes by sitting up) or is the typical pain of
angina relieved with nitroglycerine.

In summary, the history should note the presence of:

1. Family history of cardiac problems and hypertension
2. Heart murmur
3. Fatigue
4. Dry cough
5. Syncope
6. Dyspnea
7. Swelling of the ankles
8. Palpitations
9. Chest pain or heartburn

THE SURFACE PHYSICAL EXAMINATION

The diagnosis of cardiovascular conditions begins long before hands are placed on
the chest or the earpiece of the stethoscope is placed into the ear. Clues to the
diagnosis of the cardiac condition can all be present on the surface examination.
What is heard and seen can indicate the state of the heart.

Patient Complexion

Look at the color of the patient. Is the complexion *pale* and *insipid,* secondary to
an anemia? This can cause profound hemodynamic changes on the cardiovascular
system, such as tachycardias, murmurs, and heart failure.

Is the patient's complexion *ruddy*? This can signal polycythemia with its
frequent accompaniment of hypertension.

Is there a *flushing reddish hue* to the face? This is sometimes found in the
carcinoid syndrome with accompanying tricuspid valvular disease, or the circumscribed coloration of the cheeks with some telangiectasia due to mitral stenosis.

Is the complexion somewhat *brownish*? This is the telltale sign of hemochromatosis and hemochromatic cardiovascular disease.

Is there a *butterfly rash* on the face of the young woman suffering from systemic lupus erythematosus, causing lupus valvular disease?

Is the patient *cyanotic,* with a blue discoloration of the lips, nailbeds, and
mucous membranes? Cyanosis can signal cardiac disease, pulmonary disease, or
both. See if there is cyanosis of the feet, or sometimes of the left hand, with no
cyanosis in the face and right arm, which may suggest a patent ductus arteriosus
accompanied by pulmonary hypertension and a shunt from the pulmonary artery
to the descending aorta. Is there cyanosis only of the upper part of the body and
upper extremities? This may suggest transposition of the great vessels with shunt-
ing of blood from the pulmonary artery to the patent ductus arteriosus into the
systemic circulation.

Inspection of the Head, Neck, and Facies

Clues to the presence of heart disease may be found by looking at the *shape of the head.* The enlarged head and the lantern jaw of acromegaly is associated with enlargement of the heart and heart failure. The long, thin skull of Marfan's syndrome (with associated spider fingers) will alert the physician to accompanying cardiac abnormalities, such as atrial septal defects, aortic aneurysms, dissecting aneurysms, and degeneration of the cardiac valves, as in mitral regurgitation and aortic insufficiency. The abnormal motion of the head called systolic nodding of the head, or Musset's sign, coincident with cardiac systole, suggests severe aortic insufficiencies.

Observe the motion of the *neck.* Is it fixed to the skull like a block of cement with little motion possible, as seen in rheumatoid spondylitis? Rheumatoid spondylitis can cause aortitis with accompanying murmurs of aortic insufficiency or stenosis. A quick scan of the neck can show an obvious enlargement of the thyroid, which could signal myxedema or hyperthyroidism.

The *face* may have characteristic features of myxedema, with a pasty appearance, a partial loss of eyebrows, coarse puffy features, and dull speech, like a slow broken record. Myxedematous heart disease may be present with cardiomegaly, pericardial effusion, and arrhythmias. A round moon face, acneic features, and loss of scalp hair (with purple striae of the abdomen) may give the clue to Cushing's syndrome and its accompanying hypertension.

Congenital heart disease might be suspected on the basis of the low-set ears, epicanthal folds, and protruding lower lip of Down's syndrome. Forty percent of these patients may have congenital disorders of the heart, as, for example, atrioventricular communus (the direct continuity of the mitral and tricuspid valve substances).

Note any creases in the earlobes, which some physicians equate with a predilection for coronary artery disease.

Look at the patient's *eyes.* Bulging may be evidence of exophthalmos, which suggests thyrotoxicosis and thyrotoxic heart disease. Is there an arcus senilis present? This opaque circle in the cornea is commonly found in black persons, but in others may signal hypercholesteremia. Light yellowish-brown plaques in the creases at the junction of the fold of the eye with the nose, called xanthoma palpebrarum, are sometimes associated with familial hypercholesteremia. A quick look at the conjuctiva of the eye may show the presence of small petechiae, signaling the diagnosis of endocarditis.

If there are unusual markings on the head and facies, make note of them; perhaps they can be of use later on.

Inspection of the Hands

The inspection of the hands can give important clues to the presence of heart disease. The classic rheumatoid hand, deformed at the proximal interphalangeal joints, swollen, with ulnar deviation, the hallmark of rheumatoid arthritis, sometimes is associated with rheumatoid heart disease. This "arthritis of the heart," which may consist of pericardial effusions and aortic valvular deformities, may cause subcutaneous nodules on the palmar surface of the hand—round, softish, painless, freely moveable swellings the size of a small marble. Painful, tiny, red nodules at the tips of the fingers may be seen in bacterial endocarditis.

Observation of How the Patient Breathes

Is the patient breathing normally? If the patient appears to breathe normally, start a slight conversation and notice if the patient hesitates between the words to catch his/her breath. At times, people may not be aware that they are even short of breath, especially the older patient. Dyspnea at rest can signal lung or cardiac disease.

Notice the young patient who sits quietly and starts to take breaths quickly in and out, as seen in hyperventilation. It is worthwhile at this time to ask the patient if he/she ever becomes short of breath, either at rest or while walking or climbing stairs.

If the person you are about to examine appears to be short of breath, run a quick checklist in your head of the possible causes:

1.   Dyspnea of central origin, such as depression of the respiratory center
2.   Physiologic dyspnea, caused by oxygen intake insufficient to meet the individual's needs
3.   Circulatory causes, such as anemia and hypovolemia
4.   Pulmonary causes, such as embolism, atelectasis, and pleural effusions
5.   Metabolic causes, such as diabetic acidosis, uremia, and hepatic coma
6.   Cardiac causes

A gem of a question to ask is if the patient becomes short of breath when sitting up, but the dyspnea disappears when he/she is lying down. This is a definitive clue to the presence of an atrial myxoma.

Edema

Bilateral swelling of the ankles and feet is an important sign of a failing heart. A cardiac examination is not complete unless the feet and legs are inspected. Ask a simple question, if the patient has difficulty putting on their shoes, which may mean their ankles are swollen. Inspect the feet to see if there are marks left by stockings and shoelaces on the skin from edema.

For the patient lying in bed, swelling in the ankles and feet may be gone, but there still may be some swelling left in the sacral area, called sacral edema. Sometimes the inner portion of the thighs may be swollen; edema may be present in the abdominal wall or chest wall, and even the upper extremities. Naturally, there are many other causes of edema besides heart failure, such as venous insufficiency and obstruction, allergic reactions, kidney failure, liver disease and severe malnutrition. Edema of the face and eyelids is seen in angioneurotic edema and in children with heart failure.

**EXTERNAL EXAMINATION
OF THE CIRCULATORY SYSTEM**

The cardiovascular examination entails finding signals and clues sent out by the complicated hemodynamic events of the cardiovascular mechanism. The physician's senses will be trained to find abnormalities resulting from the contraction of the left and right sides of the heart, the flow of blood into and out of the heart, the complicated motions of the valves that direct the flow of the blood, the pressures that are generated inside the cardiac muscle motor, and the state of the muscle of the heart and its coverings. All of these elements must be working in a harmonious manner to keep the organism alive. The system works well until it ages and loses some of its efficiency, or its balance gets set off by diseases. How can we possibly appreciate when something has gone awry unless there is a total under-standing of what the normal mechanisms are like? Physicians are diagnosticians, detectives, engineers, mechanics, scientists, chemists, and humanists who must understand both the normal function of the system and the signals sent to indicate that one of the complicated mechanisms is malfunctioning.

Visualizing Pulsations

Pulsations of the Venous System

The veins of the body, especially those found in the neck, the thorax, and the hands, give us a picture of the events that occur on the right side of the heart, and indirect evidence of what is happening on the left side of the heart. When the patient lies flat on his/her back, the neck veins, ie, the internal jugular veins, which are in contiguity with the superior vena cava and the right atrium, may be seen to be distended and pulsating. The right jugular vein is inspected rather than the left, because the left vein may be distended as a result of a kinked innominate vein and give false evidence of distention of the vein. When examining the neck, one looks at the external jugular vein, but the pulsations will come from the in-ternal jugular vein beneath the sternocleidomastoid muscles. The carotid artery also lies underneath, and both can cause pulsations. In normal cardiovascular status, if the patient sits up the veins will empty and become less pronounced, even dis-appearing. Light pressure from a finger over the vein just above the sternal end of the clavicle will cause the venous pulsation to disappear. It will do nothing to stop the pulsation of arterial origin. Also, the pulsations will diminish with inspira-tion in a normal person if they are from the internal jugular, but they will not be affected by inspiration if they are from the carotid. Likewise, elevation of the patient to 45 degrees may make the normal pulsations disappear while carotid pulsations are unchanged.

This is not an easy examination and takes a great deal of experience. The pulsations of the internal jugular vein are sometimes difficult to see and may not be seen at all, because the pressure in the venous system in a normal person is low and is not palpable. It is much easier to examine venous pulsation in somebody who has an elevation of the right atrial pressure when the veins are full and pulsating. If the patient is grossly obese and has a fat neck, and the internal jugular vein is deeply imbedded, this part of the cardiovascular examination may be nonproductive unless the patient is in severe heart failure, especially right-sided heart failure. The internal jugular vein lies deep to the muscle mass. The pulsations look like fine, transparent waves and may be seen adjacent to the insertion of the sternocleido-mastoid muscle to the clavicle. A light shined perpendicular to the supraclavicular area behind the sternocleidomastoid muscle can make them more visible.

A venous pressure tracing can be used to illustrate the relationship between jugular vein pulsations, heart sounds, and the electrocardiogram (Figures 5.1 and 5.2). When the right atrium contracts it produces an A wave, and, as the atrium relaxes, there is a fall of this wave. The A wave begins prior to the first heart sound, and is followed by the X descent, atrial relaxation, and flow of venous blood into the atrium. The V wave is the normal pressure rise in the right atrium and corresponds to atrial venous filling. During the Y descent right atrial blood pas-sively flows into the right ventricle in early diastole. Think of the letter M; the upstroke is the A wave followed by the X descent, then comes the second peak of the letter M, the V wave, followed by the Y descent. Careful auscultation reveals that the A wave is synchronous with the first heart sound, the X descent falls between the first and second heart sounds, and the V wave coincides with the second heart sound (V).

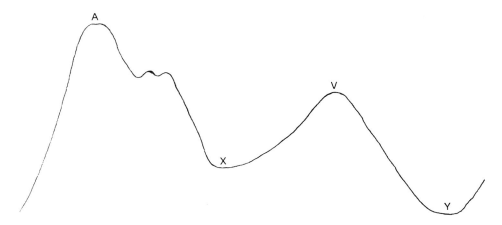

**FIGURE 5.1   Venous pulsations. A wave: Atrium contracting, tricuspid open;
X descent: Atrium filling, tricuspid closed; V wave: Atrium tense, full, tricuspid
closed; Y descent: Atrium emptying, tricuspid open.**

Abnormal Venous Distention (Figure 5.3). Abnormalities in distention of the
jugular vein have many diagnostic implications.

The A wave disappears in atrial fibrillation.

Increase in A waves is seen in tricuspid stenosis and in advanced cor pul-
monale, tricuspid atrasia, Ebstein's anomaly, and elevated ventricular and diastolic
pressures, as occurs with pulmonic stenosis or pulmonary hypertension.

Large or giant A waves indicate an increased resistance to right ventricular
filling, as in right ventricular hypertrophy (Figure 5.4).

**FIGURE 5.2   Normal venous pulse coordinated with the heart sounds and elec-
trocardiogram.**

Normal Venous Pulse

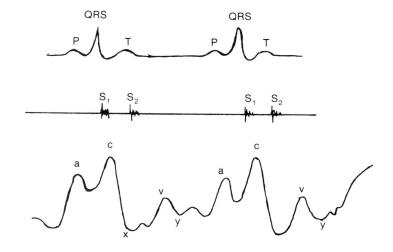

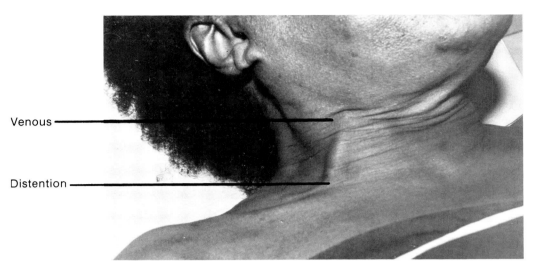

FIGURE 5.3   Abnormal venous distention.

Cannon A waves, which are intermittent large A waves, result when the right atrium contracts at a closed tricuspid valve, as seen in complete atrioventricular block or during a premature ventricular contraction.

The jugular veins may be distended in patients with obstructive lung disease; distention will be present predominantly on expiration and then collapse on inspiration. This finding does *not* indicate congestive heart failure.

Venous distention on inspiration (Kussmaul's sign) indicates congestive heart failure. Also, venous distention that appears or increases if pressure is applied to the upper right quadrant of the abdomen for a period of 30 to 60 s, an increase of 1 cm or more in the jugular venous filling, is considered positive for congestive heart failure. Forewarn the patient that this maneuver, if there is congestive heart failure, may be attended with some discomfort.

Bilateral venous distention is recognized in cardiac tamponade and constrictive pericarditis, giving the impression of an M-shaped venous pulse wave.

Prominent V waves are present (Figure 5.5) in tricuspid regurgitation, which causes a systolic expansion of the internal jugular vein. *A Diagnostic Pearl:* Tricuspid regurgitation may cause the patient's head to move from side to side (the "no-no" sign).

FIGURE 5.4   Prominent V waves in tricuspid stenosis.

Tricuspid Stenosis

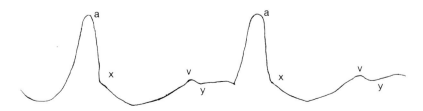

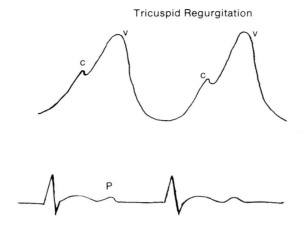

FIGURE 5.5   **Prominent V waves of tricuspid regurgitation.**

Estimating Central Venous Pressure. The pulsations of the jugular vein can
be used to obtain a fairly accurate estimate of central pressure. With the
patient raised to 45 degrees from the horizontal, observe the highest point of the
pulsations of the internal jugular vein. Measure with a ruler the vertical distance
between that point and the sternal angle (the sternal angle, or the angle of Louis,
is the manubrium of the sternum). The simple technique is to take a horizontal
piece of paper, place it against the height of the maximum point of distention of
the jugular vein, run it to a ruler placed on the sternal angle vertically, and read
the point of intersect in centimeters. A venous pressure reading greater than 3
to 4 cm above the sternal angle is considered elevated. Simply doubling the reading
(in centimeters) will give an approximation of the actual central venous pressure.

Pulsations of the Arterial System

Inspection of the cardiovascular system is not complete until arterial pulsations
are surveyed. If present, they may be felt as thrills.

Look in the second interspace to the right of the sternum in the aortic area for
pulsations that may be seen in aortic aneurysms.

Look in the second left intercostal space and above the third left intercostal
space (the pulmonic area). Pulsations observed here result from increased pressure or flow in the pulmonary artery.

Pulsations may be visualized in the right lower portion of the neck beneath
the sternocleidomastoid muscle. Prominent, bounding pulses are seen in aortic
insufficiency, thyrotoxicosis, anemia, hypertension, and coarctation of the aorta.
Faint pulses can result from aortic stenosis, bradycardia or induced by medications.

Check for any pulsations of the abdominal aorta, which are often seen in normal thin persons.

The Italian surgeon Giovanni Lancisi, physician to the Pope, observed a 55-year-old man, in the year 1728, who was fond of
singing and who harbored a large aortic aneurysm protruding
from his chest. The aneurysm was so large that it made the
chest bulge each time he hit a high note. The surgeon concluded
it was an aneurysm from the constant pulsations. He constructed
an iron belt with a spring, not unlike the spring truss worn by a

patient with a hernia, to retain the protrusion within the chest. With this belt the aneurysm was kept within the chest, and the patient continued to sing merrily until he died many years later.

Heartbeat-related Impulses on the Chest

In patients who are quite thin, the heart can be seen to lift and rise toward the apex (so that it strikes the chest at the moment of maximum impulse and the beat may be seen on the chest), as first noted by William Harvey. In obese patients, or in patients who are emphysematous, this may be difficult to observe. Have the patient lie flat on the back in a slightly left lateral position as you stand on the right side of the patient. This normal maximum impulse can be seen in the fifth intercostal space inside the left midclavicular line, usually referred to as the PMI (point of maximum impulse). In thin patients, a slight systolic retraction can also be seen. Next ask the patient to take a deep breath and hold it; the PMI will move downward from the fifth to the sixth intercostal space. Deep inspiration brings the lungs over the heart and the impulse moves or disappears, especially in patients who have emphysema.

Question: When is the cardiac impulse on the right instead of the left side of the chest? *Answer:* In dextrocardia.

When the left ventricle becomes enlarged, it will displace the PMI to the left outside the midclavicular line and downward.

The apex of the heart can sometimes be seen beating furiously against the chest wall in normal hearts or in individuals who are nervous during the examination. The apex movement is due to ventricular contractions, and sometimes corresponds to the A wave of the venous pulse. In a similar fashion, the apex may reveal a third heart sound, to be described later.

An impulse seen in the left parasternal area may be caused by a right ventricle that is suffering from volume overload or hypertrophy. Right ventricular hypertrophy is seen in mitral stenosis, which causes a sustained heave or a lift during systole. To make things even more confusing, a left ventricular impulse can be seen close to the sternal border and may be confused with the right ventricular parasternal impulse. Turning the patient to the left will cause the left ventricular impulse to move laterally, while the right ventricular heave remains near the sternal border.

A Diagnostic Pearl: Bulging in the epigastrium can be caused by a large pericardial effusion, known as Auenbrugger's sign.

It should be noted that the female breast may cover the apical impulse and must be gently pushed aside.

Palpation

The human hand is incredibly sensitive; it is probably one of the most complex components of the entire body with its multitudes of entanglements of nerves and arteries. The hand can sometimes perceive better than the ear. Cardiologists of bygone days whose hearing had failed could feel fourth heart sounds, third heart sounds, gallop rhythms, and murmurs, without the aid of the stethoscope.

Not all hands are created equal; undoubtedly, some are more sensitive than others.

Just as hearing has to be trained, the hand needs to be educated. The art of palpation requires experience, and should be part of the routine examination of the cardiovascular system. Too often, physicians rush with the stethoscope to listen to the chest before going through inspection and palpation.

The hand should be clean and the nails well groomed. Before the hand is used for the cardiac examination, it should be thoroughly warmed and comfortable.

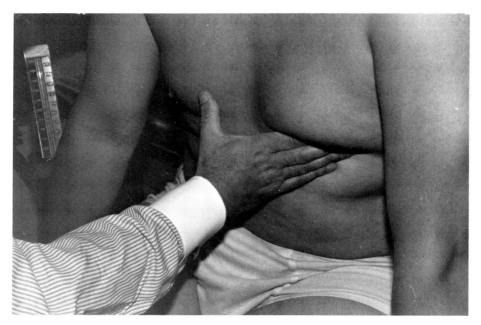

FIGURE 5.6   Palpating the apex of the heart.

There is nothing more disagreeable than to place a cold, clammy hand on a sensitive, anxious body. A useful technique is sometimes to take the patient's hand to warm your own. You can introduce this point of the examination by simply stating, "My hands are a little cold. Why not let me warm them up with yours?" This will relax the patient, who will find it amusing and perhaps even touching (no pun intended).

Which part of the hand is most sensitive depends on the individual examiner. For some people, the ball of the hand (the surface at the base of the fingers) is most sensitive to vibration and useful in detecting motion and thrills. The finger-pads are allegedly more helpful in detecting and analyzing pulsations, but this may not always be the case. There may be individual variations that depend on nerve distribution, vasculature, and musculature.

Left ventricular activity is normally palpable in adults and normal young subjects who are thin. If there is a hyperdynamic circulation, normal right ventricular motion can occasionally be detected. The palpable apex impulse that is felt represents contraction of the left side of the interventricular septum and the medial anteroseptal wall of the left ventricle.

The examination is best conducted when the patient is lying down, with the physician sitting at the patient's right side with the palm of the hand extended over the precordium. Palpation of the base of the heart should be performed with the patient sitting up, and of the apex with the patient lying flat.

Locating the Apex of the Left Ventricle (Figures 5.6 and 5.7)

Locating the apex of the left ventricle is sometimes easier said than done. If the patient is thin and your eyes are keen enough to observe the pulsation of the apex in the fifth intercostal space, or just medial to the midclavicular line, then place the palm of your hand gently below the nipple. Once you have felt the

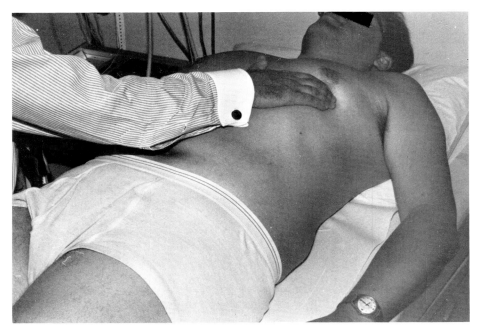

FIGURE 5.7   Palpating the apex of the heart.

location of the apex, then move your fingers to make a final assessment of its location. If you do not feel the apex beat, even after you have searched in the
fourth and fifth interspace, move the patient onto his/her left side. This maneuver
will separate the lung from the heart and bring the heart closer to the chest wall.
In females, this examination may be more difficult. With a nurse assistant at your
side, either have the patient move the breasts herself, or gently move the left
breast with your left hand and, with the right hand, palpate the apex. The same
maneuver can be tried with the patient turned onto her left side.

Some physicians state that the apex of the left ventricle is only felt in half of
adult patients. A careful search should be made in the majority of patients who
are not emphysematous or grossly obese. An extra aid is to have the patient sit
upright or lean forward. In the patient who has emphysema the apex can be felt
in the subxyphoid area.

Quickly run through your mind the following questions when feeling for the
apex. Is it located in the fifth intercostal space, on left midclavicular line, or has
the apex moved over toward the axilla, as is found in left ventricular hypertrophy?
Assess the amplitude. Does it just touch the fingers, or does it lift it vigorously
off the chest wall? Is it easy to compress the beat? The greater the amplitude and
the force, the more likely left ventricular enlargement is present.

The first heart sound is synchronous with the apical beat. The apical impulse
may have an increased amplitude when the cardiac output is increased (see further
details below under "Advanced Precordial Palpation").

Place your hand next to the sternum on the right. A heave may represent right
ventricular hypertrophy, also known as right ventricular heave or volume overload.
The right ventricular area, which includes the lower half of the sternum and the
parasternal area, especially on the left, may have a diffuse lift or heave. This can
be felt in normal thin adults and in children.

Advanced Precordial Palpation

In this section, I will discuss the more fruitful areas derived from palpating the heart. It is not enough to locate the point of maximum intensity. The normal impulse can be felt as a brief outward movement in early systole without any palpable diastolic movements. Early systole can be identified by the first heart sound, and extends to the second heart sound. The apical impulse normally is felt only during the first half of systole, or right after the first heart sound. A sustained impulse, heave, or thrust that is felt during the second half of systole up to the second heart sound means there is an increase in left ventricular mass and volume, which may be found in hypertension and aortic stenosis (ie, pressure overloading of the left ventricle). Patients with large ventricles and a decreased left ventricular ejection fraction have a sustained impulse. A plateau or large impulse is a sensitive indicator that there is something wrong with the left ventricle.

A hyperkinetic apical impulse may also be a sign of left ventricular enlargement. The impulse lifting the palpating finger with a normal contour is characteristic of volume overload, as in aortic or mitral insufficiency and ventricular septal defects.

Lateral Displacement of the Apex. As the left ventricle dilates, it displaces the apex out toward the axilla and downward. Palpation of the apex during a heart attack can be fruitful. Before the first heart sound, there may be presystolic distention of the left ventricle, which corresponds to the fourth heart sound on auscultation. These atrial sounds, as I will describe later, are sometimes felt better than heard and sometimes even seen better. The atrial, or presystolic impulse, results from a vigorous atrial contraction against a ventricle that is reduced in compliance, as noticed in an ischemic or infarcted myocardium. Ischemic hearts have diastolic and filling pressure abnormalities, which may be regional or global.

As the left ventricle fails, an outward movement of the apex may be detected after the second heart sound in early diastole. This corresponds to the third heart sound, or a gallop. This early diastolic outward movement can be felt in ventricular septal ruptures and mitral regurgitation.

Ectopic Areas of Apical Impulse. During systole, occurring with the first heart sound, a systolic outward impulse or a bulge may be seen representing a weakened infarcted segment of the heart expanding in systole. This can be felt in the third to the fifth intercostal spaces between the lower left sternal border and the cardiac apex. These are called ectopic areas of pulsation. This impulse is palpable medial and superior to the usual apical impulse. Thus, there is the apical impulse and the ectopic impulse. If you use two hands, the left hand to palpate the apex and the right hand to feel the ectopic area, you will see that they are not contracting at the same time—there is an asynchrony between the two areas. Sometimes, these ectopic impulses are located more medially in superior to normal apical beats. Similar findings may be noted in cardiomyopathy.

Ventricular Aneurysm. A systolic outward bulge that is palpated in the third to fifth intercostal spaces may also represent a ventricular aneurysm. Turning the patient on the left side will increase the cardiac output and the force of the contraction.

Right Ventricular Enlargement. A lift adjacent to the sternum, called the parasternal lift or heave, is maximum in the fourth and fifth intercostal spaces along the left sternal border directly beneath the lower sternum. Right ventricular enlargement can cause the entire anterior precordium to thrust upward, with the right ventricle now producing the apical beats. If this is found, there may also be a palpable second pulmonic sound, and a pulmonary artery impulse in the second or left interspace.

A very large left ventricle, as in severe mitral regurgitation, can also result in a left sternal parasternal impulse. The heart thrust is forward, coinciding with the peak of a left atrial V wave. The large left atrium causes the heart to thrust forward. Differentiating between right ventricle enlargement and left ventricle enlargement is not easy; the stethoscope will be of help. If the patient has mitral stenosis and significant pulmonary hypertension, it is an enlarged right ventricle that is heaving underneath the sternum. The left ventricle in pure mitral stenosis is small.

Palpating a Thrill. It was Laennec who described the thrill as a cat's purring: "It may be compared quite accurately to the vibration which accompanies the sound of satisfaction which a cat makes when one strokes it with the hand." Laennec also noted that a similar sensation can be produced by stroking the palm of a gloved hand with a toothbrush. The purring sound that you feel as a thrill should not be confused with a rough rubbing sensation, like two pieces of leather, over the precordium, as seen in pericarditis, which corresponds to a friction rub.

Usually, if a thrill is palpated, there will be an accompanying murmur underneath. If you think you feel a thrill and there is no murmur, then it probably was not a thrill. A thrill is always accompanied with a loud murmur, usually of Grade 4 intensity.

Place your hands over each of the cardiac areas. (Some examiners find the heads of the metacarpal bones detect a thrill better than the fingertips.) First palpate in the aortic valve area, which is best detected with the patient leaning forward and with the breath held in expiration. A thrill that is felt in the second right intercostal space is suggestive of aortic valvular disease. The same thrill from aortic stenosis can be felt at the left of the sternum or at the cardiac apex.

A thrill felt in the second left interspace is suggestive of pulmonic valvular stenosis, and one felt further down, in the fourth left intercostal space, could mean a ventricular septal defect. A systolic thrill felt at the cardiac apex is produced by mitral regurgitation, sometimes accompanied with mitral stenosis.

A thrill felt before the first heart sound, which is called a presystolic or diastolic thrill, is probably mitral stenosis.

A continuous thrill heard throughout the first heart sound up to the second heart sound suggests a patent ductus arteriosus, or an atriovenous communication.

RECORDING THE BLOOD PRESSURE

Every office visit should begin with a blood pressure reading. Blood pressure readings are obtained with a sphygmomanometer, either mercury or aneroid. A proper cuff size should be used with an inflatable bag. The width of the bag should be approximately 40% of the circumference of the limb where the cuff is placed. Using an average blood pressure cuff on an obese arm will lead to a false diagnosis of hypertension.

The blood pressure should be measured on the right arm. However, it may be helpful to take both a left arm and a right arm reading with the patient sitting and standing for several minutes. The normal person has a 5- to 10-mm difference in blood pressure between the left and right arm. It is recommended that future readings in a given patient be made on the arm with the higher blood pressure.

Place the inflatable bag over the brachial artery on the inside of the arm, being certain that the antecubital crease is well exposed. The cuff should be at at least 2.5 to 3 cm above this crease. It was in 1905 that Korotkoff introduced the auscultatory method of estimating the blood pressure, giving rise to the Korotkoff sounds, which may be heard by placing the stethoscope over the brachial artery in the antecubital fossa.

Pump the cuff up gently to the point where the pulsations of the brachial artery disappear. Deflate the cuff slowly until the pulse reappears. At the point that two consecutive beats are heard with the stethoscope, read the systolic blood pressure. Be certain that the cuff is inflated sufficiently so that the peak pressure is not missed. As the blood pressure cuff is further deflated, the Korotkoff sounds become muffled. At the disappearance of the sounds, read the diastolic blood pressure. It may be difficult to ascertain the diastolic blood pressure reading in patients with aortic regurgitation because the diastolic pressure will be quite low, giving rise to a large pulse pressure (the difference between the diastolic and systolic blood pressure).

As of 1985, normal blood pressure is considered to be 140/90, and readings above or below that are considered abnormal. The blood pressure should be taken at least twice, and, if found to be elevated, it behooves the physician to have the patient return at least on one occasion within a week for a second reading. However, if the diastolic pressure is greater than 110, it is my choice to start treatment at this time.

The blood pressure may vary from minute to minute. The patient may first arrive in the office with a blood pressure reading of 160/110. As the physician begins to talk with the patient, carrying on lightly and reassuring the patient, the blood pressure may then settle down to a normal level.

The patient is entitled to know his or her blood pressure readings, as reported by the Joint National Committee on the Detection, Evaluation and Treatment of High Blood Pressure of the United States Department of Health, Education and Welfare in 1978, although I do recommend that should be the choice of the physician at the particular time. If the patient is to be told his/her blood pressure, the physician should explain what this means in terms of its variability and follow-up. It is of no use to tell a patient his/her blood pressure is 160/100 and not to worry about it. As one of my patients said, "It's easy for you to say, Doctor, not to worry about it; it's not your blood pressure." Explain why the patient should not worry, why the blood pressure must repeatedly be measured, and, if it is elevated, that you will normalize the blood pressure with an active treatment program.

MEASURING THE ARTERIAL PULSE

I know of no other branch of the cardiovascular system so intimately studied historically as the arterial pulse. As far back as 3,500 years ago a connection was found between the heart and the pulse, as described in the papyrus scrolls. It was in ancient China where the art of pulse-feeling had its origin.

Herophilus, in 300 BC,, was the first to describe extrasystole. It was he who introduced into medicine an instrument to count the pulse, known as the water clock. He recognized that the pulsations of the arteries are caused by the heartbeat, and that "they may be rhythmic and in relation to age and disease."

Galen, in the year 132, noted the grave significance of an intermittent pulse, which we now know as pulsus alternans. Famous paintings of the Dutch and Flemish schools portray physicians seated in a chair discovering the ills of the patient by clasping the pulse. However, in the 1980s the diagnostic importance of the pulse seems long forgotten.

Location and Measurement of the Pulses

The best way to feel the pulse is to try to feel your own radial pulse. Elevate your right forearm slightly (I find that elevation of the arm makes the pulse easier to feel). With the fingers of your other hand, trace along down the edge of the thumb; invariably, the pulse will be found with the index finger pointing in the direction of the heart. Count the rate. A simple method is to count the number of beats in 15 seconds and multiply by four.

It has been my experience that the clinician should get in the habit of feeling for the pulses of the right and left arms simultaneously by merely elevating both wrists. This will automatically determine that the pulse is present in both wrists. A decreased or diminished pulse in one arm could mean that there is a vascular obstruction in the arterial trunk in the arm or at the periphery. For example, the pulses may be different in their strength because one has an aberrant route, or because of the presence of a scalenous anticus syndrome, a thrombosis embolus involving one of the subclavian or brachial arteries, a dissecting aneurysm, or a local obstruction, as sometimes occurs after cardiac catheterization or arterial puncture.

To learn the quality of the arterial peripheral pulse requires a repeated auto-matic reaching to feel the pulse, which, in a sense, is a gauge of the heart's action. The flow of blood through the arteries depends on the viscosity of blood, cardiac contraction, the elasticity of the vessels, and the resistance—all give character to the pulse. If the ventricular systole is weak, it is possible the pulse may be weak; however, the pulse may be feeble even though the heart contracts well. THE FORCE OF CONTRACTION OF THE HEART IS NOT REFLECTED BY THE FORCE OF THE PULSE.

The femoral pulses (Figure 5.8a) should be included in the examination of the cardiovascular system prior to listening to the heart as part of the total examina-tion of the heart. The femoral pulses are a necessary portion of the examination. However, it is important that you forewarn the patient that you are going to feel for the femoral pulses before reaching into the pelvic area. The femoral pulse is located below the inguinal ligament, midway between the anterior superior iliac spine and the symphysis pubis.

Other arterial pulses that should be examined at this time include the popliteal pulse (Figure 5.8b), which is difficult to feel, and the pedial pulses, which are lo-cated on both feet on the dorsum. Place your fingers gently on the dorsum of the foot to feel these pulses (in men, the absence of hair on the toes sometimes sig-nals severe peripheral vascular disease).

The posterior tibial pulse (Figure 5.8c) is felt in the following manner: place your thumb over the lateral malleolus of the foot and your hand around the top of the foot with the fingers reaching below the medial malleolus where the posterior tibial artery is located.

The normal pulse rates in adults can vary from 60 to 90 beats per minute. The pulse becomes slower in the elderly and more rapid in young children, where it ranges from 90 to 130. It is useful to note the following:

1. Qualitative characteristics of the pulse
2. Is it of large or small size?
3. Is it quick or prolonged?
4. Is it hard or soft?
5. Is the pulse rate rapid or slow?

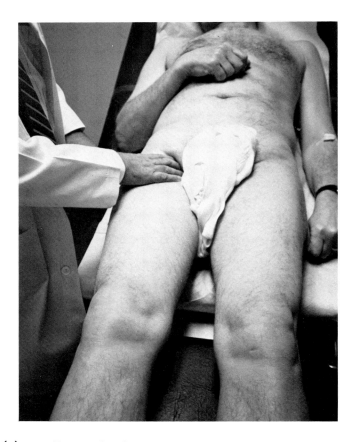

FIGURE 5.8 (a)   Femoral pulse.

Is the pulse regular? There should be at least 6 to 10 beats that follow one after the other. One hundred pulsations per minute is the upper limits of normal, and above that is called sinus tachycardia. A fast heartbeat, or tachycardia, may be the only finding in early congestive heart failure, chronic myocardial disease, and hyperthyroidism. Temperature increases the pulse, five beats for every degree Fahrenheit (eight beats for every degree Centigrade). Tachycardia can occur in anemia, dehydration, and medical student excitement.

A pulse of 60 or less is called sinus bradycardia, a common finding in medical students who jog 5 miles or more per day   It is also found in myxedema, viral infections, jaundice, and heart blocks, and with β-blockade and calcium blocker medications.

Medical Trivia: What is Merseburg triad? Exophthalmos, tachycardia, and goiter found in Grave's disease. (The thyroidologist, Dr. Basedow, lived in Merseburg, Germany.)

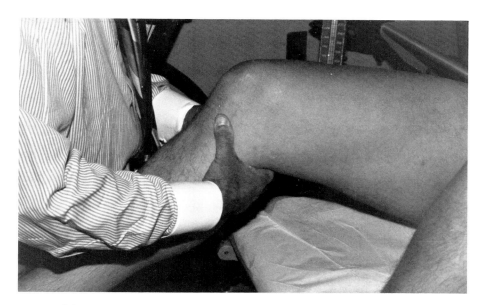

FIGURE 5.8 (b)   Popliteal pulse.

FIGURE 5.8 (c)   Posterior tibial pulse.

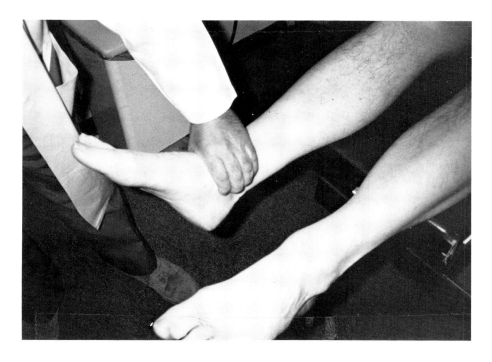

Abnormal Pulse Findings

Pulsus Alternans

Pulsus alternans is a much forgotten and important sign of a failing heart, first described by Dr. Ludwig Traube in 1872. This is the kind of pulse that at one moment is full and high, and then changes to weak beats alternating with stronger beats. Simultaneous cardiac auscultation may reveal an alteration in the intensity of the heart sounds—weaker, alternating with stronger beats. Beware of bigeminal rhythms, which sometimes can sound like pulsus alternans. Have the patient take a deep breath; if the pulse diminishes or disappears during the height of inspiration, there may be the presence of a paradoxical pulse, as seen in severe asthmatics or in emphysema. It is also a clue that constrictive pericarditis or cardiac tamponade may be present.

Pulsus Bisferiens

A double pulse, entitled pulsus bisferiens, could signal that aortic stenosis and aortic insufficiency are present. Sir James Mackenzie, through his diligent observations in practicing general medicine and cardiology, made an accurate description of the pulse found in premature contractions and atrial fibrillations. Premature contractions, as Sir Mackenzie so elegantly described, may be perceived by the examining finger as the impression of a pause followed by resumption of a normal rhythm. Premature contraction can originate from the ventricle or above the ventricle.

Sinus Irregularity

As the patient breathes normally, the pulse may vary according to the respirations, a common finding in healthy individuals and in infants. This does not indicate heart disease—the pulse rate merely speeds up during one moment of the respiration cycle and then slows. When the pulse is totally irregular, it probably represents atrial fibrillation. A *Diagnostic Pearl:* If less than six successive beats occur together, the possibility of atrial fibrillation has to be entertained. The A wave of the venous pulsation occurs almost about the same time as the first heart sound; it will be seen that the A waves have disappeared in atrial fibrillation.

The Generous Pulse

The generous pulse is full and is related to the degree of arterial distention during systole, and arterial collapse during diastole. If the pressure difference between systole and diastole (the pulse pressure) increases, the generosity of the pulse increases. The sudden rise and then the collapse of the pulse is characteristic of aortic insufficiency.

The Corrigan Pulse

The Corrigan pulse is characteristically seen with a high pulse pressure, systolic blood pressure of 180, and diastolic over 40. It is also found in anemias, coarctation of the aorta, patent ductus arteriosus, ruptured sinus Valsalva, and arteriovenous fistula.

Pulsus Parvus/Pulsus Tardus

The pulse that feels small and firm is sometimes found in aortic stenosis as a result of low pulse pressure (blood pressure of 100/85).

Examination of the Carotid Pulse

It is important to learn how to palpate for the carotid artery both for the general physical examination and during the examination of the unconscious patient, when the peripheral pulses may be too weak to feel. The carotid arteries give information not only about the heart but about the cerebral blood flow. The pulsations arising from the carotid artery may be visible medial to the sternocleidomastoid muscles. It is best that the sternocleidomastoid muscle be relaxed by turning the patient's head slightly toward the side being examined. Follow with your fingertips the medial border of the sternocleidomastoid muscle of the lower half of the neck, which might lie just below the thyroid cartilage. Press gently, because directly above the carotid artery is the carotid sinus, and toward the angle of the neck pressure on this carotid sinus can cause a reflex drop in the pulse rate or blood pressure.

Pulsations of the internal jugular vein, which lies deep to the sternocleidomastoid muscle, can be confused with those of the common carotid artery. In the normal person, deep inspiration will collapse the jugular pulse in the neck. This will not occur with the carotid pulse. Gentle light pressure over the vein and above the sternal end of the clavicle will also eliminate venous pulsation. A little more gentle pressure is required to eliminate the pulses of the carotid artery.

The normal upstroke of the carotid artery is smooth and rapid (Figure 5.9). It follows after the first heart sound. The downstroke is normally less abrupt than the upstroke. A rapid upstroke with a quick descent is found in hyperthyroidism anemia, and in nervous individuals. A thrill may be palpated over the carotid

FIGURE 5.9   Normal carotid pulse coordinated with phonocardiogram and electrocardiogram.

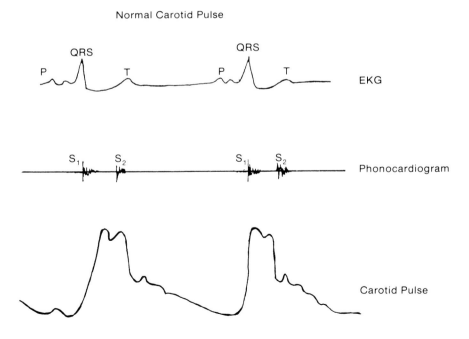

Normal Carotid Pulse

EKG

Phonocardiogram

Carotid Pulse

artery, as commonly seen in aortic valvular stenosis, and also in thyrotoxicosis anemia and other conditions where there is a high cardiac output.

A weak pulsation can also be caused by decreased stroke volume. Local factors, such as arterial narrowing or occlusion, as in carotid artery stenosis, can cause weak pulsations. There may be a variation of the amplitude from beat to beat, which can be due to pulsus alternans, bigeminal pulse, or paradoxical pulse. Low amplitude of the carotid pulsation, as with small upstroke and a small volume, is indicative of aortic valvular stenosis.

WHAT ABOUT PERCUSSION OF THE HEART?

Although it is traditional to describe the method of percussion of the heart in most textbooks of physical diagnosis, it is so antiquated and worthless that there is no need to burden you with a maneuver that will only lead you astray.

AUSCULTATION OF THE HEART

Cardiac auscultation is the piece de resistance, the eclair of physical diagnosis. It is almost an act of snobbery to hear the sounds of the heart and piece them together into an anatomic or pathologic presence.

A Thirty-Second Review of the Characteristics of Sound

There are three characteristics of sound: frequency or pitch, amplitude, and quality. The **frequency** or **pitch** is the number of vibrations per second. The human range of hearing is between 20 and 20,000 vibrations per second. Heart sounds arise from the lower end of the range of human hearing. The first and second sounds have frequencies of less than 70 cycles per second, and the third and fourth heart sounds have frequencies of 30 cycles per second. **Amplitude** is the measured intensity of a sound and is a reflection of the force that produced it. **Quality** refers to the softness or the coarseness of a sound.

A combination of the vibrations and harmonics determines the quality of the sound. Harmonics are called the higher frequency components. Sounds also have loudness and intensity. For practical purposes, these will be regarded as one quality, which depends on the sensation produced and also on the sensation perceived. Transmissions of the sound that you hear in your ear can be influenced by the chest wall, the surrounding muscles, and the lung fluid. As sound passes from one medium to another a portion is reflected and the rest passes through. In media of the same intensity, most of the sound goes through and only a small part is reflected. For example, blood and muscle have about the same density, and sound passes through them without much reflection, whereas lungs, with their air spaces, cause a great deal of reflection and sounds are not well transmitted.

The Stethoscope

The stethoscope remains the stamp of the physician. Whether you wear it wrapped around your neck, dangle it from your pocket, hold it in one hand, or just let it gently protrude out of your pocket, it is unmistakable. The only person I have ever seen with a stethoscope who wasn't a physician was my pool repair man. He was trying to locate a leak. From his box of tricks, he pulled out a black stethoscope, placed the earpieces into his ears, and began to crawl along the lip of the pool, listening for that unmistakable telltale sign of the leaky pipe—the rushing turbulent noise of the pipe that was breached.

Choosing a Stethoscope

Buying your first stethoscope is a thrilling experience. Choosing the correct one is not that difficult. The internal tubing should preferably be plastic, it should be small in diameter, and the length should not exceed 16 inches. There should be a bell, a diaphragm, and earpieces that fit comfortably.

I have known students to buy different types of stethoscopes because they do not "hear as well with one." It reminds me of my search for the proper tennis racquet to improve my stroke, which is of no avail. Your stethoscope will become a very personal, endearing belonging throughout your medical training. It will not disappoint or fail you if you learn to use it correctly and trust it. Remember, it requires intensive training and practice. Each time you listen to the heart, it should be like a new experience, concentrating on every component and not omitting one step. It will be useful to you in every specialty, even orthopedics (listening to the motion of a joint). Even psychiatrists and dermatologists may have an occasional use for it.

How to Listen With the Stethoscope

The ideal setting is in a quiet, soundproof room; clothing should be removed from the chest. When examining women, I use a towel to cover their breasts while they are lying down, and uncover only the area to be examined. It is best not to carry on a conversation while you are examining the heart. You should introduce your examination by telling the patient, "I am now going to listen to your heart, and I would like you to breathe naturally."

The heart examination is accomplished with the patient lying flat, turned to the left side, and sitting up and forward. Be sure that the stethoscope diaphragm is well warmed, especially if you just arrived from the cold outside. It is a most disagreeable sensation to have a cold diaphragm placed on your chest.

Which to use, the bell or the diaphragm? The bell of the stethoscope transmits low-frequency sounds and must be placed lightly on the skin. If you press it firmly, it will act as a diaphragm. The diaphragm listens to higher frequency sounds. If this is pressed gently on the chest, it acts like a bell, transmitting low-frequency sounds. The diaphragm of the stethoscope must be pushed firmly enough against the chest to leave an imprint in order to shut off all other sounds.

Auscultation must be performed in all areas of the heart (Figure 5.10):

The aortic area—second right intercostal space

The pulmonic area—second left intercostal space

The mitral area—fifth left intercostal space

The tricuspid area—below the sternum

The pulmonic and tricuspid valves are located near the chest walls and their sounds are transmitted close to the auscultatory areas. Because the aortic and mitral valves are deep in the chest, their vibrations are transmitted in the direction of blood flow close to the chest wall. The mitral sounds are transmitted to the apex, and the aortic sounds following upward toward the ascending aorta. The

Areas of Auscultation

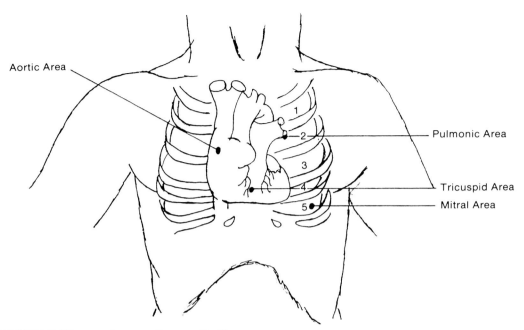

FIGURE 5.10   Areas of auscultation.

apical area of the heart is formed in part by the left ventricle, and it is here that sounds of the mitral valve and the left ventricle are best heard. The area left of the sternal end of the sternum is over the right ventricle, and here the sounds of the tricuspid valve are produced.

Place your stethoscope in your ears and try to locate each of the auscultory areas on your own chest. If you are listening to your own heart, you will hear a "lub-dub." The lub refers to the first heart sound, the dub to the second heart sound. The closure of the mitral and tricuspid valves, or atrioventricular valves, brings on the first heart sound, or the lub. The closure of the pulmonic and aortic valves causes the second heart sound, or dub. Other events of the valves and left ventricle contribute to the first heart sound, but these need not concern us at this time.

The First Heart Sound

It is best to listen to the first heart sound, or the closure of the mitral valve, at the apex—at the apical impulse. It occurs at the time of the beginning of the carotid pulse. It should not be timed with the radial pulse. With your fingers, first feel for the apex beat. The first heart sound will be directly over the outward thrust of the apex beat. As the anterior and posterior leaflets of the mitral valve come together, the first heart sound is produced. It corresponds, naturally, to the beginning of ventricular systole. It is low in frequency.

How to distinguish the first heart sound from the second heart sound: The time interval between the first and second heart sounds is shorter than that between the second sound and the subsequent first heart sound—the diastolic event is longer

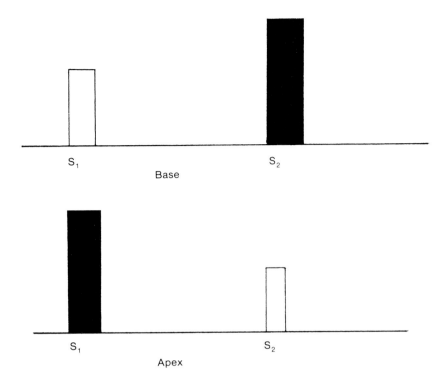

S_1

S_2

Base

S_1

S_2

Apex

FIGURE 5.11   First and second heart sounds.

than the systolic event. The first heart sound is best heard with the diaphragm of the stethoscope. The upstroke of the carotid pulse occurs immediately after the first heart sound (see Figure 5.11). The mitral valve closes approximately 0.2 to 0.3 seconds before the tricuspid valve, so, if you hear two sounds together, it is because the tricuspid valve is closing. This is commonly heard a little further up, along the left sternal border in the tricuspid area.

Causes of Increased Intensity
The intensity of the first heart sound is increased by any condition that increases the force of ventricular contraction, which will bring the heart closer to the chest wall.

The first heart sound may be accentuated in thin individuals. It is also increased in conditions that increase cardiac output, such as anemia, hyperthyroidism, and mitral stenosis.

A short PR interval causes the mitral and tricuspid valves to close from a relatively open position, which increases the intensity of the first heart sound.

In summary, causes of an increased intensity of the first heart sound include: short PR interval, mitral stenosis, and hyperkinetic states (hyperthyroidism, fever, anemia, exercise, pregnancy). This is also normally found in children and young adults with thin chest walls.

Causes of Decreased Intensity

Because the leaflets of the mitral valve and tricuspid valve are in close opposition, at the onset of ventricular contraction there is little excursion, the vibrations are small, and a faint first heart sound may result.

Decreased intensity of the first heart sound is also caused by a long PR interval, as in a first-degree heart block; diminished left ventricular contraction; acute myocardial infarction; congestive heart failure; cardiomyopathy; obesity; large breasts; and fluid and air between the heart and the stethoscope, as in pulmonary emphysema and pericardial effusions.

Splitting of the First Heart Sound

Very often, there is splitting of the first heart sound at the apex, corresponding to mitral valve closure slightly before the tricuspid closure. Splitting of the first heart sound at the apex needs to be differentiated from a systolic click and from the fourth, or atrial, sound (see below). Wide splitting of the first heart sound is always abnormal and is heard in complete right bundle branch block, because the tricuspid valve closure is delayed when there is a delay in activation of the ventricles.

The Second Heart Sound

The second heart sound is higher in pitch and shorter and sharper than the first heart sound. It means the end of systole has arrived and diastole is about to begin. Again, the diaphragm of the stethoscope is the best to use for the second heart sound. There are two components to the second heart sound, one due to the aortic valve closure and the other to the pulmonic valve closure. The aortic component comes before the pulmonic component. It is the "dub" portion of the heartbeat. The aortic component of the second heart sound is heard best in the aortic area, in the right second intercostal space, and the pulmonic component is best heard in the pulmonic area, in the second left intercostal space. The aortic component of the second heart sound is generally louder, and the pulmonic component is softer.

Thus there is a normal splitting of the second heart sound due to a delay in the pulmonic second heart sound because the aortic valve closes first (Figure 5.12). During inspiration, the interthoracic pressure increases, and venous return to the right side of the heart increases, with the result that the right ventricular stroke volume increases. It now takes longer for the right heart to eject its blood, and lengthened right side ejection time results in delayed pulmonic closure. Inspiration causes the aortic valve to close earlier, because during inspiration blood is pooled in the pulmonary bed, which will reduce the flow to the left side of the heart, shortening ventricular systole, and left ventricular ejection will end earlier than right ventricular ejection.

On inspiration by the patient, the second heart sound can be heard to split into two components. This disappears with expiration, resulting from the fusion of the two sounds. The novice may find it difficult to hear this splitting and fusion; it requires listening through several cycles. There may be a slight splitting of the second heart sound heard in expiration.

How is it possible to tell that the first heart sound is louder than the second at the cardiac apex? Clue: the second heart sound is normally louder than the first at the aortic area. If the first heart sound is equal to or louder than the second over the aortic area, then the first is probably accentuated. Using the bell of the stethoscope, inch along to the left parasternal area. Move along toward the base of the heart; the second heart sound will become louder as you arrive at the base. Keep your eyes on the patient's chest and, when he/she takes a deep breath, notice the inspiratory and expiratory movements of the chest. The physiologic splitting

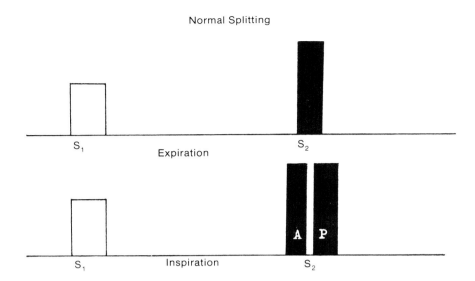

Normal Splitting

FIGURE 5.12   Normal splitting of the second heart sound.

of the second heart sound is going to be increased by inspiration because the right ventricle systole is increased slightly in inspiration with a reduction in duration of the left ventricular systole. Now that you have clearly heard the splitting of the second heart sound at the base, return to the apex.

Causes of Wide Splitting

If there is the presence of a complete right bundle branch block or a premature left ventricular beat that causes a delay in right ventricular systole (a delay of transmission of right ventricular systole electrically), there may be a wide abnormal splitting of the second heart sound. In the case of pulmonic stenosis, there is delayed closure of the pulmonic valve and wide splitting of the second heart sound is heard in the pulmonic area that will increase further with inspiration. This examination, if possible, is best performed with the patient sitting up.

Paradoxical, or reverse, splitting of the second heart sound occurs when the pulmonic valve closes before the aortic valve, which is the reverse of normal. This occurs whenever there is interference with ejection on the left side of the heart, as in electrical delays such as complete left bundle branch block, biventricular ectopic beats, and right ventricular pacing; mechanical delays, such as outflow obstructions, secondary to aortic stenosis, idiopathic hypertrophic subaortic stenosis, and severe left ventricular poor dysfunction; and at a time when the left ventricle is functioning improperly. Coronary artery disease, including large patent ductus arteriosus, may also be responsible, especially during an attack of angina. The physician must concentrate to be able to discover paradoxical splitting at the bedside. Normally, the splitting of the second heart sound increases on inspiration and fades on expiration. In paradoxical splitting, there is audible splitting on expiration, and during inspiration the sound approaches being singular (Figure 5.13). This occurs because the pulmonic valve closure occurs later than anticipated, and the two components merge into a single sound.

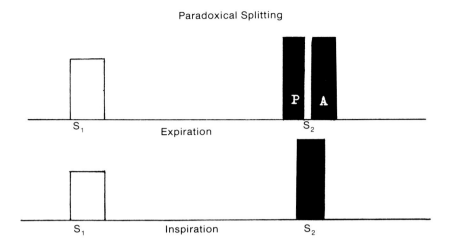

FIGURE 5.13   **Paradoxical splitting of the second heart sound.**

In summary, causes of abnormal splitting of the second heart sound include:

1. Right bundle branch block
2. Pulmonic stenosis (in severe cases the pulmonic component is delayed and soft)
3. Left ventricular ectopic beats (these are due to delay of pulmonic valve closure)
4. Mitral regurgitation
5. Large ventricular septal defect (abnormal splitting is due to shortening of left ventricular ejection time)
6. Wide splitting of the second heart sound with no change on inspiration
7. Atrial septal defect
8. Paradoxical or reverse splitting—splitting decreases on inspiration and is present on expiration
9. Left bundle branch block
10. Right ventricular ectopic beats
11. Severe aortic stenosis
12. Idiopathic hypertrophic subaortic stenosis
13. Severe left ventricular dysfunction during angina (this is due to the delay of aortic valve closure).

The Third Heart Sound

The third heart sound (Figure 5.14) is a sound that is of low frequency and is associated with the rapid flow of blood into the ventricle in early diastole. The third heart sound is caused by the sudden distention of the ventricular wall, as blood flows from the atrium into the ventricle. It is heard approximately 1.5 seconds after the second sound and can originate from either the left or the right ventricle.

This diastolic sound is sometimes difficult to hear because it is low in frequency and faint. Because this is a low-pitched sound, the bell of the stethoscope is used. Turn the patient to the left side, locating the PMI by palpation with your hand, and then place the bell of the stethoscope lightly over that area. Asking the patient to exhale will make the sound audible. The sound can sometimes also be brought out by raising the patient's legs and with coughing.

FIGURE 5.14   Third heart sound.

The third heart sound is an extraordinarily useful sound to hear in diagnosing congestive heart failure. It also represents a failing heart in an older person. However A THIRD HEART SOUND ALONE DOES NOT NECESSARILY INFER THAT THE HEART HAS FAILED, because it can occur if blood rapidly flows into the ventricle because of increased volume.

Gallop Rhythm

The first, second, and third heart sounds can sound like the gallop of a horse, or a gallop, and have come to be known as gallop rhythm. It is found in mitral regurgitation, where the third heart sound can be palpated. Similarly, a flabby stretched muscle can give rise to the gallop rhythm. The loudest third heart sound is heart in constrictive pericarditis.

A third heart sound originating from the left ventricle, (*left-sided* gallop rhythm) does not vary with respiration and is more easily audible during expiration. It is an expiratory sound. *Right-sided* gallop rhythm, occurring in the right ventricle, is heard best along the left sternal border over the xyphoid region and increases with inspiration. If the patient has pulmonary emphysema, these right-sided gallops are best heard over the xyphoid region, or even in the epigastric portion of the thorax.

Gallops are frequent during a myocardial infarction when there is an abnormally elevated left ventricular filling pressure, which means left ventricular compliance is diminished and there is marked left ventricular dysfunction.

Gallop rhythm is found commonly in cardiomyopathies. Earlier on, pulsus alternans was mentioned as an important sound of a failing heart. A diastolic gallop sound and pulsus alternans are clues to the presence of a weakened muscle. A nuclear scan of the heart will confirm your findings of a reduced ejection fraction.

Occasionally, the fourth heart sound is present along with the third heart sound, and they seem to fuse in diastole and a prominent sound results, called the summation gallop.

The Fourth Heart Sound

In recent years the fourth heart sound (Figure 5.15) has become quite fashionable to describe in a hospital chart. First described in 1840 by Clendining, it is a sound that is produced and is synchronous with atrial contraction. This sound precedes the first heart sound, is of low intensity, and is heard clearly at the apex. It is best heard with the bell of the stethoscope. It is also called the atrial gallop sound, presystolic, and generally is a sign of ventricular failure. It implies decrease in left ventricular compliance, so that the atrium must contract harder to complete ventricular filling.

Listen to the fourth heart sound by turning the patient gently to the left, feeling for the apex, and placing the bell of the stethoscope at the PMI. It can be made

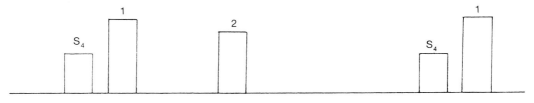

Apex

FIGURE 5.15   Fourth heart sound.

more evident after mild effort, such as gently lifting the patient or having him/
her stand up and then sit down and lie down. It is an expiratory sound. It is loudest
on expiration and corresponds to the venous return of the left heart. It is usually
heard only on expiration. A distinctive bulge at the apex that coincides with the
atrial contraction and can be felt and seen before the apical impulse corresponds
to the fourth heart sound.

How to distinguish the fourth heart sound from the first heart sound: If you
hear a split first heart sound at the apex, the sound that is heard only in expiration
is a fourth heart sound. Normally, splitting of the first heart sound is not heard at
the apex. Remember, it is a low-pitched sound. The fourth heart sound is rarely
heard along the left sternal border, but it will be heard in the tiny area of the
apical beat. Its intensity can be decreased or can disappear if the stethoscope
bell, which should be gently applied on the chest, is instead applied firmly. This
does not occur with a split first heart sound. A fourth heart sound originating from
the right ventricle is heard best in inspiration. It is important to listen specifically
for the individual fourth heart sound.

The fourth heart sound is commonly heard in hypertension, during an attack of
angina, and in almost all patients with acute myocardial infarction, because the
stiffened ischemic left ventricle welcomes the extra atrial kick to fill it with
blood. It is sometimes intermittent and may not be always heard.

In young people a fourth heart sound may be present without evidence of heart
disease.

Fourth heart sounds are heard in acute mitral regurgitation due to ruptured
chordae tendineae, or papillary muscle rupture following a myocardial infarction.
A fourth heart sound gallop is generally not present in chronic mitral regurgitation,
because the left atrium is so large and dilated it cannot generate that atrial kick.
Obviously, the fourth heart sound is going to be absent if there is atrial fibrillation.

Ejection Sounds

Ejection sounds (Figure 5.16) are heard right after the first heart sound and have
an aortic and pulmonic component. They occur at the onset of systole into the
great vessels. These sounds are best heard with the stethoscope diaphragm. Aortic
ejection sounds are heard throughout the chest, especially in the aortic area, and
are heard also at the cardiac apex. They are a useful sign for the presence of congenital bicuspid aortic valve, valvular aortic stenosis, or aortic regurgitation or
dilatation of the aortic root. An ejection sound in the pulmonic area, called pulmonic ejection sound, results from pulmonic stenosis. It characteristically diminishes in intensity with inspiration, becoming louder again during expiration.

It will help you to differentiate it from the fourth heart sound. An ejection
sound is a higher pitched sound, it is sharp, and it may actually simulate a split

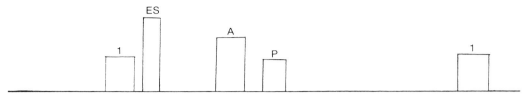

ES=Ejection Sound

FIGURE 5.16   Ejection sound.

first heart sound. If you hear a split first heart sound at the apex, it could be:
1) an atrial sound, which is low pitched; 2) an ejection sound, which is high pitched;
or 3) a split first heart sound. The atrial, or fourth heart sound, is heard predominantly on expiration; the split first heart sound will be heard over a wider area and
not in one spot; and the ejection sound will be also heard at the base predominantly.

Systolic Click

The systolic click (Figure 5.17) is another fashionable sound, described frequently
by cardiologists. It is a common sound, heard very frequently in women and in
thin-chested males, and often associated with prolapse of the mitral valve or the
click-murmur syndrome. An entire chapter could be devoted to systolic clicks. The
systolic click is not difficult to hear. It occurs between the first and the second
sounds in midsystole. It is sharp and usually single, but may be multiple.

The click followed by a murmur is a most valuable sound to diagnose prolapse
of the mitral valve. The click coincides with the maximum excursion of the anterior
and posterior leaflet of the mitral valve as it prolapses into the left atrium. Often,
the murmur that follows this click can be a musical whoop or honk secondary to
mitral regurgitation, or harsh, like a friction rub. Listen for the click in many
positions—in the left lateral, decubitis, sitting, standing, squatting, or supine. Some
are heard only during inspiration, and others only during expiration.

This is a high-frequency sound and should not be confused with the third or
fourth heart sounds or ejection sound, which is much softer. The sound that you
hear between the first and second heart sounds could be an ejection sound, a systolic click, or a murmur. A systolic click occurs later than an ejection sound. Its
timing (near the first heart sound, in midsystole, or late systolic) will vary with
various bedside maneuvers.

Intensity and timing of systolic clicks can vary with the volume of the left ventricle. Smaller ventricle size and volume causes redundancy of mitral valve leaflets
and greater prolapse into the atrium in systole. Increase in ventricular volume can
be artificially stimulated by having the patient squat, which increases venous return

FIGURE 5.17   Systolic click.

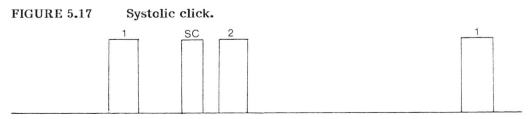

SC=Systolic Click

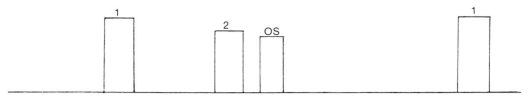

OS=Opening Snap

FIGURE 5.18   **Opening snap of mitral stenosis.**

and venous afterload; the leaflets now are prolapsed at a later time and the click will move closer to the second heart sound. In contrast, when the ventricular size and volume are reduced, as by standing up or a Valsalva maneuver inspiration, the amount of redundancy increases, the valve leaflets now prolapse earlier into the atrium in systole, and the click and the murmur appear earlier or move closer to the first heart sound.

The Opening Snap of Mitral Stenosis

The motion of the anterior and posterior leaflets of the mitral valve looks like two hands clapping together. The closing of the mitral valve is recorded as the first heart sound. When the leaflets become fibrotic and calcified, and the chordae tendineae that hold them become retracted, the opening of the valve found in mitral stenosis causes a snapping sound (Figure 5.18). This is a high-pitched sound that is heard as the opening movement of the valve, continuing to its full extent and then ending in diastole. Dr. Bouillaud, a famous auscultatologist, described the opening snap of mitral stenosis as, "the hammer which after striking the iron falls on the anvil, rebounds, and falls again motionless."

The opening snap may be the loudest sound heard during the cardiac examination. It is best heard along the left border of the sternum between the third and fourth left intercostal space. Its intensity is much less at the apex, where the mid-diastolic murmur of mitral stenosis will be heard. It has to be differentiated from a third heart sound, which is found predominantly at the apex whereas the opening snap has a wide radiation. It occurs much earlier than the third heart sound. It does not vary with respiration, and occurs 0.08 to 0.1 seconds after the second heart sound.

Picture the mitral valve during systole bulging into the atrium like a hammock. As systole ends, the pressure in the left ventricle drops below the left atrium, and the hammock of the mitral valve is snapped back and bulges into the left ventricle. As atrial pressure rises, the more forcible will be the movement of the valve and the louder the sound. The more severe the mitral stenosis, the less pliable are the leaflets, and the opening snap becomes diminished and may even disappear.

Turn the patient on the left side (the left lateral decubitis position), and find the PMI with palpation. On auscultation, an accentuated first heart sound will be heard, a second heart sound followed by an opening snap.

Pericardial Friction Rubs

Pericardial friction rubs have been reported by such historic figures as Hope, Collins, Laennec, and even Hippocrates and Stokes. The sound has been described as two pieces of leather rubbing together. Others have called it the sound of hair moving to and fro between the fingers. These leathery sounds may have three components occurring during atrial systole, ventricular systole, and early diastole.

The pericardial friction rub represents the parietal and visceral pericardia rubbing against each other. It can result from inflammation due to viral, fungal, or bacterial infection as well as trauma and tumor. It is also a common finding with an anterior wall infarction. It is an important physical finding during the cardiovascular examination, and must be sought for diligently. It may be the only clue to the presence of pericarditis, especially when changes may suggest a myocardial infarction.

As the inflammation subsides, or an effusion appears separating the two coverings of the pericardium, the rub may disappear. The sound may disappear as quickly as it appears. The intern may hear it on admission, and, by the time the resident arrives in the room 10 minutes later, the sound is no longer present. It is made more audible with the patient sitting up or leaning forward. It may be increased in the left lateral position and with the arms extended above the head during inspiration. More pressure applied using the bell of the stethoscope will increase its loudness, which is not the case with murmurs.

Heart Murmurs

In order to appreciate the timing of a heart murmur, its relation to the heart sounds needs to be clearly registered. The physician must be able to identify the first and second heart sounds, corresponding to the systolic and diastolic events of the heart. A good grasp of the normal cardiovascular cycle with the normal cardiovascular events will also help to put into proper perspective the significance of heart murmurs.

A cardiac murmur results when the normal laminary flow of the blood becomes a turbulent flow. The noise created by turbulent flow may be innocent or functional or may represent organic heart disease. The three basic mechanisms responsible for cardiac murmurs are: 1) increased flow through a normal or abnormal valve; 2) blood flowing from a smaller vessel into a dilated vessel or through a partially closed atrioventricular valve; and 3) regurgitant flow or backflow through an incompetent valve, a septal defect, or a patent ductus arteriosus or AV fistulae.

Once a murmur is heard, it must be qualified for diagnostic purposes. Qualifying murmurs also gives the ability to communicate this information from California to Main with a certain degree of consistency. Murmurs should be qualified according to the following characteristics (it would also be helpful to use this format in the write-up on the heart):

1. Timing: is it systolic, diastolic, or continuous?
2. Location and radiation: find the PMI; is it loudest at the left sternal border, at the apex, at the pulmonic area, at the aortic area, or in ectopic areas (as in back of the vertebrae prominence, over the scapula, or along the right sternal border)?
3. Loudness: grade I-VI?
4. Pitch: is it medium or high pitched?
5. Duration: is it brief, medium, or long in duration?
6. Quality: is it a crescendo (increasing in loudness), a descrescendo (decreasing in loudness), blowing, harsh, rumbling, musical, whooping, or honking?

There are some basic physical principles that you need to keep in mind.

In **timings** systolic murmurs can be early systolic, midsystolic, late systolic, or holosystolic. Diastolic murmurs can be early diastolic, mid-diastolic, late diastolic (or presystolic), and holodiastolic.

The **pitch** of a murmur will increase with the velocity of the blood. The higher the pressure differences, the higher pitched will be the murmur; for example, flow from the left ventricle to the left atrium in mitral regurgitation.

The **location** of the murmur, where it is heard best, is the PMI. This may be at the apex, left sternal border, pulmonic area, aortic area, or in ectopic areas. The vibrations of a murmur are produced downstream. In aortic stenosis, for example, the wake of flow is downstream, so the murmur will be best heard in the second and first right intercostal spaces up in the neck. In aortic regurgitation, the wake is upstream and the murmur will be heard along the left border of the heart.

The intensity of the murmur is dependent on the velocity of blood flow. At rest, the murmur of mitral stenosis may not be heard, but it becomes evident with exercise at times. Most murmurs become louder with exercise. Determine the **loudness** of the murmur according to the universal grading system. A grade of 1 out of 6 is a faint sound sometimes heard only after exercising. A grade 2 murmur is faint but readily heard. Grade 3 is loud but without a thrill; in grade 4 there is a thrill. In grade 5 the murmur is so loud that it can be heard with the stethoscope almost partly off the chest. In grade 6 the murmur can be heard with the stethoscope raised slightly above the chest, with a loud thrill.

The purpose of qualifying murmurs is to make an attempt to precisely identify the murmur, trace its origin, and enables the physician to monitor change in the murmur over time. For example, a murmur that was once a grade 2 and has become a grade 4 reflects an anatomic and hemodynamic turnover. The diastolic murmur of aortic regurgitation that becomes longer and louder may mean a worsening of aortic regurgitation. In a similar manner, a systolic murmur that is only barely audible during the course of a myocardial infarction turns from a grade 1 to a grade 4 coarse sound that occupies all of systole if there is a rupture of a cord of the mitral valve or even a perforation of the septum.

Systolic Murmurs

The timing of a systolic murmur is not difficult if you relate it to the first heart sound. If it is early after the first heart sound, it is considered early systolic (Figure 5.19). If in between the first and second heart sounds, it is midsystolic (Figure 5.20). If the murmur appears right before the second heart sound, it is considered late systolic (Figure 5.21). Does the murmur take up the entire systole between the first and the second heart sounds? If so, it is called holosystolic or pansystolic (Figure 5.22).

Determination of Anatomic Origin

Once you have decided it is a systolic murmur and have determined its pitch, its loudness, its duration and its quality, the next maneuver is to determine its location. Take the stethoscope, using either the bell or the diaphragm, whichever you hear the murmur best with, and inch it along the chest, tracing the murmur's PMI. The murmur may be loud throughout the chest, and that needs to be noted.

As mentioned earlier, murmurs should be listened to with the patient sitting forward and lying flat. See if the systolic murmur disappears when the patient lies flat, or if it increases, or is only heard when the patient sits up. Those that tend to disappear either when the patient lies flat or sits up may be known as innocent murmurs (see further below).

Systolic Murmurs Heard at the Base of the Heart. If the murmur is heard at the base of the heart, determine whether it arises from the aortic valve or from the pulmonic valve by inching the stethoscope to the right second intercostal space (the

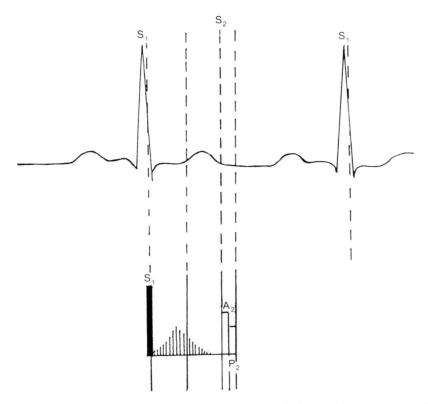

FIGURE 5.19   Early systolic ejection murmur timing with cardiac cycle.
Adapted from: Classification of murmurs according to timing in the cardiac cycle.
Clin Highlights, December 1984, p 29.

aortic valve), or the left second intercostal space (the pulmonic valve). If the
murmur is heard predominantly over the aortic valve, it could arise from: 1) a
normal aortic valve with increased blood flow through the valve as the result of a
high-velocity rate of ejection through the valves; 2) dilatation of the aortic root
beyond the valve; or 3) a narrowed valve secondary to aortic stenosis, which could
be acquired or congenital. Because the murmur arising from the aortic valve may
be transmitted along the left sternal border and even toward the apex, sometimes
the murmur may change its characteristic quality at the apex.

Prior to listening to the heart, you will have palpated for thrills. If a thrill
was present over the aortic area, at least a grade 4 accompanying systolic murmur
will be heard.

Take your stethoscope and trace the murmur along to see if it radiates up to
the neck, which is characteristic of aortic stenosis. Listen for the systolic murmur at Erb's point, the third and fourth left intercostal spaces along the left
sternal border.

The Systolic Murmur Arising in the Pulmonic Area. The murmur may be arising
from the pulmonic valve as a result of either subvalvular stenosis or dilatation of
the pulmonary artery and increased pulmonary flow, as may occur in normal young
children or in patients with atrial septal defect. The murmurs heard in the aortic
or pulmonary valve area may be early systolic, midsystolic, or crescendo/de-
crescendo, the so-called diamond-shaped murmurs.

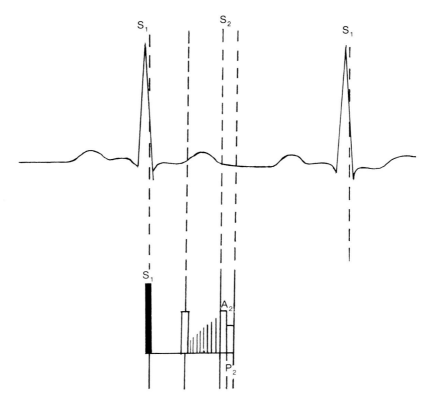

FIGURE 5.20   **Mid systolic ejection murmur timing in cardiac cycle coordinated with electrocardiogram.** Adapted from: **Classification of murmurs according to timing in the cardiac cycle.** *Clin Highlights,* December 1984, p 29.

A systolic murmur heard along the left parasternal area can arise from the aortic valve, the pulmonic valve, the mitral valve, or the tricuspid valve. This is an area of auscultation that can confuse the student. It is best, once hearing the systolic murmur along the left parasternal area, to trace it by inching your stethoscope and listening to whether it is heard maximally in the aortic area or in the pulmonic area, or radiates predominantly down to the apex, or originates from the lower portion of the sternum, which could mean a tricuspid or a mitral valve origin. Does the pitch and quality remain the same? In older persons the murmur of aortic stenosis is sometimes best heard at the apex, but originating at the aortic orifice.

Systolic Murmurs Originating From the Mitral Area. Once a murmur is heard in the mitral area or in the apex, then you will notice whether it takes up all of systole (it is holosystolic), which could be caused by mitral regurgitation and inter-ventricular septal defect with left–to–right shunt (tricuspid regurgitation). Once a murmur is heard at the apex in the mitral area, inch your stethoscope along and see if it spreads to the axillary line and beyond, which is a characteristic of a mitral regurgitation.

Diagnostic Interpretation of Systolic Murmurs. A characteristic holosystolic murmur, or pansystolic murmur, in the mitral area radiating to the apex generally,

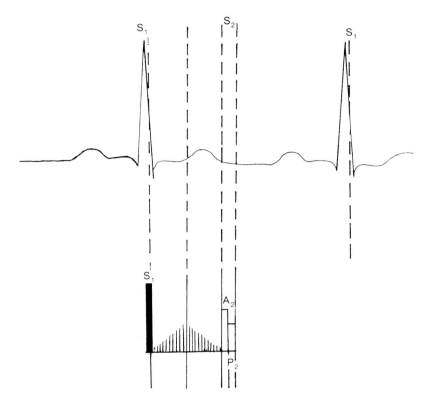

FIGURE 5.21   Late systolic murmur timing with cardiac cycle. Adapted from: Classification of murmurs according to timing in the cardiac cycle. *Clin High-lights,* December 1984, p 29.

usually means that there is a regurgitant flow through the mitral valve, or mitral regurgitation. The holosystolic murmur may be coarse and loud, which could arise from a rupture of a papillary muscle or even a ventricular septal defect.

The midsystolic murmur in the mitral area, which can fall in the category of medium pitch, increases in intensity before arriving at the second heart sound. Classically, the midsystolic murmur, when associated with a click, means prolapse of the mitral valve. A late systolic murmur heard in the mitral area with a systolic click is again characteristic of prolapse of the mitral valve.

The holosystolic murmur heard at the mitral valve, which represents backflow of blood from the ventricle to the atrium through an incompetent mitral or tri-cuspid valve, results from escape of blood from a chamber of high pressure into a lower pressure. When you hear a systolic murmur at the apical sternal area, automatically ask the patient to take a deep breath. If the murmur increases with inspiration, it means that it arises from the tricuspid valve or tricuspid insuffi-ciency; the murmur of mitral regurgitation does not change.

A rare valvular condition that causes a systolic murmur at the apex that re-sults from left ventricular outflow obstruction is entitled idiopathic hypertrophic subaortic stenosis (IHSS). It may be a holosystolic or a midsystolic murmur. Squatting will characteristically decrease the systolic murmur of aortic stenosis. Standing again increases the murmur of IHSS.

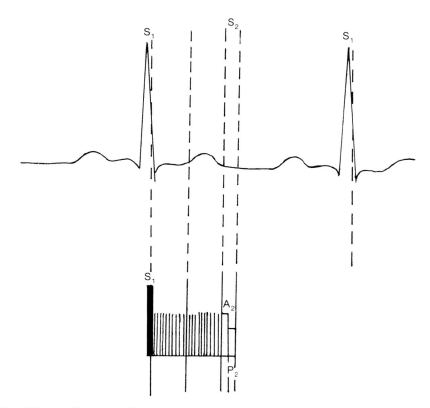

FIGURE 5.22   Pansystolic regurgitant murmur timing with cycle. Adapted from: Classification of murmurs according to timing in the cardiac cycle. *Clin Highlights,* **December 1984, p 29.**

Systolic Ejection Murmurs. Systolic ejection murmurs are the most difficult to sort out from the point of view of their origin. They may result merely from an increase of flow across a normal heart valve, or may indicate that a valve is stenotic or deformed with various hemodynamic consequences. The murmur can also result from a dilatation of the vessel beyond the valve. Systolic ejection murmurs begin at the first heart sound, generally reaching their peak in intensity during early mid or late systole, and then diminish. These murmurs can be soft, medium-pitched, or coarse.

As a general rule, a systolic ejection murmur heard at the base of the heart is heard best in the aortic area and can represent aortic stenosis, valvular and sub-valvular dilatation of the ascending aorta, increased stroke volume, or a hyperkinetic state. YOU CANNOT DIAGNOSE AORTIC STENOSIS SIMPLY BY A SYSTOLIC EJECTION MURMUR HEARD IN THE AORTIC AREA. Many other characteristics of aortic stenosis must be placed together with the systolic murmur.

Pulmonic systolic ejection murmurs may represent pulmonic valvular stenosis or substenosis, dilatation of the pulmonary artery, or increased pulmonary flow, as in atrial septal defect, and are best heard in the second and third intercostal spaces. Systolic ejection murmurs sometimes are heard in the apical area or in the apical sternal area, often as a result of radiation from the aortic or pulmonic valve.

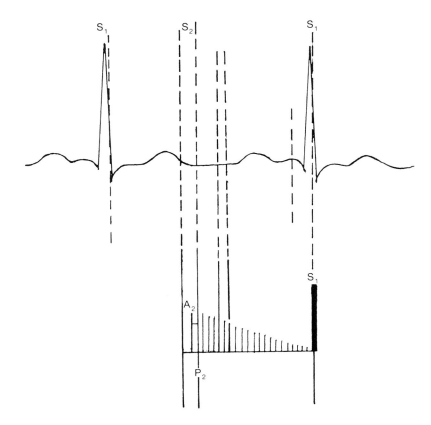

FIGURE 5.23   Early diastolic murmur timing with electrocardiogram. Adapted from: Classification of murmurs according to timing in the cardiac cycle. *Clin Highlights,* December 1984, p 29.

An apical systolic ejection murmur of medium pitch that is not holosystolic needs to be differentiated from one of aortic origin, IHSS, and mitral regurgitation. A careful inching of the stethoscope or listening for the same characteristic murmur in the aortic area will help you to decide if it arises from the aortic valve.

Diastolic Murmurs

Diastolic murmurs are heard after the second heart sound and may be of short or long duration. They are categorized as early diastolic (Figure 5.23), mid-diastolic (Figure 5.24), late diastolic (or presystolic) (Figure 5.25), and holodiastolic, occurring throughout the diastolic period. Diastolic murmurs can perhaps be best described as the sound made by blowing across the top of a bottle. Diastolic murmurs are always pathologic and reflect flow across diseased atrioventricular or semilunar valves during ventricular diastole. They can result from a high flow across a normal valve, as heard in the mitral flow rumble of a ventricular septal defect or the tricuspid flow rumble of an atrial septal defect.

Because they are the murmurs most commonly missed in everyday cardiac auscultation, diastolic murmurs need to be carefully sought. The diaphragm of the stethoscope should be used with firm pressure on the chest, enough so that a slight

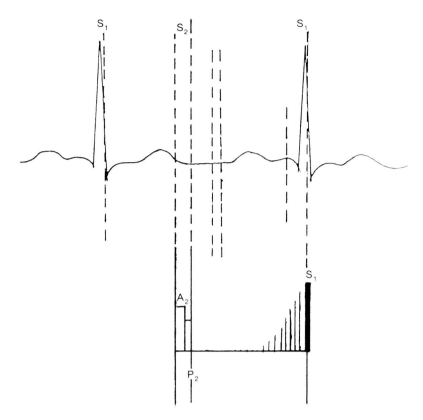

FIGURE 5.24   Mid-diastolic murmur. Adapted from: Classification of murmurs according to timing in the cardiac cycle. *Clin Highlights,* **December 1984, p 29.**

mark is left. The patient should be asked to take a deep breath, exhale, and hold his/her breath while you firmly auscultate along the aortic area, the pulmonic area, and especially at Erb's point, the area of aortic regurgitation located in the second and third left intercostal spaces along the left sternal border. The diastolic murmur is then also sought in the lower portion of the sternum and in the apical sternal and mitral area.

If, during the course of auscultation, the patient has not been leaning forward with breath held in full expiration and the stethoscope held firmly below the pulmonic area at Erb's point, diastolic murmurs of aortic regurgitation will be frequently missed. In addition, a diastolic murmur of mitral stenosis will be missed unless the patient is turned on the left side or even slightly elevated on the left elbow, and the bell of the stethoscope placed at the PMI.

Diastolic Murmurs of Aortic Insufficiency (Regurgitation). The diastolic murmur of aortic insufficiency is of high frequency and low amplitude, originating from the aortic valve and radiating down the left sternal border. It is sometimes best heard in the second and third left intercostal spaces, or Erb's point. Dr. James Hope first described it in 1821.

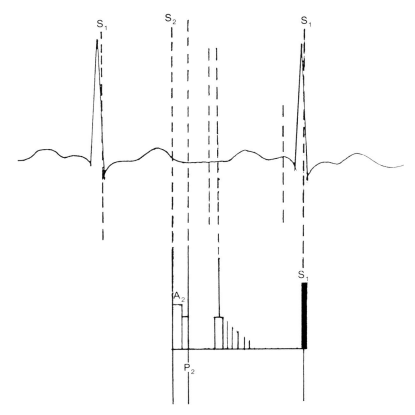

FIGURE 5.25   Late diastolic or presystolic murmur timing with electrocardio-gram. Adapted from: Classification of murmurs according to timing in the cardiac cycle. *Clin Highlights,* December 1984, p 29.

This blowing murmur begins brusquely after the aortic valve closure or the second heart sound, is loudest at its onset, then becomes a decrescendo and may disappear early in diastole. Sometimes the diastolic murmur may be of musical quality. A briefer diastolic murmur does not necessarily impart the diagnosis of mild aortic insufficiency, because acute aortic insufficiency can present with a short, trivial diastolic murmur. Conversely, when aortic regurgitation is severe the murmur may be harsh and short.

The murmur resulting from aortic regurgitation is best heard in the third left intercostal space next to the sternum. If the murmur is loudest in the right intercostal space, it usually results from an aorta that is dilated, or from unusual causes of aortic regurgitation, such as dissection of the aorta, an aortitis from lues or rheumatoid arteritis, or rupture of an aneurysm at the sinus of Valsalva.

The Diastolic Murmur of Pulmonic Regurgitation. Alas, the diastolic murmur of pulmonic regurgitation has a pitch, timing, and quality similar to that of aortic regurgitation, but it is more localized in the pulmonic area. When pulmonic regurgitation is present with severe pulmonary hypertension, the diastolic murmur is called the Graham Steell murmur. It will help to differentiate the diastolic murmur of pulmonic regurgitation by means of the second heart sound if there is pulmonary hypertension (which is usually always present). The second heart sound is then accentuated and there may be a pulmonary ejection sound.

To diagnose a diastolic murmur of pulmonary insufficiency, look for: 1) an accentuated pulmonic component of the second heart sound; 2) a pulmonic ejection sound; 3) a giant A wave in the jugular venous pulse; and 4) parasternal systolic lift secondary to right ventricular hypertrophy.

Diastolic Murmurs of Mitral Stenosis. The diastolic murmur of mitral stenosis (Figure 5.26) produces a low-pitched apical rumble best heard with the bell of the stethoscope while the patient is turned on the left side. The bell of the stethoscope should be applied lightly on the skin. If too much pressure is used the diastolic murmur may disappear. It should be sought over the apical impulse. It occurs during mid-diastole, with an accentuation before the onset of the first heart sound (presystolic). The murmur may also have an early diastolic component occurring

FIGURE 5.26   Mid–diastolic murmur of mitral stenosis. Adapted from: Classification of murmurs according to timing in the cardiac cycle. *Clin Highlights,* December 1984, p 29.

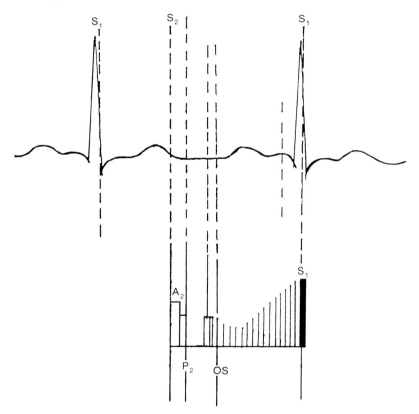

soon after the second heart sound that results from a rapid passive filling. The pre-systolic phase results from a retroflow during atrial systole. This presystolic murmur or rumble disappears once atrial fibrillation occurs. The diastolic murmur of mitral stenosis is loudest in early and late diastole. If an accentuated first heart sound is heard in the mitral area, pay particular attention to find the diastolic murmur of mitral stenosis. In addition, you should hear an opening snap (see above).

The classic sequence of events is as follows: There is a loud accentuated first heart sound followed by a second heart sound, an opening snap, and then the mid-diastolic murmur with a presystolic accentuation occurring after the opening snap and followed by the accentuated first heart sound. The diastolic murmur of mitral stenosis is usually confined within a small area above the apex. If the right ventricle begins to enlarge, the left ventricle and atrium may be pushed laterally, and the PMI will now appear in the midaxillary line, and the diastolic murmur should be sought in that region. This mid-diastolic rumble is low pitched.

As mitral stenosis becomes more severe, the chordae tendineae are more fibrosed and the cusps become more immobile, and the first heart sound as well as the opening snap are diminished in loudness.

The diastolic murmur of tricuspid stenosis has the same timing, the same pitch, and the same quality, except perhaps the murmur may be higher pitched early in diastole, resembling the murmur of aortic regurgitation. Pressing the bell of the stethoscope lightly against the chest, the murmur of tricuspid stenosis can usually be heard along with mitral stenosis. It is located, however, just left of the lower end of the sternum; it does not extend out toward the apical sternal area. Inspiration will increase the diastolic murmur of tricuspid stenosis, whereas the murmur of mitral stenosis will remain unchanged.

The presence of tricuspid regurgitation will also increase the loudness of the murmur of mild tricuspid stenosis. Tricuspid regurgitation and stenosis are almost always associated. Look for the large A wave that increases on inspiration to tell you that the murmur comes from the tricuspid valve.

Diastolic murmurs heard at the apex that do not originate from mitral stenosis include myxoma of the left atrium and the Austin Flint murmur of aortic regurgitation, causing a diastolic rumbling murmur, resulting from premature closure of the mitral valve, fluttering of the mitral valve, and regurgitant stream. Diastolic rumbling apical murmurs may also be heard in cardiomyopathy, dilated ventricles, IHSS, tricuspid stenosis, and left-to-right shunts.

Innocent Murmurs (Functional Murmurs)
A good rule to remember is that diastolic murmurs are never innocent. Most innocent murmurs are systolic ejection murmurs heard in the pulmonic area. They are commonly heard in children, young adults, and women. They are grade 1, and are sometimes heard in the left sternal border and the apical sternal area. They have a vibratory quality. They may vary with position, disappearing when the patient is sitting up and reappearing when he is lying down.

In spite of the characteristics that I have described for the innocent murmur, it may at times be deceiving, and it can be difficult to be certain that it does not arise from a diseased valve. The clinician should make a further attempt to characterize if the murmur is innocent or not by using three simple maneuvers.

MANEUVERS

Squatting. With the stethoscope on the chest placed at the PMI of the murmur, the patient is asked to suddenly squat. Hemodynamically, this will result in increased venous return and afterload. If the murmur decreases in intensity, it may be caused by IHSS. The murmur of aortic stenosis does not change in these circumstances.

Isometric Exercise. A simple hand grip exercise, which may consist of the patient squeezing a partially inflated blood pressure cuff, should result in an increase in the pulse rate, blood pressure, and cardiac output. The murmurs of mitral regurgitation, mitral stenosis, and aortic regurgitation will increase in intensity, whereas the murmur of IHSS will decrease, as will any murmurs originating from left ventricular outflow obstruction.

Amyl Nitrate. Amyl nitrate, one of the oldest drugs used in cardiology, is a volatile preparation of nitroglycerine. Amyl nitrate, when administered, can cause a precipitous drop in the blood pressure and even bring the patient into shock. Adequate resuscitation equipment should be available when amyl nitrate is given, and the physician should have a setting where the patient can be placed into a Trendelenburg position and even an intravenous fluid given. There are some patients who are highly susceptible to amyl nitrate. Prior to giving amyl nitrate the patient should be forewarned that there will be an initial rush of extreme lightheadedness with a flushing burning sensation in the face and a marked increase in the heart rate, cardiac output, and stroke volume. The patient should be told that the flush will have its onset in 5 to 10 seconds and have a duration sometimes of an entire minute.

The hemodynamic result of this sudden inhalation of amyl nitrate is that the lower systemic resistance produces either no change or a decrease in intensity of murmurs resulting from mitral regurgitation, aortic regurgitation, and ventricular septal defect. Because there is an increased cardiac output and inflow, the intensity of murmurs resulting from aortic stenosis, pulmonic stenosis, and mitral stenosis may increase, while the murmur of IHS becomes softer.

Summary of Findings of Innocent Systolic Murmurs

1. They are vibratory systolic ejection murmurs
2. They are usually crescendo/descrescendo in form
3. They are medium pitch, rough, and usually not harsh
4. These murmurs do not radiate maximally at the apex.

Innocent murmurs are usually heard with the patient lying down and disappear upon his/her sitting up. Holding the breath in expiration will increase the murmur.

Warning: Sometimes an innocent systolic murmur in the second left intercostal space can be coarse and may sound like the murmur of an atrial septal defect or pulmonic stenosis, especially in children. The second heart sound in an innocent murmur will be normally split on inspiration and disappear on expiration.

Continuous Murmurs

Do not confuse a continuous murmur with a pansystolic murmur. A continuous murmur extends from systole to diastole. Do not confuse it with a holosystolic murmur together with the presence of a diastolic murmur. The tip-off is that the continuous murmur has the same quality between the first and the second heart sound and well into diastole.

Continuous murmurs are found in patent ductus arteriosus, usually peak at the second heart sound, and are best heard beneath the left clavicle. As pulmonary hypertension develops, it becomes modified.

A continuous murmur may also indicate the presence of a coronary arteriovenous fistula, a ruptured sinus Valsalva, aneurysm of the right atrium, pulmonary systemic arteriovenous fistula, or a collateral circulation resulting from coarctation of the aorta.

An obstruction of the arterial stenosis can cause a continuous murmur sometimes heard in the carotid artery. These murmurs may be heard throughout the chest.

A Venous Hum

A venous hum is an innocent continual sound heard along the neck. It peaks in diastole. Sometimes this murmur is so loud that it can be confused with a pathologic murmur. These can be differentiated easily because compressing the internal jugular vein will make a venous hum disappear.

Famous Murmurs

The **Austin Flint murmur** is a mid-diastolic and presystolic murmur heard at the apex in patients with aortic regurgitation who do not have mitral stenosis. Since Austin Flint described it in 1862, the cause has remained unclear. Some clinicians believe that it is due to the fluttering of the anterior leaflet of the mitral valve from the regurgitant flow.

The **Graham Steell murmur** is a high-pitched early diastolic murmur of pulmonary regurgitation. It is heard in mitral stenosis associated with pulmonary hypertension.

Summary of Auscultatory Findings in Congenital Heart Disease

Patent Ductus Arteriosus

A continuous murmur of systolic accentuation begins with the first heart sound, increases in intensity to the second, and then decreases in intensity during diastole. The PMI is in the second left intercostal space, and the murmur is of similar quality in systole and diastole. As pulmonary hypertension develops, which decreases the flow through the ductus during diastole, the diastolic component disappears and only the systolic component is heard. As pulmonary hypertension increases, the murmur may disappear and the murmur of pulmonary regurgitation may appear.

Ventricular Septal Defect

The murmur is holosystolic, and is of maximum intensity in the third or fourth intercostal space, left of the sternum. With a marked shunt, a rumbling apical diastolic murmur may be heard. Ventricular septal defect occurring in an adult can result in rupture of the interventricular septum following acute myocardial infarction, but this is a rare condition occurring in 1% to 3% of patients. It is heralded by the sudden development of a harsh holosystolic murmur, grade 3 or greater, loudest in the third and fifth intercostal spaces along the left sternal border, accompanied by a thrill. The left ventricle apical impulse is hyperactive and hyperdynamic. As heart failure progresses, the murmur decreases.

Papillary muscle rupture is rare but occurs as a complication in acute myocardial infarction. Auscultatory findings consist of a loud, high-pitched holosystolic murmur with a musical or harsh quality arising from the apex and radiating to the axilla. It may be so loud that it is transmitted towards the sternum.

Atrial Septal Defect

There is fixed splitting of the second heart sound. The murmur is a medium-pitched systolic murmur, rarely harsh, and may be short.

Pulmonic Stenosis

The murmur is a systolic diamond-shaped murmur with a PMI at the second left intercostal space lateral to the sternum. It is usually accompanied by a thrill. There is delay in right ventricular ejection, and the pulmonic component of the second heart sound is widely split. There may be a systolic ejection click.

Pulmonary Regurgitation

Pulmonary regurgitation is usually seen in the presence of pulmonary hypertension, causing a relative pulmonary insufficiency, which results in the Graham Steell murmur. It has a high-pitched frequency similar to that of aortic regurgitation.

Tricuspid Regurgitation

The murmur is similar to the murmur of pulmonary regurgitation and it may be difficult to distinguish between the two. This murmur increases in intensity on inspiration. It is usually caused by dilatation of the right ventricle and the tricuspid valve ring.

Tricuspid Stenosis

Tricuspid stenosis is part of rheumatic heart disease along with mitral valve disease. It has findings similar to those of mitral stenosis, but the murmur is increased with inspiration.

Auscultation of the Normal Prosthetic Valve

It is important that the physician become familiar with the normal auscultatory phenomena associated with prosthetic valves. Valve failure can be recognized with the stethoscope, but normal prosthetic valve sounds must be learned.

There are four major types of prosthetic valves. The **ball valves** (eg, the Starr-Edwards) have distinct audible opening and closing sounds, which coincide with the excursion of the ball. These are high pitched and easily distinguished from the normal cardiac sounds. In the mitral position, there is a very prominent opening click which follows a second aortic sound by 0.07 seconds. There is a similar relationship between the second aortic sound and the opening snap of mitral stenosis. It is best heard at the apex. It is a louder sound than the closing sound and obscures the first heart sound. It is common to hear a midsystolic murmur in the left sternal border, and is not considered abnormal to suggest dysfunction of the prosthetic valve. In the aortic position, the aortic valve produces a loud opening click. This sound is best heard at the apex or lower left sternal border. The second heart sound or closure sound is much less prominent and generally precedes the pulmonic component of the second heart sound. These valves will also have systolic ejection murmurs.

Tilting **disc valves** (eg, the Bjork-Shiley) do not produce an opening sound. Distinctive closing sounds are heard. When the disc valve is in the mitral position, systolic ejection murmur may be heard as well as a diastolic murmur. In addition, there is a closing sound that is clearly audible. If it is diminished in intensity, it could signal valve failure secondary to fibrosis or thrombosis. In the aortic position, the opening is rarely heard with the stethoscope but there is a distinct closing sound with a mid-systolic ejection murmur.

Porcine valves have opening sounds that are crisp and high-pitched, but much less evident than in **mechanical valves.**

The **bi-valve** prosthesis, or St. Jude valves, produce distinctive opening sounds with a high-pitched metallic closing sound. No diastolic murmurs are heard.

Auscultation of Arrhythmias

I am including a special section on auscultation of arrhythmias because they can be very useful in diagnosing cardiac arrhythmias. It goes without saying that the gold standard for the diagnosis of an arrhythmia is an electrocardiogram, and it also sometimes may be necessary to do electrophysiological testings. However, there can be some clues as to the type of arrhythmia present to the auscultator.

Rhythm is considered as being regular or irregular. The average heart rate of a person is generally between 50 and 100 beats per minute; below 50 beats, we speak of sinus bradycardia, and above 100 beats is sinus tachycardia. If the rhythm is normal and the heart rate is greater than 100, it could represent sinus tachycardia, supraventricular tachycardia, atrial flutter, or ventricular tachycardia (slow ventricular tachycardia can also occur). A regular rhythm with a pulse between 60 and 100 could be a normal sinus rhythm or flutter with a regular ventricular response. A regular rhythm with a pulse less than 60 could be a second-degree heart block, or a complete heart block. If the rhythm is irregular, interspersed with regular beats, this could represent premature atrial or ventricular contractions.

Irregular beats can be a sinus arrhythmia alternating with normal rhythm. Total irregularity of the heart is seen in atrial fibrillation or atrial flutter with varying block. Sometimes it is quite difficult to differentiate atrial fibrillation from multiple premature beats. I find that six beats in a row consecutively is generally a sinus rhythm.

It should be emphasized that the heart rate will not differentiate between supraventricular tachycardia, as a rule, and ventricular tachycardia or flutter with varying ventricular response. In supraventricular tachycardia, the auscultation will reveal a rapid rate, between 160 and 200, and the heart sounds are normally split. Ventricular tachycardia generally has abnormally split sounds.

In summary, if the heart sounds are single or normally split, the rhythm generally is supraventricular tachycardia; if there is wide splitting of the second heart sound with varying intensity of the first sound and an irregular occurring A wave, the tachycardia is most often ventricular in origin. Sometimes it may even be extraordinarily difficult to differentiate between supraventricular tachycardia and ventricular tachycardia, especially supraventricular tachycardia with aberrant conduction, on the electrocardiogram.

The rules that I have given here need to be interpreted cautiously, but are helpful.

SUMMARY OF CARDIAC PHYSICAL EXAMINATION

Aortic Stenosis

Pathophysiology
Progressive aortic orifice narrowing leads to chronic increase in afterload and increase in chronic wall stress, followed by ventricular hypertrophy and a stiff compliant left ventricle with dilatation, deterioration of the ejection fraction, and, finally, overt left ventricular failure.

When the ventricle becomes noncompliant, left ventricular failure may occur. This occurs with pulmonary edema, syncope, and anginal coronary insufficiency.

Pulse
Palpation of the carotid pulse will show a small volume, delayed upstroke (pulsus parvus and tardus); the radial pulse is of small volume. The jugular pulse is unremarkable.

On palpation, there may be a thrill in the aortic area.

On palpation of the precordial motion, sustained apical systolic heave due to increased interventricular pressure and hypertrophy of the left ventricle may be noted.

Heart Sounds

S1: normal or decreased

A2 (aortic component of S2): may be accentuated, absent, or single

Paradoxical splitting of S2: splitting heard during expiration diminishes during inspiration.

S4: especially in young adults, if there is a large ventricular aortic gradient.

S3: with left ventricular failure

Murmurs

Timing: midsystolic ejection murmur.

Location: if loud enough, all throughout the chest, but maximal in the aortic area; frequently radiates to the neck and to the apex.

Loudness: grades 2 to 6.

Pitch: higher frequency at the apex.

Duration: The peak occurs late in systole if obstruction is mildly severe; sometimes the murmur may be holosystolic in severe stenosis. In severe aortic stenosis the murmur is harsh, and reaches its intensity late in systole.

CAUTION: A coarse loud murmur in the aortic area can occur in individuals who have markedly calcified cusps, causing a turbulent flow, and may not indicate severe aortic obstruction.

A soft murmur in the aortic area can be present even if there is severe aortic stenosis, if the patient is obese. As the narrowing becomes more severe, special maneuvers (amyl nitrate) will cause the murmur to increase after the first 20 seconds. In mitral regurgitation, the murmur decreases with amyl nitrate.

CAUTION: The carotid pulse can have a delayed and decreased upstroke in a patient who has carotid artery stenosis, as seen in elderly patients.

Aortic Regurgitation

Pathophysiology

A rheumatic deformity of the aortic valve causes incompetence and a diastolic regurgitant flow. The left ventricular filling pressure rises. A large forward stroke volume causes forceful and prominent carotid pulses and pounding of the heart, followed eventually by myocardial hypertrophy and decompensation.

Pulses

Carotid pulses exhibit an abrupt rise and collapse due to increased pulse pressure and increased volume; there is associated head nodding (Musset's sign), pounding pulses, peripheral artery pistol shot pulses, and nailbed pulses (Quincke's pulse). Jugular pulses are normal, except when ventricles fail, causing elevation of the A and V waves.

Blood Pressure
The aortic diastolic pressure decreases and the systolic pressure increases.

Heart Sounds

S1: may be soft

2: (the other component of S2): may be accentuated or tambourlike

S3 or S4: may be heard

Murmurs
The murmur is high pitched, and is best heard with firm pressure on the stethoscope, using the diaphragm, with the patient leaning forward, breath held in expiration. The larger the leak, the louder the murmur. It usually extends throughout all of diastole, is loudest in the aortic area, and can be transmitted along the left sternal border to the apex. A diastolic rumble at the apex, called the Austin Flint murmur, may occur in severe aortic regurgitation. An additional finding is that the left ventricle is hyperkinetic and enlarged and displaced to the left and downward. The French called it coeur en sabot.

An early decrescendo diastolic murmur can be heard immediately following the aortic closure.

An ejection systolic murmur is common in pure aortic regurgitation with roughening of the leaflets, dilatation of the ascending aorta, and increased stroke volume.

An ejection click is often heard.

Hypertrophic Cardiomyopathy

Pathophysiology
There is a decrease in left ventricular compliance secondary to left ventricular hypertrophy and intraventricular septal hypertrophy. There is difficulty in ventricular filling and small diastolic volume. The thickened left ventricle has a small cavity and is hypercontractile, with a high ejection fraction. Systolic anterior movement of the mitral valve occurs, and it is set opposition to the hypertrophied intraventricular septum.

Pulses
The carotid pulse is a rapid initial upstroke, then a percussion wave followed by small tidal wave.

Heart Sounds

S1: normal

S2: normally split; it may vary

S3: may be present

S4: present

Murmur
A harsh, crescendo/descrescendo murmur begins well after the first heart sound, is heard between the apex and the left sternal border, and radiates to the left sternal border, the axilla, and the base of the heart but not to the neck vessels. The murmur may be holosystolic and blowing at the apex. The murmur is due to turbulence through the narrowed left ventricular outflow tract and to mitral regurgitation. A diastolic rumble may be heard.

The murmur disappears on squatting and increases with Valsalva maneuver.

Mitral Stenosis

Pathophysiology
Progressive fibrosis, scarring, calcification of the mitral valve, fusion of the commissures, and chordae tendineae are present. Narrowing of the valve to 1.5 to 2 cm results in persistent gradient across the valve and a holodiastolic murmur. Left atrial pressure becomes elevated at rest and further with exercise. Transmission of increased atrial pressure into pulmonary capillary circulation results in dyspnea and orthopnea. Further stenosis of the valve to less than 1 cm results in moderately severe pulmonary hypertension and the cardiac output decreases.

Pulse
Carotid pulses are normal. Jugular venous pulse is normal, unless the right ventricle fails, with tricuspid insufficiency producing larger V waves. The A wave of atrial contraction is absent. Atrial fibrillation may be present. The precordial motion is a small and tapping apical pulse.

Heart Sounds
A parasternal lift is felt when pulmonary hypertension is present. You may feel a loud S1 opening snap and a part of the component of S2. S1 is increased due to forcible closure of the thickened mitral valve and delayed closure. The pulmonic component of S2 is loud when pulmonic hypertension exists. There is an opening snap heard in early diastole, and a narrowed 8-second heart sound–opening snap interval signifies high left atrial pressure and results in early opening of the mitral valve. The auscultation is as follows: loud accentuated heart sound followed by an S2, an opening snap, and then a mid-diastolic murmur with a presystolic accentuation occurring after the opening snap, following up an accentuated S1. As mitral stenosis becomes more severe, the chordae become more fibrosed, the cusps more immobile, and the first heart sound diminished.

Murmurs
The diastolic murmur is usually confined within a small area above the apex.

Mitral Regurgitation

Pathophysiology
A large portion of the left ventricle stroke volume is injected into the low-pressure left atrium, and chronic volume overload results. There is left ventricular enlargement, hypertrophy, and elevation of left atrial and pulmonary artery pressures. Right ventricular failure may follow. Poor left ventricular function will cause a fall in forward stroke volume.

Pulses
Carotid pulse is normal. If the mitral leak is severe, it may resemble the quick rising pulse of aortic regurgitation. If ventricular failure follows, the venous pressure is elevated and prominent V waves will be noted.

With regard to precordial motion, there may be a hyperdynamic apex, a sustained beat from left ventricular enlargement, and modest lateral displacement. Parasternal heave may suggest pulmonary hypertension and right ventricular hypertrophy if the left atrium enlarges. Although the right ventricle may be normal, it is pushed forward.

Heart Sounds

S1 is normal to soft. S2 may be loud in the pulmonic area due to pulmonary hypertension, and S3 may be present along with an early diastolic rumble, especially when the regurgitation is severe. There is no S4 because of a large left atrium that cannot contract.

Murmurs

The murmur is classic pansystolic; it begins with S1 and goes to S2. It is best heard at the apex with transmission to the axilla down to the left sternal border, and has medium pitch and a harsh buzzing sound. A thrill may be present.

Acute Mitral Regurgitation

The sudden disruption of the mitral valve apparatus can cause a distinct clinical picture of sudden dyspnea and a loud murmur.

The five integral components of the apparatus are:

1. valve leaflets
2. the chordae tendineae
3. the annulus fibrosus
4. the papillary muscle
5. adjacent ventricular wall

For example, the rupture of the chordae tendineae in patients with long-standing prolapse of the mitral valve can cause a coarse, loud, grade IV/VI pansystolic murmur, with a thrill, soft first heart sound, and a hyperdynamic left ventricular apex.

LYMPHATIC SYSTEM

A detailed examination of the lymphatic system will be made in Chapter 11. During the general physical examination, look for lymph node enlargements in the following areas: 1) the regions of the neck, the anterior and posterior cervical chain, and the occipital area of the skull; 2) the right and left axillary regions; 3) both the right and left olecranon area at the elbow; and 4) the right and left inguinal area. The size and character of the lymph nodes needs to be ascertained. Are they soft, tender, hard; are they freely moveable? Is the patient aware of their presence?

Check the **cervical nodes.** Gently run your hand along the front and side of the neck, beginning at the upper margin of the sternocleidomastoid muscle for the anterior chain, proceeding downward to the sternoclavicular joint. Lymph node enlargements may have been present for years and the physician should be certain not to unnecessarily cause alarm until a thorough investigation is performed. Small nodes may be missed if too vigorous pressure is used by the examining hand.

The **posterior chain of nodes** is traced from its beginning behind the ear to the anterior border of the trapezius muscle. Gently place your fingers in the retroclavicular area, because metastatic nodes are often found here, in particular, Virchow's node, which represents metastatic disease from malignancy of the abdomen.

The **axillary nodes** are searched for by having the patient raise his/her arm above the head, then placing the fingers of one hand into the axilla while taking the patient's hand with your other hand and bringing the arm gently down. It is essential that you go deep into the axilla lest you miss a small node.

Inguinal nodes are best found with the patient lying flat. These nodes, which drain the rectal and urogenital areas, are easily palpable and are often present.

Keep in mind that lymph node enlargement may represent infections, lymphomas, and metastatic disease, and today the public is well aware of lymph node enlargements being an early sign of the acquired immune deficiency syndrome and its variants.

A good rule to follow is, if you find one node proceed to search for others. You are obligated to answer the question, what is the cause of the enlargement?

REFERENCES

1. Basta L, Bettinger JJL: The cardiac impulse: A new look at an old art. *Am Heart J* 1979;97:96-111.

2. Basta LL, Wolfson P, Eckberg D, Abboud FM: The value of left parasternal impulse recordings in the assessment of mitral regurgitation. *Circulation* 1973;48:1055-1065.

3. Conn RD, Cole JS: The cardiac apex impulse: Clinical and angiographic correlations. *Ann Intern Med* 1971;75:185-191.

4. Constant J: Inspection and palpation of the chest, in *Bedside Cardiology,* ed 2. Boston, Little, Brown, and Co., 1976, pp 100-103.

5. Craig E: Clinical value of apex cardiography. *Am J Cardiol* 1971;28:116-121.

6. Deliyannis AA, Gillam PMS, Mounsey JPD, Steiner RE: The cardiac impulse and the motion of the heart. *Br Heart J* 1964;26:393-411.

7. Eddleman EE: Examination of precordial movements, in Hurst JW, Logue RB, Schlant RC, Wenger NK (eds): *The Heart,* ed 4. New York, McGraw-Hill Book Co., 1978, pp 201-217.

8. Eddleman EE: Kinetocardiographic changes in ischemic heart disease. *Circulation* 1965;31:650-655.

9. Gibson C, Madry R, Grossman N, McLaurin LP, Craige E: The A wave of the apex cardiogram and left ventricular diastolic stiffness. *Circulation* 1974;49:441-446.

10. Hurst JW, Schlant RC: Inspection and palpation of the anterior chest, in *Examination of the Heart, Part 3.* Dallas, American Heart Association, 1972, pp 1-28.

11. Mills RM, Kastor JA: Quantitative grading of cardiac palpation. *Arch Intern Med* 1973;132:831-834.

12. Mounsey JPD: Inspection and palpation of the cardiac impulse. *Prog Cardiovasc Dis* 1967;10:187-206.

13. Stapleton JF, Groves BM: Precordial palpation. *Am Heart J* 1971;89:409-427.

14. Sutton GC, Prewitt TA, Craige E: Relationship between quantitated precordial movement and left ventricular function. *Circulation* 1971;41:179-190.

15. Voigt GC, Freisinger GC: The use of apex cardiography in the assessment of left ventricular diastolic pressure. *Circulation* 1970;41:1015-1024.

16. Crawford J, O'Rourke R: A systematic approach to bedside differentiation of cardiac murmurs and abnormal sounds. *Curr Probl Cardiol* 1977;1:1-24.

17. Davies H, Nelson WP: *Understanding Cardiology.* Woburn, MA, Butterworth, 1978.

18. de Leon AC Jr: *Heart Sounds: What They Teach Us.* Los Angeles, Humetics, 1975.

19. de Leon AC Jr, Harvey WP: Clinical approach to the patient with suspected heart disease, in Spitell JA (ed): *Clinical Medicine.* New York, Harper & Row. 1983, vol 6, chap 3.

20. Fowler N, Marshall W: Cardiac diagnosis from examination of arteries and veins. *Circulation* 1964;30:272.

21. Tavel ME: *Clinical Phonocardiography and External Pulse Recordings,* ed 3. Chicago, Year Book Medical Publishers, 1978.

22. Harvey WP: Technique and art of auscultation, in Segal BL (ed): *Theory and Practice of Auscultation.* Philadelphia, FA Davis Co, 1963.

23. Leatham A: Auscultation of the heart. *Lancet* 1958;2:793.

24. Leonard JK, Kroetz FW (revised by Leon DF, Shaver JA): *Auscultation, Part 4: Examination of the Heart.* Dallas, American Heart Association, 1974.

25. Levine SA, Harvey WP: *Clinical Auscultation of the Heart,* ed 2. Philadelphia, WB Saunders Co, 1959.

26. Perloff JK: *Physical Examination of the Heart and Circulation.* Philadelphia, WB Saunders Co, 1982.

27. Stapleton JF, Harvey WP: Systolic sounds. *Am Heart J* 1976;91:383.

28. Craige E: On the genesis of heart sounds: Contributions made by echocardiographic studies. *Circulation* 1976;53:207.

29. Barlow JR, Bosman CK, Pocock WA, et al: Late systolic murmurs and non-ejection ("mid-late") systolic clicks. *Br Heart J* 1968;30:203.

30. Leatham A, Leech GJ: The first and second heart sounds, in Hurst JW (ed): *The Heart,* ed 5. New York, McGraw-Hill, 1982.

31. Ronan JA Jr, Perloff JK, Harvey WP: Systolic clicks and the late systolic murmur: Intracardiac phonocardiographic evidence of their mitral valve origin. *Am Heart J* 1965;70:319.

32. Leon DF, Shaver JA (eds): *Physiologic Principles of Heart Sounds and Murmurs.* AHA Monograph, No. 46, 1975.

33. O'Rourke RA, Crawford MH: The systolic click-murmur syndrome: Clinical recognition and management. *Curr Probl Cardiol* 1976;1.

34. Ronan JA Jr: Cardiac sound and ultrasound: Echocardiographic and phonocardiographic correlations. *Curr Probl Cardiol* 1981;6.

35. Harvey WP: Mitral valve prolapse, in *Conferences on Clinical Auscultation of the Heart.* Nutley, NJ, Hoffmann-LaRoche Inc, 1983.

36. Stapleton JF, Harvey WP: Heart sounds, murmurs and precordial movements, in Sodeman WA, Sodeman TM (eds): *Pathologic Physiology: Mechanism of Disease,* ed 6. Philadelphia, WB Saunders Co, 1979, chap 11.

37.   Fontana ME, Wooley CF, Leighton RF, et al: Postural changes in left ventricular and mitral valvular dynamics in the systolic click–late systolic murmur syndrome. *Circulation* 1975;51:165.

38.   Abrams J: Current concepts of the genesis of heart sounds: First and second heart sounds, third and fourth heart sounds. *JAMA* 1978;239:2787-2791.

39.   Harvey WP, de Leon AC Jr: The normal third heart sound and gallops, ejection sounds, systolic clicks, systolic whoops, opening snaps and other sounds, in Hurst JW (ed): *The Heart,* ed 5. New York, McGraw-Hill, 1982.

40.   Chizner MA: Bedside diagnosis of the acute myocardial infarction and its complications. *Curr Probl Cardiol* 1982;7.

41.   Harvey WP, Stapleton J: Clinical aspects of gallop rhythm with particular reference to diastolic gallops. *Circulation* 1958;17:1007.

42.   Harvey WP, Ronan JA: Bedside diagnosis of arrhythmias. *Prog Cardiovasc Dis* 1966;8:429.

43.   Harvey WP, Perloff JK: The auscultatory findings in primary myocardial disease. *Am Heart J* 1961;61:199.

44.   Shaver JA, O'Toole JD: The second heart sound: Newer concepts. *Mod Concepts Cardiovasc Dis* 1977;46:7.

45.   Mounsey P: The opening snap of mitral stenosis. *Br Heart J* 1952;15:135.

46.   Leatham A, Gray I: Auscultatory and phonocardiographic signs of atrial septal defect. *Br Heart J* 1956;18:193.

47.   Wood P: An appreciation of mitral stenosis. *Br Heart J* 1952;15:135.

48.   Chizner MA: Valvular aortic stenosis in adults. *Primary Cardiol* 1981;7.

49.   Mounsey P: The early diastolic sound of constrictive pericarditis. *Br Heart J* 1955;17:143.

50.   Hancock EW: The ejection sound in aortic stenosis. *Am J Med* 1966;40:561.

51.   Wood P: Chronic constrictive pericarditis. *Am J Cardiol* 1961;7:48.

52.   Hultgren HN, Reeve R, Cohn K, et al: The ejection click of valvular pulmonic stenosis. *Circulation* 1969;40:631.

53.   Harvey WP: Auscultatory findings in diseases of the pericardium. *Am J Cardiol* 1961;7:15.

54.   Sosman MC: Quotation, in Shamroth L (ed): *Diagnostic Pointers in Clinical Electrocardiography.* Bowie, MD, Charles Press, 1978.

55.   Levine SA: Coronary thrombosis: The variable clinical features. *Medicine* 1929;8:245.

56.   Levine SA: *Clinical Heart Disease.* Philadelphia, WB Saunders Co, 1951, p 98.

57.   Lofmark R, Nordlander R, Orinuis E: The temperature course in acute myocardial infarction. *Am Heart J* 1978;90:153.

58.   Cooper HR: Atypical symptoms in myocardial infarction. *J Fla Med Assoc* 1964;51:581.

59. Frink RJ, James TN: Intracardiac route of the BeFold–Jarisch reflex. *Am J Physiol* 1971;221:1464.

60. Gibson TC: Blood pressure levels in acute myocardial infarction. *Am Heart J* 1978;96:475.

61. Schlant RC, Felner JM: The arterial pulse: Clinical manifestations. *Curr Probl Cardiol* 1977;2.

62. Ewy GA, Groves BM: Venous and arterial pulsations, in *Famous Teachings in Modern Medicine.* New York, Medcom, 1973.

63. Marx JH, Yu PN: Clinical examination of the arterial pulse. *Prog Cardiovasc Dis* 1967;10:207.

64. O'Rourke RA: Physical examination of the arteries and veins, in Hurst JW (ed): *The Heart,* ed 5. New York, McGraw-Hill Book Co, 1982, p 188.

65. Silverman ME, Fowler NO, Hurst JW, et al: *Examination of the Heart,* pts 1-4. Dallas, American Heart Association, 1975.

66. Vanden Belt RJ, Ronan JA, Bedynek JL: *Cardiology: A Clinical Approach.* Chicago, Year Book Medical Publishers, 1979, p 8.

67. Gordon MS: Cardiology: A scholarly bedside examination. *Med Student* 1981, p 188.

68. Ewy GA: Precordial pulsation, in *Famous Teachings in Modern Medicine.* New York, Medcom, 1972.

69. Ewy GA: Bedside evaluation of precordial pulsations. *Med Times* 1972;100 (suppl 1):156.

70. Cohn JN, Guiha NH, Groden MI, et al: Right ventricular infarction: Clinical and hemodynamic features. *Am J Cardiol* 1974;33:209.

71. Stapleton JF, Groves BM: Precordial palpation. *Am Heart J* 1971;81:409.

72. Abrams J: Precordial motion in health and disease. *Mod Concepts Cardiovasc Dis* 1980;49:55.

73. Benchimol A, Dimond EG: The apexcardiogram in ischemic heart disease. *Circulation* 1965;32:650.

74. Mounsey JPD: Inspection and palpation of the cardiac impulse. *Prog Cardiovasc Dis* 1967;10:187.

75. McGinn FX, Gould L, Lyon AF: The phonocardiogram and apexcardiogram in patients with ventricular aneurysm. *Am J Cardiol* 1968;21:467.

76. Harvey WP: Some pertinent physical findings in the clinical evaluation of acute myocardial infarction. *Circulation* 1969;39(suppl 4):175.

77. Delman AJ, Stein E: *Dynamic Cardiac Auscultation and Phonocardiography: A Graphic Guide.* Philadelphia, WB Saunders Co, 1979.

78. Eddleman EEJ, Langley JO: Paradoxical pulsation of the precordium in myocardial infarction and angina pectoris. *Am Heart J* 1962;63:579.

79. Price WH, Brown AE: Alteration in intensity of heart sounds after myocardial infarction. *Br Heart J* 1968;30:835.

80. Harvey WP: Abnormalities of the first and second heart sounds in the diagnosis of heart disease, in Segal BL (ed): *The Theory and Practice of Auscultation.* Philadelphia, FA Davis Co, 1963.

81. Tavel ME: *Clinical Phonocardiography and External Pulse Recording,* ed 3. Chicago, Year Book Medical Publishers, 1978.

82. Burggraf GW Craige E: The first heart sound in complete heart block. *Circulation* 1974;50:17.

83. Stept ME, Heid CE, Shaver JA, et al: Effect of altering PR interval or the amplitude of the first heart sound in the anesthetized dog. *Circ Res* 1969;25:255.

84. Ronan JA Jr: Cardiac sound and ultrasound: Echocardiographic and phonocardiographic correlations. *Curr Probl Cardiol* 1981;6.

85. Rytand PA: The variable loudness of the first heart sound in atrial fibrillation. *Am Heart J* 1949;37:187.

86. Yurchak PM, Gorlin R: Paradoxic splitting of the second heart sound in coronary artery disease. *N Engl J Med* 1963;269:741.

87. Harvey WP, Roana JA: Bedside diagnosis of arrhythmias. *Prog Cardiovasc Dis* 1966;8:429.

88. Curtiss EI, Matthews R, Shaver JA: Mechanisms of normal splitting of the second heart sound. *Circulation* 1975;51:154.

89. Perloff JK: Auscultatory and phonocardiographic manifestations of pulmonary hypertension. *Prog Cardiovasc Dis* 1967;9:303.

90. Cobbs BW Jr: The second heart sound in pulmonary embolism and pulmonary hypertension. *Am Heart J* 1966;17:843.

91. Hill JC, O'Rourke RA, Lewis RP, et al: The diagnostic value to the atrial gallop in acute myocardial infarction. *Am Heart J* 1969;78:194.

92. Sutton G, Harris A, Leatham A: Second heart sounds in pulmonary hypertension. *Br Heart J* 1968;30:743.

93. Riley CP, Russell RP, Rackley CE: Left ventricular gallop sound and acute myocardial infarction. *Am Heart J* 1973;86:598.

94. Perloff JK, Harvey WP: Auscultatory and phonocardiographic manifestations of pure mitral regurgitation. *Prog Cardiovasc Dis* 1967;5:172.

95. Heikkila J: Mitral incompetence complicating acute myocardial infarction. *Br Heart J* 1967;29:162.

96. Harvey WP, de Leon AC Jr: Auscultation of the heart: The normal third heart sound and gallops, in Hurst JW (ed): *The Heart,* ed 5. New York, McGraw-Hill Book Co., 1982, p 203.

97. Harvey WP, Stapleton J: Clinical aspects of gallop rhythm with particular reference to diastolic gallops. *Circulation* 1958;17:1007.

98. Chizner MA: Cardiac auscultation: Heart sounds. *Cardiol Prac* 1984;1:141-156.

99. Smith ND, Raizada V, Abrams J: Auscultation of the normally functioning prosthetic valve. *Ann Intern Med* 1981;95:594-598.

6
Examination of the Abdomen

Sherwin B. Nuland, M.D.

INTRODUCTION

The examination of the abdomen is an artful demonstration of eliciting information from the surface of the body. Careful history taking, along with the examination of the abdomen, as so precisely outlined by Dr. Nuland, should enhance the possibilities of a precise diagnosis. Through the use of the techniques described in this chapter, drawn from Dr. Nuland's many years of experience as a teacher and practicing surgeon, the student should have the gratifying experience of being able to elicit findings that later are confirmed by imaging examinations and surgical procedures.

The student must imagine that he does not have multiple diagnostic examinations available and is left only with his hands and brain to arrive at a sensible diagnosis. The student can diagnose such conditions as an acute gallbladder attack, appendicitis, duodenal ulcer, perforated stomach, peritonitis, pancreatitis, and/or kidney stones if a proper history and abdominal examination are performed. Abdominal aneurysms should be readily felt with gentle probing. Sometimes masses can be outlined, and a large liver and spleen should not be missed even if the patient is obese.

This chapter is divided into inspection, auscultation, percussion and palpation of the abdomen, and the rectal examination. After studying this chapter thoroughly, and performing many examinations, the student should have obtained enough competence to do a thorough abdominal examination.

As sensitive clinicians, we should never allow ourselves to suppose that the physical examination is a one-way street. At its very best, this particular form of laying on of hands can become a transaction between patient and physician in which each learns a great deal about the other. Just as the examiner is seeking out clues that may lead him to a diagnostic judgment, his every touch and word transmit messages by which the seemingly passive patient can become informed about the qualities of his doctor. It is our duty to convey reassurance, concern, and capability, as much as it is our duty to treat disease. It is, in fact, essential to the treatment that we do so. There is no part of the doctor-patient relationship that is more crucial to the success of such an obligation than the physical examination. It can, in its own way, begin the therapeutic process.

To this end, it behooves each of us to become so thoroughly skilled in this most subtle of the physician's arts that we transmit to our patients a feeling of confidence that allows their maximum cooperation with our efforts. The diagnostic touch must not be tentative, just as it must not be harsh. There must be no hurry and there must be no distraction. During the period of the examination, the observations being made must be at the central focus of all of our intellectual energy. It is no time to be thinking about the problems of any other patient; at this moment there lies before us the most important person in the world. The proper mood is well described in the words of a famous prayer attributed by some to the 12th century physician-theologian, Moses Maimonides: "May no irrelevent thoughts divert my attention at the bedside of the sick, or disturb my mind in its silent labours."

In no part of the body is the foregoing as true as in the examination of the abdomen. We deal here with a large, yielding expanse of warm, sensitive tissue through which can be felt, under varying pathologic conditions, virtually every underlying organ. The covering itself includes areas so different from each other that two-point discrimination is found to be dulled within a hand's breadth of zones of such specialized sensitivity that we call them erogenous. The emotional connotation of palpating some abdominal foci is so charged for many patients that examiners of both sexes must never, in their own clinical objectivity, forget its potential significance. But perhaps the most important thing to remember is that when we, as physicians, see an abdomen we see an old friend whose counterpart we have encountered many times before, albeit every one is somewhat different than its predecessor. On the other hand, when a patient sees his physician for the first time, he is seeing a stranger, and an authoritarian stranger at that. It is our obligation, and perhaps our most rewarding challenge, to show the patient that the stranger brings comfort and the hands of the healer. This is the hidden agenda of the physical examination.

Our fingers must be tactile and tactful, simultaneously. It goes without saying that both the hands and the heart must be warm. It is well to spend a few moments in physical and mental preparation, so that we can enter the room with a clear head, de-chilled fingers, and a sense of concerned competence that is transmissible to a frightened fellow creature. Thus can begin the history taking.

As the story of the illness unfolds, the clinician can attempt to "reconstruct the crime," as it were, gradually putting himself in the situation of the patient like a good actor reliving an episode in the life of the character he is playing. Although the clinical history will lead him into seeking certain specific findings on the physical examination, the physician must be careful not to let its apparent direction deter him from carefully and systematically completing the quest. In physical diagnosis, thoroughness can have unexpected rewards.

OBSERVATION

There is no part of the examination of the abdomen so commonly underestimated in importance as is simple observation. Observation may, in fact, begin even before one has met the patient, if the structural arrangements are such as to allow the examiner a glimpse of him as he enters the room. It is at this time that such significant findings as splinting can be appreciated, as the victim of peritoneal irritation walks bent forward to one side or the other to protect a tender quadrant. The jarring of ordinary locomotion causes some persons to tread very gingerly and slowly. Those with renal colic may occasionally hold a hand up on the flank, or even be observed to massage that area as they move. I have seen a patient holding his shirt away from his body while he walked down the corridor of a surgical clinic; he proved to have herpes zoster. A middle-aged man with perforated ulcer was wheeled in one day, willing only to move his eyeballs, lest even the turning of his head increase his abdominal pain. There are many such anecdotes to be told; gait, bearing, and movement may be the first clues to the underlying disease process.

It is difficult to control the impulse to begin the examination of the abdomen with palpation. Not only is palpation usually the most rewarding of the four modalities we use, but it is such an active thing to be doing that it is well-nigh irresistible to the fledgling examiner. But resist it he must, or remain a fledgling until the end of his days. It is a quirk of which we are all victim that the least intrusive technique proves to be the one most commonly trivialized, a state of affairs that is not in the best interest of the patient, and does not help the physician much, either.

There may be another reason that inspection is so often skimmed over: the first view of a bare and vulnerable belly can be an embarrassment to patient and doctor, creating an awkward moment for both. For this reason, one must learn to see a great deal at one glance; do not linger in the looking.

Some authors recommend viewing the trunk from various angles, shifting the lights and shadows, even dropping down on one knee to get a grazing tangential view. I have never found any of this to be very useful. Quite the contrary, such maneuverings only serve to introduce an element of embarrassment to what is already not an easy moment. If the doctor is of one sex and the patient of the other, the strain may be even greater. In decades past, the doctor-patient relationship was treated as though it exists on a plane that makes it immune to the intrusions of sexuality. It is not.

In spite of an occasional finding that can be made more visible by shadowing, the best kind of lighting is direct, downward daylight. Since the latter is not often possible, a white light approximating 75 foot-candles is a reasonable substitute. Most modern emergency wards and medical examining rooms are so equipped, although, oddly enough, most hospital rooms are not.

For the briefest possible moment at the very beginning of the inspection, there must be a suspension of modesty and an interval during which some of the foregoing admonitions about the patient's sensitivities are ignored. All the garments and bedclothes should be removed from caudal to the nipple line while the examiner stands at the foot of the bed for the period of approximately half a dozen breaths. Those 30 seconds will provide ample time to assess symmetry and contour, which are so important in the diagnosis of abdominal disease. There are a number of abnormalities that may be found in this way. The slight scoliosis that is caused by splinting an irritated psoas muscle will be readily apparent when the axis of the body is seen from the perspective of the feet, as will the minimal protrusion of either side of the abdomen such as may be secondary to dilated bowel adjacent to an inflammatory process. A ballooning of the cecum, a distended stomach, a flank that is a bit fuller than its opposite number, the slight bulging of the right upper quadrant caused by a wad of omentum wrapped around an inflamed gallbladder—all of these are most visible from below, and easy to miss when looked down upon from a height 2 feet anterior to the umbilicus.

Having taken in all that is available from this vantage point, the examiner can now move to the side of the bed, and cover the patient enough to leave exposed just the area from the lower chest to the upper thighs. From such a less distant observation post, one can again be in a position to carry on a more human transaction with his examinee, both by conversing and by occasionally glancing up to make eye contact. There are many things to look for, and they can be appreciated without hurry in less than a minute. It will take longer to read the appropriate few paragraphs below than it will to make the observations they describe.

Of course, the patient is by now lying flat on his back, as straight and symmetrical as his condition will allow. His arms are at his sides, and his head, if supported at all, rests on the smallest of pillows. However, the patient very likely was not in this position when the examiner first entered the room. A golden opportunity for finding important clues will have been missed if a general impression has not by now ingrained itself in the clinician's mind, concerning the overall appearance presented by the patient. It takes a great deal of experience for embryonic physicians to consistently remember to ask themselves just how sick an individual looks at the moment he presents himself. Failure to appreciate the "big picture" is one of the most common reasons why junior house officers send undiagnosed patients out of hospital emergency rooms only to have them return severely ill on the next resident's shift.

This is less the house staff's fault than it is the fault of the way we teach medicine in the late 20th century. It was the emergence of pathologic anatomy almost 150 years ago that began the process by which we now direct our attention to ever more submicrodimensional parts of sick people. Before then, diseases were thought to be primarily constitutional, and etiologies were sought that invoked such global instigators as miasmas, morality, and tight bowels. Then, along came Giovanni Morgagni, in 1761, and with one simple statement the stage was set for the birth of modern clinical medicine. Having studied the autopsy findings of more than 700 persons whose premortem complaints had been recorded, the Italian anatomist pointed out to all the believers in ill winds and phlogistic diatheses that they were sniffing the wrong ground. Symptoms, said Morgagni, "are the cries of the suffering organs"; it is only in the study of organ pathology that disease can be understood.

The next several generations of investigators sought out, while their patients were still living, the pathologic processes that caused those cries, and tried to determine ways of identifying from which viscera they arose. Thus began the early salad days of physical diagnosis, as the Auenbruggers, the Corvisarts, and the Laennecs began to correlate their percussing and their palpating and their auscultating with the inner workings of the disordered machinery. After the middle of the 19th century, clinicians began to spend more time in laboratories, realizing that the evidence of the naked eye was not enough. Rudolf Virchow demonstrated to them that the real answers to the understanding of the disease process were to be found on a cellular level. Later workers, particularly in Germany, came to investigate the biochemical and physiologic determinants of bodily function. Gradually there arose the concept of what is called pathophysiology, a term we use in recognition of the multiple etiologies and expressions of disease. If you want to gain some appreciation of just how far this two-century course of events has taken the clinical diagnostician, spend a morning making visits to each of the laboratories to which you send drops or bits of your next complicated patient. From looking at whole people who are sick, we have reduced ourselves to being experts in the study of flecks and specks of humanity.

An evolving process that resulted in the magnificent attainments of modern clinical medicine should not be disparaged. The reductionism and specificity that began with Giovanni Morgagni brought science into medicine, and changed our role from that of useless philosophers to true healers. As researchers focused on ever more abstruse workings of the organism, they created an edifice upon which to support increasingly skillful diagnosis and effective therapy. It was only when physicians abandoned the whole-patient approach and replaced it with studies of individual parts and specialized functions that order was created from clinical chaos. The segmentation of the sick into abstract cells and molecules is the Rosetta stone that is decoding the hieroglyphics of disease.

Paradoxically, a by-product of this scientific progression has been that it has removed us ever further from our patients. The cells and molecules are no longer seen as abstractions; they are the contemporary reality we teach our students. Somewhere along the way we have allowed the sick to become the abstractions. Ethicists, clergymen, and humanists try to find ways to help us return to them.

Of the several paths that will bring us close to those who come to us for help, there is one that leads directly and most naturally back. It is the comforting reassurance of a well-conducted, sympathetic physical examination. It begins with a warm greeting, and is preceded by a caring history taking and an all-encompassing look, once again, at the whole patient, who is, after all, the only unchanging reality.

The all-encompassing overview serves not only to provide some sense of the degree to which the patient's illness has affected his/her constitutional state, but also as a point of comparison with later examinations that may be necessary. Particularly in the diagnosis of acute abdominal disease, it is often more than a little helpful to repeat certain parts of the evaluation at appropriate intervals of time, such as 6 or 8 hours. As a pathologic process evolves, there is nothing that changes as dramatically as the patient's general appearance and the effects he makes to ease discomfort. The facial expression, the breathing, the cast of his complexion, the position assumed in the bed, his speaking voice (and even willingness to speak at all) all convey messages about the patient's condition and its cause. The classic description of the appendicitis subject who lies on the right side with knees drawn up is seen as commonly as the textbooks claim, and so is the thrashing about of the victim of pancreatitis. An elderly lady with an incarcerated femoral hernia may refuse to straighten out her leg.

As may be imagined, it is a safe rule of thumb that the more one's parietal peritoneum is being irritated the less one will be willing to change position. The more generalized the irritation, the more painful the movement; it is easy to understand why the man whose peritoneal cavity is awash with hydrochloric acid lies as still as a mummy. The more localized the peritoneal process the more specific the findings, and the more likely they are to be referred in certain well-described patterns. A little extrapolation makes it clear why the lacrosse player with a splenic hematoma does not want to lie down, or why he grabs his left shoulder before agreeing to take a deep breath.

These are the kinds of things that can be taken in at a glance, providing that the examiner has schooled himself to see them and appreciate their significance. Having taken a good look, and committed the scene to memory, he is now ready to gently encourage the patient to relinquish his defenses enough to allow the rest of the evaluation to be carried out. Occasionally, an acutely ill person will not be able to cooperate, which in itself can usually be interpreted as evidence of the advanced state of the disease process. Occasionally, however, a patient's refusal to assume the requested posture may arise more from psychosocial than from physical factors. This, too, becomes a test of the clinician's skill and patience.

INSPECTION

Having arranged the proper position, and after the evaluation from the foot of the bed, the time has come for the direct inspection of the abdominal wall. As pointed out earlier, everything that is visible can be assessed in no more than a minute, especially in view of the fact that the period of visual vigilance quite obviously extends itself into the time during which auscultation, percussion, and palpation will be carried out.

All publicity about the conjunctivae to the contrary, there is no better place to look for jaundice than on the broad white expanse of a Caucasian patient's abdomen. Because there is so much area to look at and because it is outlined by a border of white sheet, the abdominal skin will usually betray a bilirubin level as low as 2.5 milligrams percent. Unless the patient is dark-skinned or Oriental, scleral evidence will rarely improve on that figure.

While looking for icterus, observations can be made about other surface characteristics such as skin nutrition, hair distribution, hydration, pallor, and areas of discoloration due to livido or bruising. In patients who are suspected of harboring a pelvic abscess, look at the groins very carefully, lest a faint trace of erythema elude you. Particularly in the case of a pericolic mass due to diverticulitis, the inflammatory process may dissect its way retroperitoneally, producing a faint reddish blush medial to the inguinal crease. An appendiceal abscess occasionally does the same thing.

Take note of every scar, and be sure you ask for details of the operation that produced it. It is not enough to know that a transverse suprapubic incision is the result of a hysterectomy; ask why the procedure was done. Because so many people forget to mention an operation or two carried out 40 years earlier, the physical examination provides another opportunity to review or add to parts of the history.

If an appendectomy scar is found, try to ascertain whether appendicitis was confirmed; you may find a clue to the diagnosis of Crohn's disease. It is absolutely appalling to realize how little is known by many patients about the most obvious details of major operative procedures that they have allowed to be performed on themselves. This is a commentary on something, but it is difficult to divine exactly upon what.

It is important to train oneself to recognize the customary incisions that are ordinarily used for common operations. A patient's knowledge, or lack of it, may be supplemented by the examiner's awareness, for example, that a left subcostal scar is far and away most likely to be the track of a splenectomy. With the increasing use of midline incisions for such a variety of purposes, this kind of information may one day be much less useful than it is at present, but that day is still a long way off.

It is also helpful to know that certain kinds of operations are more prone to particular categories of long-range complications than are others. Small bowel obstruction, for example, is much more often the accompaniment of an old hysterectomy scar than of the wound produced by removal of the gallbladder. It is, in fact, a good general rule that previous surgery in the upper abdomen is far less likely to result in later adhesive obstruction than is an operative procedure below the umbilicus. There are cogent anatomic reasons for this.

Several facts about healed abdominal incisions may be of consequence in specific situations:

A wound that was drained is more likely to develop an incisional hernia than one that was not

The same is true of wounds that become infected

It often takes 6 months or longer for a maturing scar to lose its slight puffiness and redness, a piece of information that has on more than one occasion proven to be the downfall of a Munchausen man

A pigmented scar should raise a suspicion of adrenal insufficiency, particularly
if purplish striae can be seen on other parts of the abdomen

Eruptions, nevi, accessory nipples, spiders, and venous patterns can be taken
in with the same glance that evaluates the skin surface for color, scars, and quality. To differentiate the spider hemangioma from anything else, the well-known
maneuver of pressing down with a flat piece of glass has never been improved
upon. The bespectacled physician has a distinct advantage here, providing he is not
so myopic that the eyeglasses must be kept on his nose at all times.

Prominent venous patterns on the abdominal wall are due either to portal hypertension or obstruction of the vena cava. Even with mere inspection it is not very
difficult to differentiate between the two etiologies. The veins of caval obstruction tend to be larger and more tortuous, sometimes to the point of appearing ropy.
It is a simple matter to determine direction of blood flow by compressing a venous
channel with two separated fingers that can then be relaxed one at a time to allow
filling. An obstructed inferior vena cava always results in collateral flow that
moves cephalad, regardless of where on the abdominal wall it is tested. Moreover,
an obstructed cava causes marked dilatation of the saphenous system in the legs.
The collateral flow of portal hypertension, on the other hand, proceeds always in
the normal direction: cephalad above the umbilicus and caudad below it. The
channels are thinner, and are concentrated above the umbilicus. They commonly
occur on skin stretched so tightly by ascites that it glistens.

Having evaluated the surface of the abdomen, its contour must be assessed.
The asymmetry that may have been appreciated from the foot of the bed is here
seen from a different perspective, and other characteristics of shape and form can
be more easily identified when looking directly downward. One of these is the
natural declivity that is invariably present under the costal margin of the nondistended patient. Whatever the degree of obesity, there is always a dip in the
abdominal wall just inferior to the flare of the lower border of the rib cage. This
slight concavity disappears when upper abdominal distention supervenes. It is a
reliable way to determine whether an abdomen protrudes because it is distended or
simply because it is fat.

Abdominal masses are particularly likely to be visible in thin patients, but in
most cases the presence of a space-occupying neoplasm or inflammatory process
is much more prone to result in slight changes in contour of the anterior trunk
than in a clearly visible protrusion. Thus, a diverticular abscess will often cause
some filling out of what might otherwise be a somewhat hollow left iliac fossa,
and a distended cecum will be detectable as a modest ballooning just medial to the
right iliac crest. One cannot make much of the mere sight of a visibly pulsating
mass; even after palpation the nature of the thing often remains elusive. Many
recommendations have been made to help in the differentiation between the direct
pulsation of an abdominal aortic aneurysm and the transmitted pulsation seen or
felt through a mass anterior to it. Although some of them are quite ingenious,
none are consistently dependable.

Elderly, thin patients with intestinal obstructions will occasionally provide the
direct equivalent of a cineradiograph of their peristaltic rushes visibly outlined
through the parchmentlike tissues of a stretched abdominal wall. Infantile
pyloric stenosis can do the same thing. It must be kept in mind that normal peristalsis, in a patient who is thin enough, can sometimes be visible. However, it is
unlikely that even an inexperienced examiner will mistake the gentle undulations
of a healthy bowel for the crashing of an obstructive crescendo.

Although a hernia is ordinarily easily visible when incarcerated, it may take
certain maneuvers to demonstrate it when not protruding. These include the

time-honored coughing and straining, but anything that increases intra-abdominal pressure will do. An otherwise uncooperative child, for example, may enjoy holding his nose and trying to blow hard against the closed nostrils, while an older patient may find it easier to lift his head and shoulders than to produce a somewhat prolonged Valsalva maneuver. The latter technique is particularly helpful in seeking out incisional hernias and diastases. Telling a young child to "blow up your stomach till it looks like a big balloon" is an effective way to demonstrate an umbilical defect. It should also be pointed out, parenthetically, that this little game is particularly useful in producing peritoneal irritation, as when one is trying to differentiate between appendicitis and gastroenteritis. Its exact opposite, "Try to suck your stomach in, to make it as small as possible," is even better.

We cannot leave the discussion of abdominal inspection without mentioning certain appellations that have become attached to this portion of the physical examination. These are listed not because they are necessarily helpful, but only because they are sometimes invoked on rounds, particularly by computerized clinicians who rarely treat but often make pronouncements.

> **Caput medusae**—This term refers to a circle of collateral veins radiating from the umbilicus in cases of portal hypertension. It has been said by more than one astute wag that it is a finding that occurs only in textbooks.

> **Cullen's sign**—A bluish discoloration of the umbilicus, caused by an intra-peritoneal bleed of sizable amount. Cullen's sign is most commonly associated with a ruptured ectopic pregnancy.

> **Grey Turner's sign**—A blue-gray discoloration of the flank due to retroperitoneal blood. Although rarely seen, it can be a grave prognostic finding in hemorrhagic pancreatitis.

> **Linea nigra**—A thin midline streak of dark pigmentation running from pubis to umbilicus in many women who have borne children. Although its absence is meaningless, its presence tends to weaken the arguments of a gonorrhea suspect who insists that she is a virgin.

> **Sister Mary Joseph's nodule**—A metastatic nodularity in the umbilicus, secondary to intra-abdominal carcinoma. The finding acquired its eponym from the tradition that it was first pointed out to Dr. Will Mayo by Sister Mary Joseph.

AUSCULTATION

If inspection is that part of the physical examination that is most frequently underestimated in importance, auscultation is the part most frequently neglected completely. During my own training days in the 1950s and 1960s the pocket of the surgical resident's short white coat was considered by some to be more gainfully occupied by a nasogastric tube than by a stethoscope. That was patent nonsense then as it is patent nonsense today. Ears are as useful for examining the gut as they are for the lungs.

Apparently, not everyone agrees. That most oft-quoted of authorities on the acute abdomen, Zachary Cope, devotes only one paragraph of my edition of his classic little book to auscultation, stating that the technique "is occasionally of use in determining whether the normal sounds due to intestinal movements are to be heard." Even in his chapter dealing with intestinal obstruction, he restricts his stethoscopic commentary to one terse sentence: "Sometimes borborygmi may be heard passing along the bowel." Those sections relating to perforated ulcer mention auscultation not at all, even in the paragraphs in which are discussed the differential diagnosis between it and obstruction, pneumonia, and several other conditions. It is as though René Laennec had never lived.

In fact, auscultation can be a remarkably useful tool in the evaluation of abdominal disease. Not uncommonly, the sounds that are heard (or not heard) will be the determining factor in making a diagnosis, most particularly in acute disease. In no other area of physical examination is a familiarity with normal more important than in the interpretation of bowel sounds. Students and junior house officers are well advised to devote several minutes to eavesdropping on the abdomen of each patient they encounter whose disease is located elsewhere, so that the full range of normal can be appreciated. One's own borborygmi are a constantly available guide, and a great deal less expensive than a tape recording.

Bowel sounds are produced by the action of intestinal movement on the mixture of gas and fluid in the gut lumen. Peristalsis itself is silent; unless it has the gurgly mixture to churn and propel, it leaves no auditory evidence of its existence. This is why surgeons often see rhythmic bowel motion at the end of a long abdominal operation and yet hear no sounds for days afterward. What we are accustomed to calling a postoperative ileus is largely the product of a virtually empty gut.

Normal bowel sounds are soft, short, gentle, and low-pitched. When the intestine is distended, the pitch becomes higher as the wall is stretched and the resonating chamber becomes larger. When a normally functioning length of bowel is rolling its contents along toward an obstruction, the power of the driving force makes the sounds not only longer, but increasingly louder, reaching a crescendo as the occluded area is approached. The crescendo of sound is understandably synchronous with a rising wave of colicky pain. As the wave reaches a climax, so does the sound, until the next long roll brings it back. After a prolonged period of obstruction, the muscular coat of the intestinal wall loses its tone as it becomes overstretched. The obstructive sounds become higher in pitch and gradually less organized. The periodic spasms of noise give way to irregular tinkles and blips, the result of small amounts of gas and fluid falling from one cavernous proximal loop to another. Any condition that weakens or destroys the tone of the intestinal smooth muscle can result in such feeble sounds. They can be heard, therefore, not only in late obstruction, but also in ischemia, segmental ileus, certain neurophysiologic abnormalities, and in a bowel recovering from any adynamic period during which it has become distended or poorly perfused.

A crescendo of intestinal rushing accompanied by a crescendo of pain is, therefore, *the* definitive finding in a case of **small bowel obstruction.** It makes the diagnosis with even more certainty than does an x-ray. However, it must not be forgotten that the rushes do not go on forever. Their absence may simply mean that the patient has arrived for treatment late in his course. Therefore, late obstruction, resolving obstruction, and partial obstruction provide a whole panorama of auditory possibilities, depending on both degree and stage.

Absent bowel sounds portend an **adynamic ileus.** Possible etiologies include generalized peritonitis, certain electrolyte abnormalities, retroperitoneal hematoma, trauma, and ischemia. The latter condition can effect peristalsis in any of several ways. Many experienced clinicians will attest to having heard a gut with a segmental area of ischemia behave, rushes and all, like a small bowel obstruction.

The decision that bowel sounds are absent or hypoactive should not be reached until at least three minutes of auscultation have passed. The stethoscope should be placed lightly but snugly over the midportion of one of the lower quadrants, since this is the region under which most of the small bowel lies. If the patient is wearing a nasogastric tube, be sure that the suction is turned off to prevent the adventitious intrusions that such an apparatus can sometimes cause. If you hear sounds that fit no familiar pattern or wavelength, ascertain that your man's abdominal hair is not crinkling under your stethoscope, or that your woman is not absent-mindedly running a finger across her costal margin. And above all, never put a cold diaphragm or bell on a sick person's abdomen. Not only will the patient tighten up, but he will probably become so wary of your touch that his suspicions will extend into the period of palpation, when you most want him to be relaxed.

All hyperactive sounds are not obstructive. The blood from a rapid upper **gastrointestinal hemorrhage** will usually stimulate the bowel into increased movement, which, acting on the large amount of fluid in the form of blood, will cause a great churning and constancy of sound. This finding is so common that it is a useful criterion by which to differentiate an upper from a lower gastrointestinal bleed in those situations in which it is not otherwise clear. Gastroenteritis also, and other inflammatory diseases of bowel, may increase the volume and raise the pitch of borborygmi, sometimes making them sound enough like obstructive rushes to introduce a note (pun intended) of diagnostic confusion.

There are important sounds to listen for in the abdomen other than those that are intestinal in origin. A succussion splash is audible when a very distended air- and fluid-filled stomach is suddenly moved; it can be elicited by rocking the patient, quickly, from side to side. This sound, although rare, can be a most dramatic accompaniment of an **obstructed pylorus** or the upside-down stomach of a **paraesophageal hernia.**

More common by far are the variety of bruits that betray a degree of **vascular occlusion.** These have a blowing or whiffing quality, although they may sometimes be quite harsh. As might be expected, they occur during systole, and are best heard by listening directly over the vessel. Since such sounds tend to be transmitted along the course of the arteries, the examiner should be sure that what he is calling an iliac bruit does not actually arise from the aorta. Differentiation of one origin from another is accomplished by comparing the sounds over each of any two paired vessels. Since it is unlikely that each iliac or renal artery, for example, is producing a murmur exactly like its contralateral fellow, identical bilateral bruits tend to come from a shared origin, which is likely to be aortic or even cardiac.

Occasionally one may make a very astute diagnosis of **renal artery stenosis** in a hypertensive patient by using the stethoscope wisely, especially in the flanks and posteriorly. Interestingly, the murmur of this disease is described by some authors as being as likely to be continuous with a systolic accentuation as it is to be systolic alone. This is probably attributable to the poststenotic dilatation that is so common in the partially obstructed renal artery.

The faint, continuous, soft buzz that is heard from time to time near the midline is called a venous hum, and arises from the normal vena cava. **Portal hypertension** can also produce such a sound, which should be listened for in patients with visible abdominal wall collaterals. Venous hums are distinguishable from arterial bruits by the fact that they change in quality with respiration and posture.

Vascular sounds are sometimes heard over **intra-abdominal neoplasms.** Carcinoma of the body of the pancreas, for example, has been known to be accompanied by a left upper quadrant systolic bruit, due to encasement of the splenic artery by tumor, a characteristic angiographic finding in this disease. The harsh bruit that may be audible over the liver in cases of hepatoma, on the other hand, is thought to be due to the increased vascularity that such primary liver growths receive from the hepatic artery; the element of vascular compression seems to be absent. Although usually heard in systole, the murmur of a hepatoma may be continuous, with systolic accentuation.

Lastly, a bruit with a to-and-fro quality should raise the suspicion of **arteriovenous aneurysm,** especially in a patient with a history of major trauma or previous vascular surgery. Even more rare than this is a similar sound produced by **shunts within a tumor.**

There is a small assortment of wheezes and creaks that the careful auscultator (the feminine form of this noun must certainly be auscultatrix) may be called upon to interpret on occasion. Leathery friction rubs over liver or spleen imply that an underlying tumor, infarct, or inflammatory process is present. A similar sound lower in the abdomen is sometimes due to roughened, inflamed peritoneal surfaces rubbing across one another. A distended bowel is particularly likely to amplify or transmit this kind of noise, which is therefore ominous when it occurs in the abdomen of a patient suspected of mesenteric ischemia.

There is one more audible observation that should be mentioned, because it is easily confused with more meaningful findings: In the utter stillness of a totally silent abdomen it is sometimes possible to detect the soft ticking of a normal aorta or the heart from which it arises. Trying to hear it is a little like listening for elves in the forest.

PERCUSSION

Simply stated, the aim of percussion is to distinguish areas of different density from each other. The act of tapping sets up a vibration in the examined surface that is transmitted audibly to the observer. If the tapping is done through the intervening finger or hand of the examiner, as is usually the case during physical diagnosis, the vibration is also palpable as a tactile sensation in that finger or hand. Thus, the evidence obtainable by percussion is not limited to what is heard, but can also be appreciated by the quality of the vibrations felt by the physician.

Except for special purposes, direct percussion is rarely used. The method of tapping on the third finger of one hand (the so-called pleximeter finger) with the third finger of the other (the plexor finger) is called mediate percussion, just as listening through the indirect means of a stethoscope is called mediate auscultation. The use of mediate percussion adds to our diagnostic armamentarium, therefore, by providing an extra method of observation, the vibratory sense of the pleximeter. Unfortunately, this added advantage is rarely used.

It is well worth training oneself to appreciate the subtle differences in vibratory sense that are imparted to the examining hand by tissues of varying densities. Not only do such differences serve to confirm the impressions of one's hearing, but there are occasions on which they are more reliable. There are examiners so highly skilled in this technique that they deliberately tap very softly so as not to obscure the evidence transmitted to their digits; forceful tapping may confuse the vibration that the plexor produces in the pleximeter with that which is coming in to it from the abdominal wall.

When the abdomen is being inspected or auscultated, the examiner is using what amounts to a technique of scanning; he looks or listens for anything that may come, before focusing his attention on individual findings. In percussion, on the other hand, one is more often seeking specific information right from the start. Hepatic size, for example, is reliably assessed by tapping out the superior and inferior borders of the liver. This is because the dull note that emanates from the underlying solid parenchyma provides such a marked contrast to the sounds produced from the resonant lung above and the tympanitic bowel below. Because it represents so large and distinct a difference from its surroundings, in fact, the liver is the ideal structure on which to become familiar with the strictly tactile results of percussion. It is probably safe to say that the organ is enlarged if it measures more than 12 cm from top to bottom.

Percussing the liver can be useful in determining whether free air is present in the abdominal cavity, since under these circumstances the usual dullness is absent or lessened. Although this is most comfortably assessed in the ordinary supine mode, tapping along the midaxillary line of a patient while he lies in the left lateral decubitus position is likelier to provide definite findings. Because it creates such a long area of adjacent differences in density, this is also an ideal angle for an x-ray, particularly in a patient suspected of having perforated a duodenal ulcer.

The tympanitic percussion note that resounds from the distended cavity of an **obstructed stomach** sends out a warning to insert a nasogastric tube with all possible dispatch. A markedly distended air-filled cecum is similarly resonant and tells a tale of equal or greater urgency. Even when not fatal, **cecal perforation** enormously complicates the management of the obstructing colonic carcinoma, which is its usual cause.

Intestinal obstruction of any sort may result in segments of tympanitic gut, particularly if the obstructive process is of the closed-loop variety, as in small bowel or sigmoid volvulus. A resonant note is also characteristic of any paralytic ileus, increasing as the degree of distention increases. The rapid loss of tone in an ischemic gut is capable of increasing intestinal diameter so quickly that the term "meteorism" has been applied to the process and its outcome. In such cases, the act of percussion produces not only increased resonance but significant tenderness as well. This percussion tenderness is, in fact, a finding that is similar to rebound, being present in situations characterized by marked peritoneal irritation. When tenderness is accompanied by an absence of liver dullness, the generalized peritonitis of perforated ulcer is virtually diagnosable by percussion alone.

Because air-filled loops of bowel tend to float on the surface of collections of intraperitoneal fluid, there are several percussible signs of **ascites.** When a patient with this condition lies flat on his back, a central area of tympany surrounded on all sides by dullness becomes quite significant, especially when accompanied by bulging flanks that are also dull. Turning the patient on his side at an angle of about 45 degrees will allow the resonant gut to float toward the uppermost flank as the fluid shifts to the lower, a phenomenon appropriately called shifting dullness.

Detection of a fluid wave, although not as easy as is often claimed, is helpful in those few instances in which it can be elicited with certainty. To do this one must enlist an assistant, who presses the ulnar side of his hand firmly but not deeply into the subcutaneous tissues of the midline to steady the jiggling of fat. With the palm or fingertips of one hand the examiner smartly taps the lateral abdominal wall on one side while holding the flat of his palm against the other. In the presence of significant ascites, a fluid wave is transmitted with enough force to be felt by the examining hand. Like so many other of the findings of physical diagnosis, and more so than most, this one is of value only when positive.

Percussion is quite reliable in determining **bladder size,** where recognizing the smooth symmetry of the distended organ will sometimes save the embarrassment of describing what is misinterpreted as a lower abdominal tumor. **Neoplasms** are, in fact, difficult to outline in this manner, even when easily palpable; no time should be wasted in trying to tap out the margins of a deep-lying intra-abdominal mass. The one exception may be metastases on the lower edge of the liver, whose size and shape can sometimes be very accurately determined by soft percussion and the use of the vibratory sense. The same can be said of a spleen that is markedly enlarged.

There is a maneuver that is dignified by calling it **fist percussion,** and therefore it will be included here, as well as for want of any other suitable category into which to put it. The hypothenar side of the clenched fist is brought down smartly on to the dorsum of the opposite hand, which lies on the right lower costal margin of a patient who is suspected of having cholecystitis. As brutal as it sounds, this kind of jolt can pick up a relatively slight degree of tenderness when it is not easily elicited by direct palpation. For this reason, fist percussion is also worth using in the physical examination of patients who may have inflammatory diseases of the liver. A less pugilistic way of accomplishing the same thing is to forcefully compress the right lower rib cage with one good squeeze.

PALPATION

Anatomy of the Abdomen

Skill in the art of abdominal palpation cannot be acquired without a secure knowledge of three-dimensional anatomy. It is a paradox of modern medicine that the very technology that makes some physicians neglect physical diagnosis should bring once more to the forefront the absolute necessity of anatomic expertise. Indeed, a radiologist can no more read a computed tomography or NMR scan or ultrasound study than can a clinician pretend to interpret the evidence at his fingertips, without each of them having an accurate understanding of organ relationships.

It is not enough to have a generally good idea of which organs are most commonly found in each of the four quadrants of the abdomen; the diagnostician who wishes to squeeze (another forgettable pun) the most information out of his probings must appreciate the importance of such factors as topographical landmarks, the cross-sectional appearance of the trunk at various levels, and the depth at which certain of the internal structures lie. Attention will be paid in the following paragraphs to factors that determine the palpability of viscera, vessels, and variegated tissues.

To begin with, a transverse section through the abdominal cavity is not ellipse-shaped, as so many would suppose. A glance at Figure 6.1 will show that it is much shallower along its vertical axis than it is out in the lateral gutters. Further caudad, as the pelvis is entered, the cavity becomes like a deep scoop in which all manner of abnormalities may be hidden to any but the deepest touch (see Figures 6.2 and 6.3). The surprising thing to many who have forgotten the lessons of the first months of medical school is the location of the topographical point under which the dropping off begins. It is the umbilicus. A needle passed directly through the umbilicus will enter the aorta at its bifurcation or a bit above, and become impaled approximately at the L4-5 level, just cephalad to the entrance to the obliquely tilted bowl that we call the pelvis. The aortic bifurcation lies at the midpoint of a transverse line that can be drawn joining the uppermost margins of the iliac crests.

In other words, there are two distinct parts of the abdominal cavity, which can be differentiated reasonably well on the body surface by drawing an imaginary transverse line at the level of the umbilicus. This line runs from the top of one iliac crest to the other, and crosses the aortic bifurcation. It marks the boundary between the upper quadrants and the lower. Above this line, the vertebral bodies lie relatively close to the abdominal wall, with a deep parallel trough running the length of each side; below the line, the abdomen is a backwardly tipped basin, the bottom of which becomes progressively deeper as the end of the coccyx is approached (see Figure 6.3).

Failure to know these structural facts has led many an examiner astray. The close proximity of the lumbar vertebral bodies to the anterior abdominal wall, for example, seems to be little appreciated by examiners who insist that they feel a mass, and often a pulsating one at that, in the normal epigastrium. The pulsating bulge of an aortic aneurysm is often searched for in the lower abdomen, since so many physicians are certain that the bifurcation lies much more caudally than it

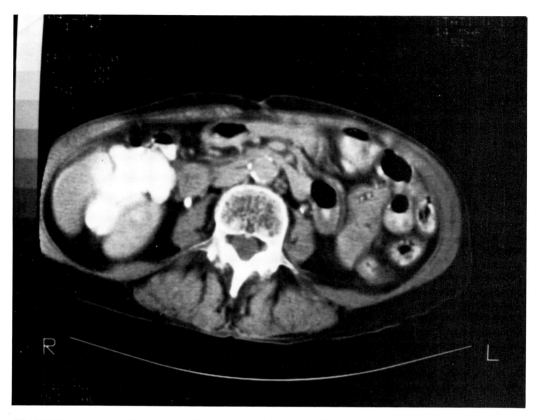

FIGURE 6.1   CT scan at the level of the umbilicus, demonstrating the considerable difference in depth between the central axis of the abdominal cavity and its lateral gutters. The plane of the image lies at L-4, just cephalad to the aortic bifurcation and the iliac crests. Note the closeness of the aorta to the anterior abdominal wall.

actually does. The finding of a palpable splenic tip is commonly interpreted as signifying just a bit of enlargement; in fact, the normal spleen lies so deep in the lateral gutter and so well tucked up under the costophrenic recess that its tip cannot be felt until the organ is approximately three times enlarged.

Having reviewed enough anatomic diagrams, schedule a trip to the autopsy room to become familiar with the positions of the various structures as they lie in situ. Do not trust vague memories from freshman anatomy courses. It may be surprising to note how close to the midline is the first duodenum, or how low in the peritoneal cavity is most of the small bowel. The deeply hidden position of the pancreas must be seen to be fully appreciated, as must the thickness and wide expanse of that much ignored structure, the omentum. Traction will demonstrate that the splenic flexure that is seen radiographically is actually the distal transverse colon rising up into the left upper quadrant; the true flexure lies attached inferior to the spleen.

A great deal of lip service is paid to the variability in position and form of the appendix, but only the morgue or considerable surgical experience will make the point unforgettable. With the abdomen open, put a gloved finger high up into the

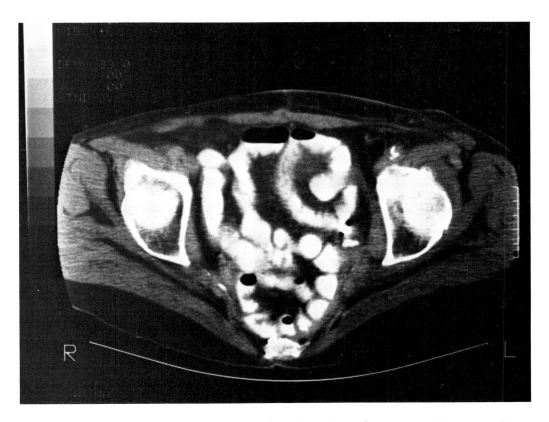

FIGURE 6.2   CT scan at the level of the junction of sacrum and coccyx, deep within the hollow of the pelvis. There is a vast difference in contour between Figure 6.1 and this figure.

rectum and observe from anteriorly which structures are palpable in this way. Do the same for the female pelvic organs by examining through the vagina. After the pathologist has removed the peritoneal contents, look carefully into the empty shell of the hollowed-out abdominal cavity. This step alone may prove to justify the entire excursion.

Methods of Palpation

Surface Touching
The word palpate is derived from the Latin *palpabilis,* referring to touch. Touch means touch; it does not mean press, or probe, or push, or any of the several other manual maneuvers that we must use in this part of the examination. It is important to remember that before those more invasive things are done, ordinary touching is still the first step. The flat palm is placed on that part of the abdominal wall least likely to be tender. Observations are made in each quadrant before proceeding to light pressure and then to deeper probings. There is a great deal that can be determined about contour and symmetry by a gentle sweeping motion over the abdominal wall, which can supplement what has already been observed visually. Areas of bulging distention, disparity between the two flanks, the

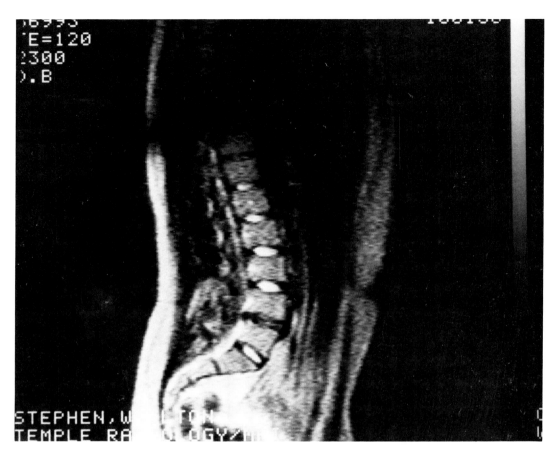

FIGURE 6.3   NMR study to demonstrate the marked changes in depth that occur in passing from the upper quadrants of the abdomen to the pelvis.

subcostal dips described earlier, the texture of the subcutaneous fat—these are clues worth tracing. A hand placed between the iliac crest and costal margin on each lateral abdominal wall will sometimes detect the subtle difference in length between the two flanks that is due to the scoliotic posture of a patient with an acute abdomen, particularly in conditions that irritate the psoas muscle, as in iliac or retrocecal appendicitis.

The flat palm lying lightly on the skin may detect borborygmi. In patients thin enough and obstructed enough to make intestinal rushes visible, they are sometimes palpable as well. Vascular thrills can occasionally be felt, and the throbbing of an aortic aneurysm will often pulsate against the hand with enough force to make it bounce rhythmically. Theoretically, a transmitted pulsation should cause a bouncing that is felt only anteriorly, whereas a direct aortic pulsation should be felt as a rhythmic expansion along a semicircle. As noted earlier, this is not very dependable, and various mechanical attempts to enhance the difference have not been of much help.

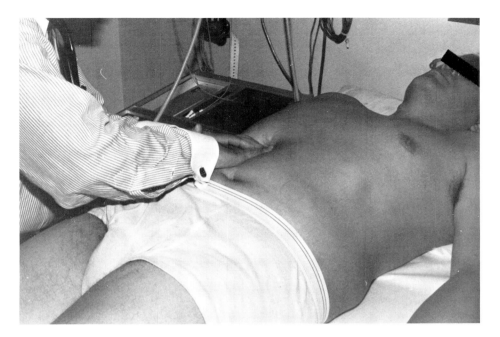

FIGURE 6.4   Deep palpation, as well as the identification of muscle spasm, are best carried out by using the flats of the fingers, particularly the pads. Sometimes a greater degree of control can be achieved by pressing on the palpating hand with the other hand's fingertips, as shown.

Although the back of the hand is more sensitive to temperature, the palm is also useful in detecting fever. Noting that the abdominal skin is hotter than it was on the last sequential examination is an important sign in following the progress of an acute disease, and may lead to the detection of rising fever hours before the nurses are scheduled to next insert the thermometer.

Gentle Palpation: Herniation
Having felt the surface, information can then be gathered about the tone of the musculature by using gentle pressure. This is best done by the flats of the fingers, particularly the pads (Figure 6.4). Pressing directly in with the fingertips should be avoided at this stage, since it is unnecessary, and serves only to make the patient tighten up. A general decrease in muscular tone may be a by-product of a chronic disease such as cirrhosis, but is also seen in many patients whose symptoms are of more recent onset. Metastatic carcinoma, for example, or ongoing sepsis, lead to a more or less rapid process of malnutrition and tissue wasting.

This is a good point at which to check for ventral or incisional hernias. The fingers should be placed along the length of each scar, while one of the maneuvers previously described is used to induce increased intra-abdominal pressure. Healed drain sites, or any other areas that are dimpled, are to be treated with particular suspicion, as is any wound that once harbored a postoperative infection. The recti may separate in the midline to reveal a diastasis that is both visible and palpable, particularly in women who have borne several children. Feel the umbilicus, and put the pads of the fingers over the inguinal canals during straining or coughing.

To evaluate the inguinal rings and posterior canal walls is a special skill in itself, and not easy to learn without a great deal of practice. One good method is to invaginate the scrotal skin at the point at which it is in contact with the most proximal portion of the penile shaft. By passing the tip of the index or fifth finger upward, the pubic tubercle becomes palpable. Alongside it lies the spermatic cord, which can be identified by rolling it with the finger across the bony surface behind it. The cord can then be followed up through the external ring. By pressing posteromedially, the canal wall can be assessed for strength as well as for the presence of the rounded bluge that indicates a direct hernia. An indirect hernia, on the other hand, should feel more like a fingerlike process coming down the length of the canal from above. There are many prescribed criteria for differentiating between direct and indirect hernias, but I have found this technique to be the most useful: if it seems to be coming down from above and to feel somewhat tubular, it is probably indirect; if it is rounded and bulgy, and seems to push in from the posteromedial direction, it is probably direct. No matter what technique or teaching you swear by, be prepared to be proven wrong more than once in a while. An incarcerated hernia, of which more will be discussed below, is virtually always indirect. The same may be said of any hernia that descends into the scrotum.

It is helpful to practice entering your own inguinal canal. If you are a woman, you may have forgotten that you have one, as well as a round ligament that is almost as good a guide into it as is your male colleague's spermatic cord. Begin directly at the pubic tubercle. Probing one's own inguinal canal is not only valuable for learning anatomy, but it is an infallible way to find out just how uncomfortable the process can be. This will make you gentler when intruding yourself into someone else's groin.

Many physicians have the idea that feeling a strong inguinal impulse against the exploring finger when the patient coughs will indicate the presence of a hernia. This is not so. A palpable impulse is not evidence of a hernia nor does it mean that the person being examined is about to develop one. It is a nonfinding. A thickened spermatic cord, however, may indicate an indirect hernia that the examiner is not able to feel. This is particularly true of small children, whose only physical evidence of hernia on any given day is not infrequently a cord that feels thicker on one side than the other, although the child's mother has, on occasion, seen the bulge.

Deeper Palpation: Spasm and Guarding

Actually, because evaluation of the inguinal rings can be so unsettling to patients, it is usually best delayed until later in the examination. Once such surface characteristics as contour, tone, and movement have been determined, it is best to proceed to the slightly deeper level of palpation that is required to determine muscular resistance, specifically whether or not spasm or guarding is present.

Spasm and guarding must be differentiated from each other. **Spasm,** or rigidity, is a reflex behavior of muscle that is caused by somatic peritoneal irritation. It is constant, it cannot be induced by the examiner, and the patient has no control over it. Stimuli from the afferent fibers in the irritated parietal peritoneum set up a reflex arc that results in the activation of spinal motor efferents. The muscle overlying the inflamed peritoneum is thereby thrown into spasm, and it stays that way until the inflammatory process is relieved.

Guarding, on the other hand, is completely voluntary, in the sense that the abdominal muscles tense up in response to a conscious cerebral message. The patient either feels pain or expects to do so momentarily, and so guards to protect himself. As opposed to spasm, which is a totally objective finding, guarding must be thought of as a subjective response. Its significance, therefore, varies from situation to situation, and from patient to patient. It must be interpreted; it should never be taken at face value.

Raising the question of differences between subjective and objective introduces an important element that bears on the entire field of physical diagnosis. There are certain findings on examination over which no patient or physician has an iota of control. Spasm, the presence of a mass, absent bowel sounds, and the like cannot be created by the most determined of actors. These are clinical clues that are completely dependable. Once an element of voluntary control can be introduced however, the clues become less reliable, and subject to personal influence, either by patient or physician. The possible significance of guarding, for example, may vary from being a true response to severe tenderness to something as far removed from reality as malingering, with a host of way stations in between. All rigidity is the same, but each person guards in his own way.

The difference between subjective and objective is particularly significant in the diagnosis of the acute abdomen, where important decisions must be made on very short acquaintance. It is easy to confuse the reliability of pain and tenderness, which are subjective, with that of intestinal rushes and palpable masses, which are objective. Equal weight in decision making must not be given to findings that are on different levels of patient control. Each of us has attended complications conferences at which negative explorations were reported; too often they are the result of relying on findings that, at least in retrospect, were unreliable. This is not to say that only patients who seek secondary gains present us with such fallacious clues; anyone who is sick enough will quickly lose his usual ability to withstand stimuli that, under ordinary circumstances, would produce no pathologic response. To be able to separate the meaningful from the misleading is a precious clinical skill.

Tenderness. An area of guarding or spasm will always overlie an area that is tender. The tenderness may be so marked that it can be detected merely by light percussion, or it may require deep palpation. Although the focus of the disease process usually lies in the tender area, the tightness of the overlying muscle may prevent the examiner from palpating as deeply as he would wish. For this reason, an inflammatory mass is easily missed by even the most experienced of physicians. This is why surgeons like to repalpate an abdomen after anesthesia has been induced prior to embarking on laparotomy.

As pointed out earlier, the area in which one anticipates eliciting the greatest tenderness is the last place that should be examined. While moving around the abdomen, getting closer and closer to the suspected focus, it is sometimes noticed that pressing down in some other quadrant causes discomfort that is referred to the location at which the pathology is expected to be found. An example is acute diverticulitis, in which pressure on the cecum will often produce pain in the left iliac fossa. For obvious reasons, this is called **referred tenderness.**

Another kind of remote control of elicited pain is what is called rebound tenderness, or simply **rebound.** This is induced by pressing down firmly at some more or less distant point and then quickly letting go. In patients with an intraperitoneal inflammatory process the sudden release of pressure causes a brief burst of intense pain in the location of the pathology. Persons with various types of enteritis are particularly sensitive to this form of peritoneal insult. Not only is the information obtained in this way rather gross and nonspecific, but many clinicians, the present one included, consider testing for rebound to be a form of cruel and unusual punishment. Whatever information is gained from it can be obtained just as well by the other methods of palpation. Although textbooks of physical diagnosis recommend it and junior house officers often seem to feel some perverse pride in proving its presence, it is mentioned here only to be condemned.

As might be expected, the anatomic location of direct tenderness is, in many cases, the single most important clue to diagnosis. It is easy to say this about such structures as the gallbladder or the sigmoid colon, whose location is relatively constant, but what about the appendix, which is loose and shaped like an elongated worm? After all, the tip of this skinny organ may be located down in the depths of the pelvis or lying high alongside the ascending colon, if not behind it. How, then, can an examiner know where to look for the tenderness of appendicitis? Well, the answer is that clinicians have been grappling with this problem ever since Reginald Fitz brought the disease to the world's attention almost exactly a century ago.

The diagnosis of appendicitis, thought by most laymen to be the simplest of medical tasks, can be one of the most challenging obstacles to a physician's diagnostic ingenuity. It does help to know that Charles McBurney proved to be more often right than wrong when he wrote in 1889 that "the seat of greatest pain, determined by the pressure of one finger, has been very exactly between an inch and a half and two inches from the anterior spinous process of the ilium on a straight line drawn from that process to the umbilicus." These days, we determine McBurney's point by moving one third of the way medially along that line, and we credit the New York surgeon with providing us with one of the most reliable of the eponyms that are scattered through the annals of diagnosis. The basis of the finding is the fact that the point at which the offending organ takes off from the cecum usually lies under the point of McBurney. The problem arises in those not uncommon appendices whose inflammatory process is limited to the distal segment of a particularly long or unusually placed worm. The difficulty is compounded when the clinical history is atypical, as it so often is. Accordingly, one must be prepared to seek the tenderness of appendicitis anywhere in the right lower quadrant, while remembering that there is scarcely an experienced surgeon alive who has not found it in the right upper or left lower quadrant. There are even a few grizzled veterans who can document a left upper quadrant appendicitis, not necessarily accompanied by a malrotation.

Rigidity. Spasm has thus far been described as though it occurs always in relatively localized areas of the abdominal wall, directly over the primary focus of the pathology. Actually, since it is due to irritation of the parietal peritoneum, it can be detected wherever the disease process has produced such a condition. If peritonitis is generalized, as in perforated duodenal ulcer, the entire abdominal wall is likely to be in such spasm that the term "boardlike rigidity" is used to describe it. Boardlike rigidity is one of the most dramatic findings in clinical diagnosis; once encountered, it will never be forgotten. It is as striking as is the radiographic presence of free air that so often accompanies it.

Patient Relaxation

As might be imagined, it is not always easy for a person with severe pain to sufficiently relax his abdominal wall for unhindered palpation to be carried out. For some, complete relaxation is impossible even under conditions of robust health. It is the responsibility of the examiner to create an atmosphere, insofar as it is possible, of enough reassurance and comfort to allow the maximum degree of co-operation. The charged surroundings of an emergency room, the apprehension of the unknown to come, the well-meaning intrusions of a newly met physician, what-ever psychosocial baggage the patient carries, the childlike helplessness induced by the illness itself—all of these are factors that intrude themselves into the process of optimal diagnostic collaboration between patient and doctor.

In those cases in which patience, gentleness, and a soothing manner are to no avail, a few physical methods are useful. Asking the patient to breathe slowly and deeply through the mouth will produce at least a minor degree of softening of the tightened musculature; I have found that requesting that the patient count up to a certain number of breaths seems to concentrate his attention away from me and my doings just a bit better than deep respiration by itself. Distracting the patient with idle conversation may contribute a bit more of a sense of ease, especially if the topic is something as innocuous as sports or morning traffic. Pain produced by coughing is a peritoneal sign that can be elicited in even the most recalcitrant patient, but only once. Drawing up the knees will always take some of the tight stretching out of the rectus muscles, and also seems to have the added advantage, at least for some patients, of letting them feel less exposed.

If all else fails, use the old stethoscope palpation trick, otherwise known as the furtive feel. Although particularly useful in those cases where you suspect the validity of a patient's history, guarding, and motives, it is also of considerable value for an unusually apprehensive person. While pretending to be deeply involved in auscultation, gradually and surreptitiously press the diaphragm of the stethoscope deeper and deeper into the tissues of the abdomen. Fortunately, the practice of medicine is not yet inhibited by some kind of Miranda law of physical diagnosis—evidence obtained in this way is not only admissible, but may prove to be crucial to solving the case.

Abdominal Texture and Tone
As the palpating hand is exploring ever deeper into the abdominal wall, an increasing sense of its texture and tone will become apparent. The symmetrical firm bulging of tense fluid in the cirrhotic patient is usually distinguishable from the more irregular enlargement produced by distended intestine. The abdomen of a patient with acute pancreatitis will sometimes feel like a large mound of unbaked bread, hence the term "doughy" that is applied to it. These observations can be made while evaluating for muscular quality, tone, spasm, and tenderness.

Visual Correlates of Palpation
It is easy to become so absorbed by the patient's abdomen that his face is forgotten. Look at the patient frequently, for several reasons. In the first place, empathetic eye contact is a continuing reinforcement of that most important message a doctor can give to one who has come to be healed: caring. Second, changes in facial expression bespeak responses to the stimuli induced during the physical examination. A wince or a grimace will betray what may otherwise be yielded up only with reluctance by a stoic patient, or one who feels that it is necessary to appear brave. Holding the breath may have the same significance. Attention should be paid to the rhythm of respiration, which may be interrupted when a sudden pain occurs or tenderness is unexpectedly induced. There is a sign named after Chicago surgeon John Murphy, which is elicited by pressing the fingertips upward under the right costal margin and asking the patient to take a deep inspiration. If he has acute cholecystitis his breath will catch in the middle of its course. Unfortunately, the diagnostic value of Murphy's sign is lessened some-what by the sensitivity of Glisson's capsule, which will cause many normal subjects to have the same response.

Deep Palpation: Organs

Having evaluated tenderness and spasm, the next level of depth is used to determine the palpability of organs. The **liver** is a good place to begin. The simplest technique involves the same maneuver as has just been described. The examiner's fingertips are held steady, somewhat deep under the costal margin, as a long breath is taken by the patient. At the very end of inspiration, the leading edge of a normal liver is barely, if at all, felt. Anything more than this connotes enlargement. It may be possible to "flip" the edge under the examining fingers, to confirm the fact that it is sharp and healthy. Nodular, irregular livers are found in cirrhotics and in patients with metastatic malignancy, in whom the nodules tend to be quite hard. Actually, the liver of the long-standing cirrhotic patient is likely to be shrunken, fibrotic, and impossible to feel. If the right lobe is easily felt, and especially if it is irregular, try to outline the left as well. Although I hesitate to describe a finding I have never encountered, it is said that the liver of a patient with tricuspid insufficiency can be felt to be pulsating.

There are times when it may be rewarding to feel for the hepatic edge from above. To do this, stand alongside the patient's right hemithorax and curl the fingers of either hand under the costal margin. A deep inspiration may bring the liver edge down to your fingertips.

A distended **gallbladder** is most prominent at the point where the lateral margin of the right rectus muscle reaches the costal arch (see Figure 6.4). If the gallbladder feels like a smooth, well-rounded light bulb that is minimally or not at all tender it is far less likely to be the site of cholecystitis than it is to be a hydrops or a Courvoisier effect. Courvoisier pointed out that a gallbladder that is chronically inflamed cannot easily dilate when the pressure rises within the biliary tree. Therefore, he reasoned, a jaundiced patient whose gallbladder is dilated will have an obstruction that is neoplastic in nature, rather than a common duct stone. Although this "law" is helpful, especially on teaching rounds, it is not even reliable enough to call it a rule of thumb.

Modern hepatobiliary imaging (HIDA) scans confirm a long-standing clinical impression that acute cholecystitis is almost always accompanied by an obstructed cystic duct. This means that the patient with this disease, providing his common duct is normal, will dilate the gallbladder to some degree. The more attacks the patient has had or the greater the chronicity of his condition, the more scarred the organ becomes and the less it can enlarge. Therefore, the person with acute cholecystitis can have any of a number of physical findings in the right upper quadrant, the only shared one being tenderness. A simple example is the presence of a tender, rounded flasklike structure in a patient with relatively recent onset of disease. If protected by omentum, the mass may be large and irregular. If chronic changes are marked, the organ may be shrunken and impalpable, particularly if there is not much omentum near its fundus. As noted, the only unifying factor is the presence of right upper quadrant tenderness, which should always raise the suspicion of cholecystitis.

Although it is important to know how best to detect splenomegaly, the opportunity to do so does not come often. Usually, we feel for the **spleen** to assure ourselves that it is *not* enlarged, rather than to demonstrate that it *is*. As noted earlier, it requires an increase in size of approximately three times before the organ descends below the costal margin. Because its hilar structures function mechanically like a pedicle, and because it has no dorsal or superior attachments, the spleen, when a bit heavy, can sometimes be made to pitch forward when the patient assumes the correct position, which is similar to that introduced by Marion Sims for vaginal delivery or examination 125 years ago. The patient lies on his right side, not in the true lateral but pitched forward so that the weight is largely supported by the bent left knee resting on the bed just anterior to the right. The examiner stands behind, with the fingers of either hand curled around the costal margin while a deep breath is taken. The hand should be moved along the entire expanse of the bony rim, breath after breath, because a spleen that cannot be felt anteriorly is sometimes palpable as the flank is reached. In the dorsal recumbent position, in fact, splenomegaly is often most apparent laterally.

There is an interesting difference between the effects of deep inspiration on the liver and the spleen, respectively. As the diaphragm descends, its pressure on the wide expanse of the liver's dome forces that organ to descend with it, directly downward. The spleen lies against the lowermost reach of the left costophrenic recess; when a deep breath is taken, this posterior curve of the diaphragm moves not only downward, but anteriorly as well, since the recess is enlarged by the process. The result of this is to project the spleen forward and inferomedially, making it somewhat easier to feel when advantage is also taken of the relative laxity of its attachments by using the Sims position.

Although bimanual methods for hepatic and splenic palpation are often recommended, I have never been able to convince myself that they have any substantial advantage over what has been described in the foregoing passages. For finding the **kidneys,** however, bimanual examination is essential. One hand is placed behind the flank and pressure is applied in an anterior direction, between the posterior rim of the iliac crest and the short projections of the lowermost ribs. By pushing the kidney forward in this way, it may be possible in thin patients to feel it against the other hand placed anteriorly. Because the right kidney lies lower than the left, this is the one more commonly identified, although if conditions are optimal the lower pole of the left will be similarly found. It is helpful to know that a kidney does not move with respiration.

There are other things to feel in the upper abdomen. The thick knot at the gastric outlet of an infant with pyloric stenosis really does feel like an olive, and describing it so is one of the few allowable exceptions to a rule that will be expounded below. An elderly patient who presents with painless jaundice very likely has carcinoma of the pancreas, a diagnosis that is supported by finding a fixed, nontender, poorly defined mass in the right upper quadrant. Cancers in the distal stomach are not infrequently palpable, and are even found to be movable if they have not yet become fixed to surrounding tissues.

Abdominal masses should be described by clear, unambiguous words. It is not very helpful to speak of a tumor that is "plum-sized" or "like a baby's fist," when one can just as easily speak in centimeters. This brings up one of the most common traps into which English-speaking physicians fall: We talk in centimeters but we think in inches. The next time you are about to describe something as being 5 centimeters in size, pick up a ruler; 5 centimeters is a much shorter distance than you think. What we call 5 centimeters is usually very close to 5 inches. The best way to circumvent this cross-cultural mensural madness is to once and for all take a measurement of the width of the distal or middle phalanges of your second and third digits lying side by side. You will then have an accurate gauge right at your fingertips, as it were. Waste no energy being amazed at how much bigger the numbers become in your admission work-ups thereafter.

To describe a mass precisely, it is necessary to use a string of adjectives that tell a great deal about its characteristics in a minimal number of words. Texture, fixation, size, degree of tenderness, location, and consistency are some of the most common qualities that need to be recorded. It is a good habit when palpating any structure to go through the whole drill of trying to determine as many features as possible. Put yourself in the position of someone reading your clinical notes. Your objective is to transmit to that person an impression so clear that he can mentally feel what you are feeling, and duplicate in his imagination the sensations imparted to your palpating fingers.

The muscular tone in the lower abdomen of most people is more lax than it is in the upper. Accordingly, a mass that is caudal to the umbilicus is easier felt than if it were higher, even though, for the anatomic reasons given earlier, most upper abdominal structures in general lie closer to the anterior parietes. Thus, a fixed, tender mass is usually palpable in the left iliac fossa in cases of acute diverticulitis, and is easily distinguishable from a sigmoid colon filled with hard stool. An appendiceal abscess may be prominent enough so that it can not only be felt, but also seen bulging out prominently in the right lower quadrant. Peritoneal carcinomatosis is sometimes palpable, as are large retroperitoneal lymphomas.

Since the sac of an incarcerated hernia lies just deep to the subcutaneous tissue, it presents as a visible, palpable, fixed, often tender structure protruding through its ring. A sensation of crepitus in the overlying or surrounding skin is a portent of strangulation and necrosis.

Before taking leave of the subject of palpation, there is a significant fact about **abdominal fat** distribution to which attention should be called, because it affects an examiner's ability to discriminate, and sometimes influences his interpretation of findings. The adipose tissue of adult females is predominantly subcutaneous, whereas that of males is much more heavily concentrated in the omentum. That is why an elderly obese man walking on a beach looks like he has swallowed a watermelon, whereas his equally overweight wife quivers like a bowl of jelly. It is a predictable surgical observation that, regardless of degree of obesity, few males have a great deal of subcutaneous fat. At the same time, even slender women have a significant layer that must be traversed before the fascia is reached. The opposite is true of the omentum. Moreover, the fat of women tends to be softer and, when present in large amounts, even a bit fluffy. That of men is more firm, and its less yielding character presents far more difficulty when dissecting in the abdominal cavity. These differences in distribution and texture mean that the challenges of palpation are sufficiently different in the two sexes that they must be taken into account.

RECTAL EXAMINATION

Some of the most valuable information to be learned about the abdominal organs is obtained by an examination of the rectum. There is no part of physical diagnosis where gentleness and tact are more important. Not only will a patient feel degraded by a brusque, plunging digit thrust rudely into his body, but he will, with good reason, resist it enough to make examination difficult. First, it is necessary to assure the patient concerning the routine nature of what is about to happen, using words that soothe rather than alarm. There are multiple variations on this theme, but it is usually not very threatening to say something like, "Now I'm going to slide a finger gently into your rectum. It may feel a little strange, but it usually doesn't hurt. If it does, it is important for you to tell me, so that I don't keep touching the painful spot."

Several different positions have been described for intrarectal palpation, and each has its advantages. For example, the prostate is best felt when the patient is standing with legs slightly spread, leaning over the examining table; the knee-chest position allows the more movable viscera, such as bowel loops, to fall away, thus getting rid of extraneous structures that sometimes cause confusion as they are felt through the rectal wall; a squatting posture, with the examiner's finger inserted directly upward, does just the opposite, so that higher structures come down in such a way as to extend the limits of the exploration—a tumor high in the rectum may thus become palpable.

However, considering all factors, as well as the relative immobility of some patients, particularly the elderly or the acutely ill, the most useful positions are the true lateral and the Sims. A right-handed examiner will do best to stand behind the patient, who is lying with his left side down. The opposite obviously applies for physicians who are lefties.

The first step is to simply lift the uppermost buttock and look. Pilonidal sinuses, condylomata, external hemorrhoids, skin tags, or a sentinel pile may be seen and perianal infections evaluated. The gloved finger is then heavily lubricated and its pad (most emphatically *not* its tip) is placed against the anal opening, with the extended digit held in the axis of the intergluteal fold, pointing anteriorly. The finger is gradually worked through the external sphincter mechanism with a bit of a rotatory motion, most of the gentle pressure being exerted posteriorly. If the patient tightens up in spite of all the physician's efforts, he should be asked to push down as though moving his bowels. This relaxes the sphincter and usually allows the finger to slide in as easily as promised.

Once inside the copious rectal ampulla, the extended digit may be turned in any direction. Anteriorly, it will pass over the prostate, whose normal condition is smooth, firm (it is often described as "rubbery"), and nontender. A clean central groove separates the two lateral lobes, either one of which may harbor the hard nodule that signifies cancer.

Palpate each quadrant of the rectum in sequence, taking plenty of time if no objection is heard from the patient. In women, the cervix is felt as a ballotable, smooth, rounded structure high against the fingertip anteriorly. Put firm pressure on it to be sure that it moves enough to stretch the peritoneal folds to which the female genitalia are attached. A woman with pelvic inflammatory disease will complain of severe discomfort at this point, some of which comes from the cervix itself. Patients with appendicitis, diverticulitis, or other causes of pelvic peritonitis may exhibit tenderness of varying degree.

Push the fingertip firmly against the rectal wall on all sides, as high as you can go, in order to identify any tenderness, masses, or abscess pockets that are present. To reach maximum height it is helpful to turn the hand sideways in order that the gluteal tuberosities do not catch against the palm. Remember that the rectum lies in a plane directed toward the umbilicus. Having the patient push down will bring another centimeter or two into your reach, and may reveal the edge of a rectal tumor or pelvic mass that might otherwise be overlooked.

There are several specific pathologic findings for which one should look. Tenderness has already been mentioned, as has abscess. The pelvic phlegmon that accompanies sigmoid diverticulitis is often felt as a tender, boggy fullness high on the left side. If palpable, it becomes a useful finding by which to follow the course of the disease process when it is being treated nonoperatively. The same type of thing is sometimes felt high on the right or in the midline in cases of appendicitis or Meckel's diverticulitis. An acute flare-up of Crohn's disease can likewise be manifested by a tender, thickened posterior peritoneum. A pelvic abscess from whatever cause is rounded and fluctuant, and may be "pointing" into the anterior rectal wall.

A rectal cancer is nodular and hard, especially at its attachment to the mucosa. It may be found in such a state of advanced infiltration that it has fixed the bowel wall to surrounding tissues. A small lump, perhaps on a stalk, is probably an adenomatous polyp. A villous adenoma is a soft, rather billowing structure that lies sessile on the mucosa.

It is important to distinguish between growths that arise from the mucosa of the rectum and those extrarectal masses that are palpable through its wall. A uterine or ovarian tumor, a retroperitoneal lymphoma, a sigmoid cancer, or even hard stool in adjacent bowel loops can usually be recognized by the fact that the mucosa at the tip of the probing finger is easily movable across the lump in question when it arises from elsewhere. In cases of metastatic intra-abdominal carcinoma a hard, nodular mass is sometimes felt anteriorly in Douglas' pouch or just cephalad to the prostate. Because the exploring digit can usually be hooked over its top, it is called Blumer's shelf, after the Yale physician who first described it near the turn of the 20th century.

Just before completing the examination, ask the patient to squeeze the anal opening tightly around your finger. This will provide a good estimate of sphincter tone, which is impaired not only in certain chronic neurologic conditions, but is often found to be reflexly inhibited in acute disease processes that result in peritonitis low in the pelvis. When the exploring digit has been removed from the rectum, carefully look at any stool that adheres to the glove. Examine it for color, gross blood, mucus, tissue shreds, and particles. A chemical test for occult blood ends the examination, and this chapter.

REFERENCES

1. Clain H: *Demonstrations of Physical Signs in Clinical Surgery,* ed 17. Chicago, Year Book Medical Publishers, 1980.

2. Browse NL: *An Introduction to the Symptoms and Signs of Surgical Disease.* London, Edward Arnold, 1978.

3. Burnside JW: *Physical Diagnosis,* ed 17. Baltimore, Williams & Wilkins, 1986.

4. DeGowin EL, DeGowin RL: *Bedside Diagnostic Examination,* ed 4. New York, Macmillan, 1981.

5. Delp MH, Manning RT: *Major's Physical Diagnosis,* ed 9. Philadelphia, W.B. Saunders, 1981.

6. Judge RD, Zuidema GD, Fitzgerald FT: *Methods of Clinical Examination: A Physiologic Approach,* ed 4. Boston, Little, Brown, 1982.

7. Prior JA, Silberstein JS, Stang JM: *Physical Diagnosis,* ed 6. St. Louis, C.V. Mosby, 1981.

8. Sreenivas VI: *Acute Disorders of the Abdomen.* New York, Springer-Verlag, 1980.

9. Walker HK, Hall WD, Hurst JW: *Clinical Methods,* ed 2. Boston, Butterworth, 1980.

7

Examination of the Breasts

Sherwin B. Nuland, M.D.

A thorough examination of the breast is essential. It can save the patient's life if a lesion is located early. Mammography has now enabled us to find lesions that are not felt during a breast examination, but this does not preclude a very careful clinical examination.

The incidence of breast cancer is on the increase, currently being reported as 95,000 cases per year. The earlier the cancer is found, without involvement of lymph nodes, the greater the chances for prolonged survival. Rightfully, women have great trepidation in anticipation of this examination that something will be discovered. Dr. Nuland has given us his experience on the most judicious and tactful way to perform a breast examination in order to elicit suspicious signs that require careful clinical assessment and follow-up.

The female patient, and, for that matter, the male one, too, will be greatly assured if a thorough examination is performed in a step-by-step fashion, as outlined in the text, rather than just a sloppy, quick exam that serves no purpose for the patient or the physician.

For a woman having her breasts examined, there is no possible way to feel calm. Whether she expresses it overtly or somehow manages the outward appearance of composure, nothing less than a physician's reassurance that all is well can put a halt to the frightened wanderings of her imagination. She has read too much, and perhaps experienced too much, to approach this part of the physical examination with anything resembling a serene mind. Whether or not she is aware of the dreadful statistic that 1 of 11 American women will at some time in their lives be found to have breast cancer, she will certainly know that the disease is very common and that its course can be devastating. At the very least, she will fear surgery, disfigurement, and the discomforts of therapy. Her anxieties may reach much further, to terrifying fantasies that involve the loss of self-esteem, love, and life itself.

It should not surprise the physician that even the most routine of breast examinations will evoke such mental meanderings. Whether it is the yearly checkup, the pre-employment physical, or the scrutiny of a breast surgeon, there is no such thing, from the patient's point of view, as a fear-free ride. This is one of the several reasons that there must also be no such thing as a cursory "going over" of the breasts. There is too much at stake ever to relegate this part of the evaluation of any patient to the realm of the superficial or hurried. We must be even more sensitive and attentive to detail when we evaluate a woman's breasts than we are in other aspects of our relationship with her.

One need not be blessed with a superabundance of empathy to appreciate the foregoing statements. It is only necessary to read the contemporary lay press to acquire some comprehension of the fears, both realistic and groundless, that are attached by modern women to a diagnosis of breast cancer. As if that were not enough, the disease and its treatment have become one of the battlegrounds in the perennial war between the sexes, the struggle being not the least bit mitigated by the fact that, in increasing numbers, the breast surgeons are themselves women. The result of all of this brewing-up of the pathologic with the sociologic is that physicians of today need an emotional armamentarium in which skill and training are matched by equivalent measures of tact, kindness, and forebearance.

Even if we are prepared to neglect our role as complete physicians, there are some obvious cold facts to think about, chief among which is that simple statistic of 1 out of 11. Consider the care lavished on the routine sigmoidoscopy, a procedure of much lower yield than that which we are discussing. Although the likelihood of finding a cancer of the rectosigmoid in an asymptomatic patient is far less, we are never satisfied unless every square centimeter of visible bowel mucosa has been peered at both going in and coming out. We listen carefully to each little noise and squeak made by the lungs, although a chest x-ray is usually much more accurate a diagnostic tool than even the most astute pair of ears. Yet, a quick pass of the hand over the breast is often the sum total of the physical examination of a structure in which palpation and inspection are far superior to all other diagnostic techniques combined.

Another virtue of careful breast examination is the opportunity it gives to follow sequential changes that may occur in the palpable tissue. In no other organ of the body is it more valuable to have careful records that may be compared to later findings. The quick pass does not allow such detailed observations to be made. Later comparisons are rendered useless by a vague memory that "I'm sure I would have noticed something there last time," if there are no recorded facts to which to refer. Remember that, although cancer is only one of the abnormalities that may be found in mammary tissue, its discovery is often made possible by recognizing that significant changes have occurred during the course of follow-up of a benign condition.

Because the breast is so directly drained by certain well-defined lymphatic pathways, the complete evaluation covers a much wider area than that of the mammary tissue alone. The field of examination stretches from the leading edge of one latissimus dorsi to the other, and from the lower neck downward almost as far as the costal margins. This wide expanse of tissue must be inspected in various positions and from various angles; it must be felt and probed, and must sometimes be moulded between the fingers, squeezed, or even pinched. It is not a job for an examiner who feels rushed, and it is certainly not a job for an examiner who has no sense of the emotional implications of his/her touch and words.

Fortunately, most modern hospital gowns are so made that it is possible for a woman to expose only that part of her body that is being evaluated, without a great deal of rearranging of clothes and sheets. Advantage should certainly be taken of this fact if it is the physician's sense that minimal exposure will best serve the patient's needs. However, in all frankness, it must be stated that it is quite difficult

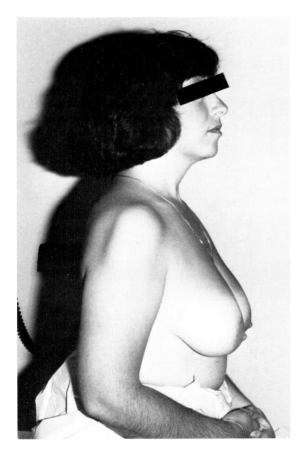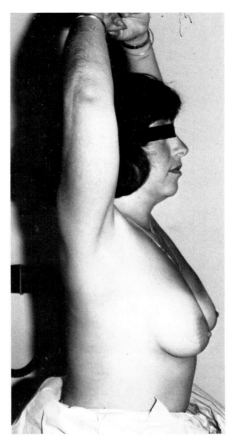

FIGURE 7.1   Breast inspection from an upright lateral angle: (a) in a resting position and (b) with arms elevated.

to carry out an adequate inspection if the patient is clothed above the waist. In practice, it is rare that this condition cannot be achieved without undue discomfiture.

INSPECTION

It is best to commence the inspection of the breasts with the patient in the sitting position with arms at her sides (Figures 7.1 and 7.2). The entire field should be looked over, and then each individual area evaluated separately. Protrusion of a supraclavicular fat pad may be a clue to underlying lymphadenopathy in the same way that a tumor in the superficial tissues of the breast may produce a visible bulge. Asymmetry between the two sides is best appreciated in this position. A slight degree of asymmetry is to be expected in the breasts of virtually all women, but large tumors may exaggerate it to a marked degree.

Look carefully at the nipples for inversion, retraction, or the eczematoid or even weeping appearance that is characteristic of Paget's disease. Inversion and retraction are two different phenomena, and have vastly different connotations. **Inversion** is basically a normal finding, which the patient will state has been present

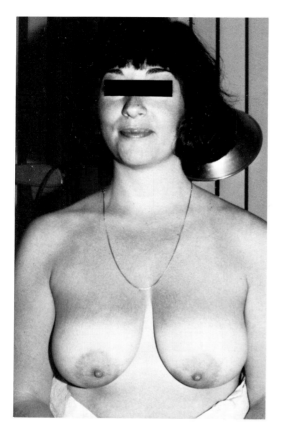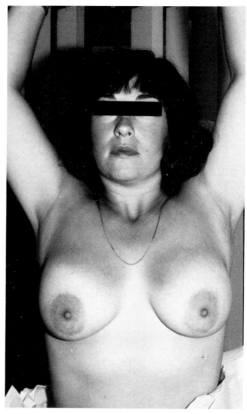

FIGURE 7.2   Breast inspection from an upright anterior angle: (a) in a resting position; (b) with arms elevated.

as long as she can remember, either on one side or both. The inverted nipple lies in a soft furrow, from which it can sometimes be withdrawn. **Retraction,** on the other hand, is the result of a pathological process by which the nipple is drawn back into the mammary tissue by a fibrosing or neoplastic process in the underlying breast. If the disease is in the retroareolar area, the nipple is pulled directly backward; if it lies to one side or the other, the retraction will be in that direction. A closely lying tumor may distort nipple symmetry in another way as well; by pulling on the tissues near the areola, it may cause that structure, even when not retracted, to point away from its normal direction.

No author has ever improved upon the description of the appearance of the normal breast and nipple written by Sir Astley Cooper in the early 19th century. It is to Cooper that we owe our knowledge of the ligaments that bear his name, suspending the breast tissue from the skin in front and the pectoralis fascia behind, and merging into the fibrous septa within the mammary gland itself. These septa and the fact that they are continuous with Cooper's ligaments will often provide a useful clue to the existence of a cancer, as will be described below. Here is Astley Cooper's appreciation of a part of the human anatomy and physiology that has fascinated poets, lovers, and scientific investigators, for varied (and sometimes similar) reasons.

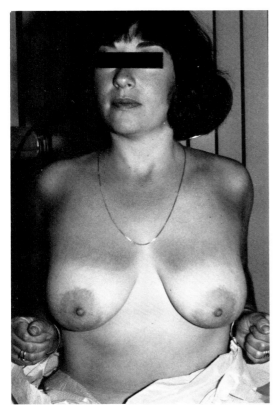 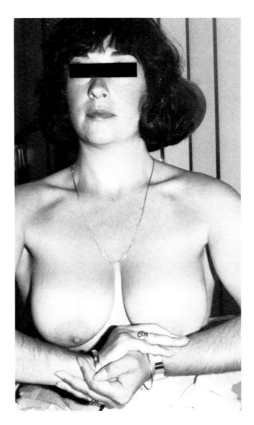

FIGURE 7.2 *(continued)*   **(c) with elbows behind back, and (d) tightening**
pectoralis major muscle.

This natural obliquity of the mammilla, or nipple, forwards and
outwards, with the slight turn of the nipple upwards, is one of the
most beautiful provisions in nature, both for the mother and the
child. To the mother, because the child rests upon her arm and
lap in the most convenient position for sucking; for if the nipple
and breast had projected directly forwards, the child must have
been supported before her by the mother's hands in the most
inconvenient and fatiguing position, instead of its reclining upon
her side and arm. But it is wisely provided by nature, that when
the child reposes upon its mother's arm, it has its mouth directly applied to the nipple, which is turned outwards to receive it, whilst the
lower part of the breast forms a cushion upon which the cheek of
the infant tranquilly reposes. Thus it is we have always to ad-
mire the simplicity, the beauty, and the utility, of these deviations of form in the construction of the body, which the
imagination of man would lead him, a priori, to believe most
symmetrical, natural, and convenient.

Local changes in skin color are usually of significance. **Erythema** may signal an inflammatory process that is either benign or malignant. The so-called inflammatory cancers of the breast are caused by mechanical obstruction of the draining lymphatics by cancer cells, a blockage that results not only in redness, but also in a characteristic type of edema, called *peau d'orange*. This appearance is due to a thickening of the skin that exaggerates the prominence of the hair follicle openings, so that the entire brawny appearance is that of orange peel. Sometimes the tumor that wreaks all of this havoc can be felt as a large mass within the tissues, but often the degree of thickness and edema is too great to allow anything but a generalized induration to be appreciated.

Erythema may also, of course, be caused by any benign inflammatory condition of the breast. In general, this type of red skin is less likely to be edematous than the malignant form, and the *peau d'orange* phenomenon is virtually never found. The margins of the erythema are more diffuse than one finds with cancer, where the edges of involvement may actually be quite well demarcated. A diffuse redness over a tender fluctuant mass in the breast of a relatively young women, especially postpartum, will almost certainly be an abscess.

A visible **bruise or ecchymosis** in the breast of a woman being evaluated for a lump should not lull the examiner into a false sense of security that he is dealing with a benign mass secondary to injury. Some breast tumors bleed with minimal trauma, including that of a recent physical examination or even a mammogram. There is an oft-told old wives' tale that spreads the fiction that breast cancer is caused by injury; the central character in the story is always a woman with a bruised skin, under which some wise consulting doctor finds a new growth.

It may be possible, with simple inspection, to detect **skin retraction.** This finding is produced by any process that results in a pulling on the fibrous septa that is transmitted to the subcuticular Cooper's ligaments, so that the overlying dermis is drawn inward. Although local inflammatory processes, like fat necrosis, may occasionally cause this, such a degree of traction will be found almost always to be due to a malignant process. Skin retraction is therefore an important physical finding when evaluating a breast mass. It is sometimes difficult to distinguish from actual invasion of the skin, which bears a much more grave prognosis.

Although retraction, when present, is sometimes seen on direct observation, it may be made more striking by any of a variety of maneuvers that enhance the degree to which the fibrous tissues pull on the skin. Raising the arms high in the air will accomplish this in some cases (Figures 7.1b and 7.2b), while asking the patient to attempt to touch her elbows together behind her back will do it in others (Figure 7.2c). Sometimes leaning far forward with the hands supported by those of the examiner will allow the breasts to hang enough to increase retraction or to demonstrate that a portion of the mammary tissue, being fixed by tumor, does not fall away from the thoracic cage as freely as the rest. Obviously, any movement that tightens up the pectoral muscles will pull on breast tissue and exaggerate the shortening of the fibrous bands. This is nicely accomplished by having the patient place the heels of the two palms against each other with one set of fingers pointing toward the ceiling and the other toward the floor. Firm pressure of one palm against the other will bring the pectoralis major muscle out in tight relief, exerting significant traction on the shortened ligaments (Figure 7.2d). The same result may be accomplished by placing the heel of each hand on the ipsilateral iliac crest and pushing inward with force. Generally, tightening the pectoralis major muscle will have its predominant effect on the upper portion of the chest. Particularly in older women, or those with large pendulous breasts, there will be little or no pull exerted below the higher portion of the upper quadrants.

Any of the maneuvers that result in traction on the tissues of the breast will also serve to increase the tendency of an underlying mass to bulge out. Thus, the above movements will not infrequently make visible a tumor that could not be seen while the patient sat quietly. Since some women present themselves with a mass they have already found, it is important for the examiner to ask its location, lest he/she miss a very subtle bit of retraction that might be seen if particular attention were paid to that spot. The false pride of the physician who wants to find a known mass on his/her own is of no help to the patient.

On the subject of pride, your own may one day get itself justifiably puffed up if you can remember the eponym of a finding so rare that it appears only once or twice, if at all, in the average clinical lifetime. This is **Mondor's disease,** a superficial phlebitis in the thoracoepigastric vein, a vessel that courses vertically in the subcutaneous tissues over the lateral aspect of the breast. The presenting symptom is a tender area or cord that, on close inspection, reveals itself to be an inflamed venous channel. When the disease has subsided, it may leave a retracted furrow of varying length that is easily mistaken for a more ominous finding.

Although far less exotic or soul-satisfying to diagnose than Mondor's disease, **accessory breasts or supernumary nipples** can provide an interesting brief conversation piece, particularly when the patient has been unaware of their presence. Most often, they are found on the chest wall just inferior to the breast. However, they have been reported in a variety of locations along the embryologic milk line that runs from the anterior axilla to the groin. A bit of mammary tissue is commonly present just deep to the rudimentary areola.

PALPATION

The ability to palpate the tissues of the breast with gentle thoroughness, so as to make some sense out of the sometimes confusing array of lumps and bumps that present themselves for interpretation, is one of the most valuable skills that a clinician can acquire. Without downplaying the great contributions of the various imaging techniques, it is safe to say that the physician's sensitive fingers remain the best defense against an undiagnosed cancer. Every experienced breast surgeon will agree that a positive mammogram is rarely wrong, but he/she will also be quick to add that a negative study in a patient with a palpably worrisome mass will often prove to be erroneous. At our present stage of technologic advancement, the mammogram is at its most useful in confirming the examiner's impression, and in the identification of lesions too small to feel. Even the addition, when indicated, of ultrasonography has not changed this state of affairs. As yet, such newer techniques as thermography and diaphanography await further development and testing.

Although most of the palpation of the various parts of the field is done with the patient supine, the upright position is most useful for examining the areas of lymphatic drainage. After careful observation of the supraclavicular fossae and lower neck, these foci are felt from the anterior position, and then again with the examiner standing behind the patient. While thus situated, a good opportunity presents itself to palpate the thyroid gland. It is not at all unusual to find a previously unsuspected nodule in this way, particularly in the gland of a young woman.

The Axillae

With the physician remaining behind the patient, the axillae should be evaluated. This portion of the examination is often rendered inadequate by a lack of appreciation of the full anatomic extent of this crucial area. Its inner margin is formed by the bony thorax, which arches away medially as one goes higher into the apex of the axilla. As a result, it is necessary to intrude the fingertips quite far up into a tight corner, in order to reach the topmost edge of the field. The moderate discomfort that may be caused by this probing is unavoidable if a thorough search is to be made. Having insinuated the digits up this high, their volar pads should be used to press the axillary contents against the ribs, in order to feel lymph nodes as distinct structures. The hand should then be turned somewhat anteriorly, with the palm side facing the anterior axillary wall, which is formed by the posterior aspect of the lateralmost section of the pectoralis major muscle. The right axilla is examined by the physician's right hand, and vice versa. The opposite hand is passed over the patient's shoulder and is used to press the pectoralis posteriorly, thereby pushing the axillary fat into a more confined space, and making it easier to evaluate. The fat of the armpit is actually somewhat fluffy, being softer than the adipose tissue in most other parts of the body, and therefore quite compressible. For this reason, it is not difficult, when palpation is carried out properly, to make accurate judgments about the presence or absence of enlarged or hard nodes. However, involved nodes are sometimes neither enlarged *nor* hard, resulting in the well-known statistic that one of four breast cancer victims whose axillae are clinically negative will be found to bear tumor in that location when the glands are studied by the pathologist.

While examining the axilla, it may be helpful to have the patient put her arm into various positions to allow easier access or to make individual nodes stand out more clearly. It is my own preference to ask that the arm be raised somewhat to allow the fingers to enter, after which the tissues are permitted to fall back into the relaxed unstretched state by lowering the extremity to the side.

The Breast

The point has now come to palpate the breast itself. The only way to identify the abnormal is to have an abiding appreciation of the extraordinarily wide range of normal. To this end, no opportunity should be lost to examine the breasts of each patient who presents herself to the clinic for whatever reason that may involve a general physical evaluation. As noted earlier, such an examination, when properly conducted, is of immense value to the woman herself, and is also of immense value to the physician and all of his succeeding patients. To put it in the form of a paradox, there is no structure in the body as atypical as the typical breast.

Having invoked Astley Cooper, perhaps this is the point at which to recall some wise words of yet another major force in medical history. Galen (131-201) wrote on a wide variety of subjects encompassing what was known of medicine in his lifetime. Until the late Renaissance, his works, with those of Hippocrates, formed the basis of all medical education, large sections of them being committed to memory by those who aspired to the acme of clinical wisdom. Living during a time of speculation and conjecture, he made many mistakes and committed many misjudgments, but he was right on the mark when, agreeing with Hippocrates, he described the ideal length of the fingernails. As we are about to launch into a description of breast palpation, it might be a good idea to think of his advice, here presented in Margaret Tallmadge May's elegant translation of his *On the Usefulness of the Parts of the Body.*

> Only nails that come even with the ends of the fingers will best
> provide the service for the sake of which they were made. It is
> for this reason that Hippocrates too has said, "The nails neither
> to project beyond, nor to fall short of, the finger tips."

It was Galen's contention that nails that are too short do not provide enough support for the finger pulp, and those that are too long are likely to dig into surfaces they touch. The application of all of this to the palpation of the delicate skin of the breast is too obvious to require amplification. It is pertinent as well to the examination of any other part of the body. Causing unnecessary discomfort not only bespeaks thoughtlessness, but smacks of a particular kind of disrespect for the patient as well. The admonition of Galen and Hippocrates should be made retroactive to the first page of this book.

Although the mammary tissues are most effectively palpated when they spread themselves flat on the chest wall of the supine woman, there is some value in examining while the patient is still sitting upright. This is particularly true when the breasts are pendulous. A bimanual technique may here be utilized, gently compressing the hanging structure between a hand which lies behind it and one that lies in front. I have seen several elderly women whose tumor could be satisfactorily felt in no other way, and one in whom it was otherwise unrecognizable.

The patient is now asked to lie flat (Figure 7.3). Some authors recommend that a small pillow be placed behind the shoulder of the side being evaluated, but I have not routinely found this to add any advantage. Before beginning to palpate, another careful inspection should be made, since the supine position tends to spread and flatten the mammary tissue enough to thin it out, thereby causing an occasional previously invisible nodule to protrude.

Taking into account the slight ridging produced by the ribs, the chest wall forms a firm background against which to compress the overlying breast. It is almost as though a loosely filled bag of mammary tissue were lying splayed out onto the curving surface of a tortoise shell. The examiner should compress the tissue gently and firmly between his hand and this underlying surface as though attempting to flatten it. This is the best way to appreciate the subtle differences in nodularity and texture that may be present in different parts of the breast. It will make a significant lump feel like a bulge that has quite a different texture from anything in its vicinity. The term "dominant mass" is often used to describe such a nodular hillock, which is palpable in a field of beads of varying sizes. It may have the hard quality of a definite cancer, or it may simply be more firm than surrounding tissue. It may be quite regular and movable, portending probable benignity, or it may be irregular and fixed, which makes it far more likely to be malignant. If it is a cyst, and of large enough size, it may convey a fluctuant sensation to the pressure of the fingers. The more well delineated it is, the more likely it is to be innocuous.

Since breasts vary so much in size, there are no hard and fast rules dictating the best way to divide the area up into convenient sections for examination. The time-honored method is to use two imaginary perpendicular lines crossing each other through the center of the nipple, in order to examine four quadrants in sequence. Having felt each quadrant, one then repeats the compressive palpation at the very center of the breast. It must be kept in mind, however, that the apparent size of a mammary gland bears very little relationship to its circumference, so that even the seemingly smallest breast may cover a wide area, requiring palpation well beyond what appears to be visible in the transverse or vertical axis. Remember also that the upper outer quadrant extends out somewhat toward the armpit, in a tongue-shaped projection called the axillary tail of Spence.

If one were to ask experienced surgeons to pay particular attention to identifying just which part of the hand is doing the palpating, almost all would report that it is the palmar surfaces of the distal and middle phalanges, particularly the former. Most would also report that they find a somewhat rotary motion to be most useful as they press the mammary tissue back against the chest wall, moving from place to place until the entire quadrant has been examined. Some would say that they

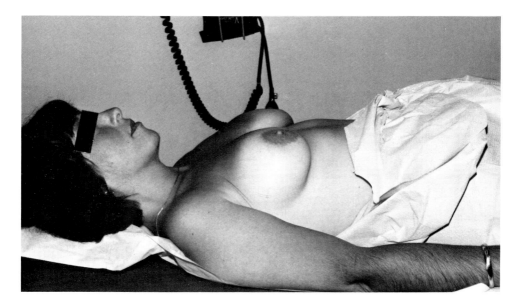

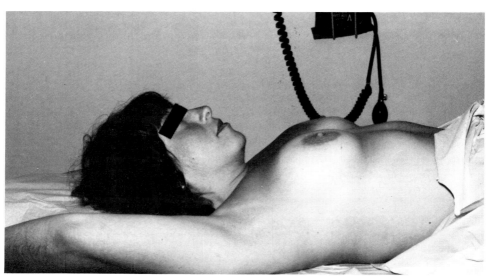

FIGURE 7.3   Breast inspection from a supine position: (a) resting lateral view; (b) arm elevated, lateral view.

use their dominant hand for both breasts, and some would change sides during the examination so that each breast is palpated by the contralateral hand.

There is no point in trying to fill up a paragraph or two describing the normal breast. In the first place, there is, as noted earlier, no typical pattern except for a generalized nodularity whose characteristics are inconsistent. It is well known and does not need emphasis that age, parity, nutrition, and stage of menses have certain recognizable effects. Also, there is the era in which we live: almost half

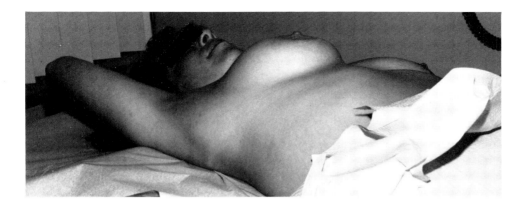

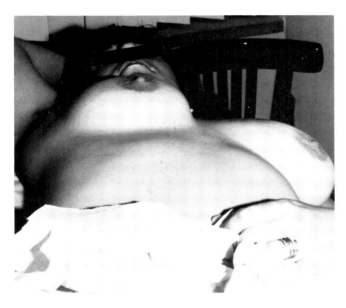

FIGURE 7.3 _(continued)_   **(c) arm elevated, oblique lateral view; (d) arm elevated, caudad view.**

of the readers of this book are women, and need only a little unhurried privacy to
become accustomed to what we call normal, if they have not already gotten used
to self-examination. The remainder are men, by whom the texture of a healthy
female breast can be learned in the clinic during the course of many physical examinations.

There is a common anatomic conformation of the mature female chest wall
that sometimes causes confusion. Because failure to recognize it has been known
to lead to unnecessary biopsy, its existence should be kept in mind. Haagensen (1)
described it as "a transverse ridge of dense nodular tissue at the caudad edge of
the breast," and attributed it to the fixation of mammary tissue to the chest wall
fascia in this location. It is his contention that the older pendulous breast presses
down upon this fixed line, while the edge of the brassiere rides over it, producing a

margin of fibrosis in the lower rim of the breast that is easily mistaken for tumor. Although the presence of this ridge is easy to verify, there is a much more straight-forward explanation for it. It has long been my impression that this inframammary ridge is caused by a prominent fifth rib, which is either a secondary sexual characteristic of females or is in some way made more overt by the pressures of successive pregnancies. Although I can identify it in the vast majority of women, I have never been able to palpate it in a man. To evaluate this further, I studied a series of dissected female cadavers in the anatomy laboratory of our medical school, and was not surprised to find, on direct inspection and palpation of the chest wall, that almost all of the specimens showed a prominence so marked that the fifth rib could be identified by a blind pass of the hand over the bared costal structures. In each case, the fifth costochondral junction was particularly bulging beyond those of the nearby ribs. Accordingly, it does seem that the inframammary ridge, so commonly thought to be a pathologic mass, is produced by nothing more abnormal than a line of breast tissue being pushed forward somewhat by the protruding rib and bulbous costochondral junction behind it.

Abnormal Findings

The following descriptions of some of the common abnormalities should be read with a caveat: Any lump can feel quite the opposite of what the examiner would expect from the disease that produces it. In other words, cancers are not necessarily hard, and all that is hard is not necessarily cancer, and so forth, and so forth, and so forth. Making the correct diagnosis is not the most important thing; the purpose of breast palpation is to identify those processes that require further evaluation. The first criterion to keep in mind is the fact that such structures feel different from anything else in that breast. There is no second criterion.

The most common breast complaints for which women seek medical attention are related to the spectrum of problems produced by the propensity of mammary tissue to become overtly cystic and to harbor a low-grade inflammatory process. This is hardly an unnatural state of affairs, but the lumps and pain associated with the processs, particularly premenstrually, can be difficult to differentiate from more serious pathologic changes. The following statements are limited to the physical characteristics that may be helpful in supporting the diagnosis of this process that has been given so many names by so many authors.

Regions of **cystic involvement** are apt to be tender, although not invariably so. The most prominent findings are usually in the upper outer quadrants and consist of rather diffuse areas of thick nodularity that merge gradually and imperceptibly into somewhat less problematic material of the same general nature. Sometimes there is an almost discrete localized clumping of particularly involved tissue that takes the form of an irregular, bumpy mass. This mass is usually rubbery, although it can be significantly harder than nearby tissues. Deep palpation with the fingertips may on occasion reveal a central area of fluctuance denoting a cyst that is large enough to aspirate. Often, a cyst may be isolated, without a lot of surrounding indurated nodularity, in which case it is relatively easy to recognize its smooth regular wall, which feels like a fluid-filled hemisphere. If there is any doubt about a locus of suspected cystic mastopathy that cannot be resolved with the help of mammography and, when indicated, ultrasound, a biopsy is indicated. This is particularly true when the mass is well localized and the patient is far enough beyond menopause that cystic problems are unusual.

The great majority of patients who present with **nipple discharge** will be found to have cystic mastopathy. This is true whether the fluid is bloody, serous, or watery, and whether it appears spontaneously or is produced by the pressure exerted during palpation. Based on published statistics, it is safe to say that no more than 10% of women with nipple discharge have a carcinoma. A persistent bloody discharge in an elderly patient may be due to a duct papilloma, which can, on occasion, be palpated beneath or close to the areola.

A lesion that ordinarily presents little diagnostic difficulty is the **fibroadenoma.** Although it has been described in all age groups, it is unusual to find it in any woman beyond the age of 35. It is rubbery in consistency and, being well encapsulated, is smooth and freely movable. It may be rounded or lobular in shape. Since it is not attached to other tissue, it is easy to delineate its borders. Although usually solitary, it may present as multiple lesions in the same breast. It does have some moderate degree of predilection for black women, in whom it sometimes grows to such a size that the term "giant fibroadenoma" is used. A well-defined, smooth, nontender, movable, solid lump in the breast of a teen-aged or twentyish woman is virtually certain to be a fibroadenoma.

The physical characteristics of **cancer** have already been described. The typical cancer is hard, irregular, nontender, more or less fixed to surrounding mammary tissue, and feels like nothing else in either breast. In most cases it will have been found by the patient herself, quite by accident and often while showering. Whatever confused and erroneous information has been imparted to the public by the mass media, a great service has been done in raising the level of knowledge about the frequency of this problem, so that we now see far more women in an early stage of disease than ever before. The awareness that they may be candidates for treatment that does not include the loss of a breast has made it easier to overcome the kinds of fears that used to keep patients away from medical attention until growths were too large to ignore or to cure. The result of these factors is that the physician must become skilled enough to appreciate a breast mass that is as small as 1 cm in size, which is a lower limit beyond which it is probably not possible to feel a tumor. Happily, the days when most breast cancer patients presented with large masses, skin or nipple retraction, and hard nodes in the axilla are forever behind us.

A HISTORY OF BREAST CANCER TREATMENT

The process of earlier and earlier medical consultation began with the introduction of the radical mastectomy by William Stewart Halsted in the penultimate decade of the 19th century. This is the same Halsted and the same radical mastectomy that are nowadays so frequently the objects of castigation by various poorly informed pitchpersons for the "patient-knows-best" approach to pathophysiology and medical history. Prior to the advent of Halsted's operation, cures were rare to the point of being, in the experience of many doctors, nonexistent. Those patients who did present themselves for surgery had a high rate of local recurrence as early as three years postoperatively, the usual figures being in the range of 80% to 90%. Those women who did not present themselves for operation were doomed to months or even years of anguish before merciful death delivered them from the misery and humiliation of the foul, ulcerated mass of rotting flesh into which the involved breast slowly became devitalized. The grim situation was best described by Halstead, himself, in a now-famous paper he wrote in 1894:

> I sometimes ask physicians who regularly consult us why they never
> send us cancers of the breast. They reply, as a rule, that they see

> many such cases but supposed they were incurable. We rarely
> meet a physician or surgeon who can testify to a single instance
> of a positive cure of breast cancer.

Halsted was not the only surgeon to recognize that the sole hope of curing the large breast cancers he did see lay in more daring resections, extending the limits of operation both wider and deeper. Meyer, Cheyne, and several others independently came to the same conclusions, and thus was born the concept of radical mastectomy. When we consider how far advanced were most of the tumors these surgeons treated, the fact that cures were at last achievable in significant numbers while excellent palliation became a possibility for many others must be looked upon as one of the greatest forward steps that has ever been taken in the treatment of neoplastic disease. For the first time, physicians felt encouraged to refer patients for operation, and women saw enough hope to seek treatment on their own. Within a few years after the general acceptance of the procedure, the entire spectrum of pessimism and despair had been replaced by a general sense of encouragement and promise.

Gradually, breast cancer became a disease that could be talked about. Women came in ever larger numbers for treatment, even though they recognized that there might be a degree of debility associated with the required operative procedure. Surgeons, seeking ways to make treatment less radical and therefore more acceptable, began to realize that lymphatic pathways do not pass through the pectoralis fascia. Halsted and the others, seeing primarily late cases with lymph duct blockage causing retrograde tumor growth, had found it necessary to remove the muscles that lay under the fascia, which they so often discovered to be infiltrated with cancer. With patients arriving at an earlier stage, it could be demonstrated that such infiltration was by direct extension, rather than through normally present lymphatics. It gradually became clear that removal of the pectoral muscles was not necessary. In 1948, Patey introduced the so-called modified radical mastectomy, which spared those structures, resulting in far better functional and cosmetic results. Although it was 15 years before the procedure caught on in this country, it finally came to replace the older methods.

As the word of modified techniques spread, it allayed some of the terror with which many women approached the idea of mastectomy. It became widely known that arm swelling was rare, immobility unusual, and fashionable clothing could be worn with much less restriction than before. This, too, contributed to the awareness that a woman who sacrificed a breast in the interest of cancer cure need not feel as though she had sacrificed her self-image as well. Then, in the mid-1970s, from a most unexpected quarter, came one of those miraculous events by which the sorrow of some individuals becomes the medium of salvation for others. Within a short space of time, two prominent American women, Betty Ford and Happy Rockefeller, became victims of breast cancer, the disease proving to be bilateral in the case of Mrs. Rockefeller. With wisdom, maturity, and the sense of obligation that has characterized the lives of both, each of these brave women allowed the details of her illness to be known by the public. The media, for once, handled the news with the kind of discretion that makes one think, in retrospect, that they must have somehow understood the enormous responsibility that had been thrust upon them, not only to Mrs. Ford and Mrs. Rockefeller, but to all women. In the ensuing weeks, clinics and doctor's offices were flooded by patients worried about newly discovered breast lumps. Some of them had cancer. As time passed, the immediate hysteria faded, but a new stage of American awareness and acceptance had been reached. There was in the selfless example of those two women the final ingredient that was necessary to legitimize, in a sense, not only the having of mammary cancer, but the loss of a breast and whatever attendant other therapy is required to achieve cure. If the saving of lives is a major criterion for a Nobel Prize in Medicine, Betty Ford and Happy Rockefeller deserve serious consideration.

Meanwhile, other things had been happening. In 1922, Geoffrey Keynes began treating inoperable breast cancers with radiation therapy. Encouraged by his results, he decided to use the technique on smaller lesions, widely excising the tumor and irradiating the breast and axilla, with promising cure rates. Others later took up the method in a more formalized manner, chief among them being Robert McWhirter of Edinburgh, who popularized the concept of simple mastectomy and x-ray treatment. In the two decades of the 1960s and 1970s, several centers began trials of what has become known as lumpectomy and radiation. Avoiding the treacherous traps of conflicting claims and counterclaims, some reasonably definite statements can be made about this approach. Based on a few good studies, it seems virtually certain that wide local resection and irradiation provides 10-year outcomes that are identical with those of modified radical mastectomy in patients with stage I cancer. Since 25% of women with clinically innocuous nodes prove to have positive pathology, axillary dissection must be part of the treatment. For stage II cancer, modified radical mastectomy seems to be distinctly superior. Several large prospective studies are now in progress to test these findings, so that the issue should be settled by the end of this decade.

The popular knowledge about lesser procedures has resulted in yet another decrease in the size of the tumors being seen by physicians. The possibility of saving a breast has made self-examination less threatening and has encouraged women not to wait to see if a lump will go away by itself. Also, it has caused women to insist upon more frequent and more thorough breast examinations by their physicians. In spite of some more than occasional shrillness and a certain naiveté about pathophysiologic reality, it must be admitted that the more radical elements of the women's movement have also helped, by publicizing lumpectomy and insisting that the usually conservative and still male-dominated medical establishment learn more about its possibilities. Ironically, the loudest spokespersons seem not to have the remotest understanding that the process by which women have gradually reached the point at which lumpectomy is a possible alternative was begun by the Halsted mastectomy, which is the subject of so much of their anger and whose author is the focus of their abuse.

EXAMINATION OF THE MALE BREAST

Throughout the foregoing discussion, the breast has been treated as though it is a structure found only in women. Since approximately 1% of breast cancer occurs in men, consideration must also be given to the physical findings in this small group. By and large, the differential diagnosis of a lump in the male breast rests between cancer and one of the forms of gynecomastia. When the patient is an adolescent, there is no problem being certain of the cause of the enlargement; the real difficulty in this situation is to find the words that might be most reassuring to a 15-year-old boy and his parents. The swelling in such cases may be unilateral, although it is usually present on both sides. It tends to be firm, and lies directly behind the nipple, being freely movable and unfixed.

Gynecomastia in the older age group has a softer, more nodular quality, and covers a wider area. Since there is commonly some hormonal alteration, this should be sought. Thus, evidence of cirrhosis or testicular atrophy can be found, when present, on further physical examination. A history of ingestion of medications that contain or are chemically similar to estrogens is often at the root of the problem. Spironolactones and digoxin are common examples. Based on my own experience, a significant number of elderly men taking the latter drug have un-suspected gynecomastia.

Any unilateral mass in the male breast for which no etiology can be identified should be suspected of being malignant. Because there is so little mammary tissue in which to hide, retraction of skin or nipple is a common finding, as is fixation to the underlying fascia. Nipple discharge of any sort in a man should raise the index of suspicion considerably.

CONCLUSIONS

The perfection of one's techniques of breast examination is a lifelong undertaking. The goal can only be approached in the career of any physician, but it is never wholly attainable. Sound training, leavened by experience and constant re-evaluation, allows us to improve our methods to the point where we can depend upon them to guide us in the care of the trusting women who come to us for treatment and counsel. The object of this chapter has been to provide some beginnings to help point the way for those who are just starting out on this quest, and for others who wish to have a little assistance along the journey. It is offered to its readers in the same spirit that motivated Astley Cooper to write his classic monograph on the anatomy and diseases of the breast 150 years ago:

> What I sincerely hope is, that this Work will have a good effect
> in inducing others to exert their best efforts to pursue the subject
> with greater zeal and ability, and to attain the grand object which
> we ought always to have in view—to exercise our profession in the
> most scientific manner, and to do all in our power to diminish
> the evils and sufferings of humanity.

REFERENCES

1.   Haagensen CD: *Diseases of the Breast,* ed 3. Philadelphia, W.B. Saunders, 1986.

2.   Haagensen CD, Bodian C, Haagensen DE: *Breast Carcinoma, Risk, and Detection.* Philadelphia, W.B. Saunders, 1981.

3.   Nuland SB: *William Stewart Halsted, Surgical Scholar.* Birmingham, AL, Gryphon Editions, 1984.

4.   Prior JA, Silberstein JS: *Physical Diagnosis,* ed 6. St. Louis, C.V. Mosby, 1977.

8
The Neurologic Examination

Arthur M. Seigel, M.D.

INTRODUCTION

Neurology has always been somewhat the orphan of internal medicine. Very few of us who practice are able to perform a thorough neurologic examination. We rely greatly on the neurologist to sort the mysterious findings and signs into an intelligible conclusion.

Dr. Seigel has taken us through a neurologic examination in a step-by-step fashion, making it a gratifying experience. A brief outline of common neurologic disorders follows, including common illnesses such as Parkinson's disease, multiple sclerosis, stroke, and cranial nerve abnormalities. This is the type of chapter that has to be read and re-read, and should be referred to periodically, It is also excellent as a refresher course.

Although we rely enormously on the computed tomography scan of the brain, and now the NMR scan, the localizations of lesions should be possible after thoroughly reading this section on physical diagnosis.

A study of the neurologic examination is best preceded by a review of basic neuro-anatomy and neurophysiology. The interpretation of observations made during the examination and the correlation between various findings depends upon an understanding of the basic science perhaps more so than in other areas of the general medical examination.

The sequence of the examination will be discussed in seven sections:

1. Mental status examination and speech
2. Cranial nerve examination
3. Motor examination
4. Cerebellar examination
5. The reflexes
6. The sensory examination
7. Autonomic function

For the student learning the technique of examination, the entire examination should be done and recorded in an organized fashion. The experienced clinician will be able to perform only those portions of the examination that are germane to the patient whom he is examining.

In the final section, examples of the findings in common neurologic disorders will be described. More detailed clinical correlation with the abnormal findings in the neurologic examination may be found in a general textbook of neurology.

MENTAL STATUS EXAMINATION AND SPEECH

Many of the pertinent observations regarding patients' mental status and speech should be made during the interview and history taking. The patient is more apt to be natural in his behavior during the history than when it is announced that his mental status is about to be examined. It is therefore important that the patient be reassured and instructed properly before beginning the formal mental status questioning. The patient should be told that some of the questions he is about to be asked may sound strange but that these questions are all part of the general examination and should be answered as well as possible. It is desirable to know some general information regarding the patient's socioeconomic background and level of education to better interpret the responses in the mental status examination. The patient and examiner should be alone during the questioning to avoid increasing the anxiety and embarrassment when answers are not known. An interpreter will be necessary, of course, if there is a language barrier. It is best to record both the question and the patient's exact answer when practical. This method will allow for comparison when the examination is repeated. Recording the patient's answers will also eliminate the need for the examiner to enter an interpretation of the answer.

The patient's level of consciousness should be observed first. Estimation of the patient's alertness, affect, intelligence, and appropriateness should be recorded. The patient's name, the current date, and the present location should be asked. Memory may be tested by stating three familiar objects (for example: baseball, automobile, and wallet) and telling the patient that you will ask him to repeat those three objects in 3 minutes. A score of 0, 1, 2, 3, or over 3 should then be recorded in 3 minutes. Digit span should be tested by giving numbers of increasing length and asking for them to be repeated immediately back to the examiner. A digit span of six to seven numerals forward and three to four numerals backward is average. Intellect and abstraction may be tested by asking that words (eg, world) be spelled backward. In each case the patient's response should be recorded rather than commenting about the response. Judgment may be assessed by asking the patient what he would do if he smelled smoke in a movie theatre or found a stamped letter lying on a sidewalk. The patient's intellect may be further evaluated by asking "What are the names of five major cities in the United States?" and "What current events are presently in the news headlines?" Although the patient's affect, including anxiety and depression, are recorded as part of the Mental Status Examination, it is best to make observations regarding affect during the history taking since the mental status examination itself often is anxiety producing. Inappropriate responses to the questions, however, should be observed and later recorded.

The common neurologic disorders of speech involve dysarthria and dysphasia. **Dysarthria** is difficulty in the articulation of speech whereas **dysphasia** is difficulty in the formulation and understanding of speech. The lesions responsible for dysphasia are usually found in the parasylvian region of the dominant hemisphere. The dysphasic patient may be mute but more commonly has speech that is disorganized and sometimes incomprehensible. Blocking may occur when the patient cannot find the right word to say. Words may be substituted for other words that are similar in sound or new words may be invented: "try" may be substituted for "tie." The dysphasic patient will also commonly have difficulty in understanding speech. This should be tested by asking the patient to do simple motor acts such as closing his eyes or lifting an extremity unaffected by illness. If this is properly done, then more complicated acts such as placing the left thumb on the right ear may be requested. Ability to write words in sentences and understand words in sentences should also be tested.

With dysarthric speech, the correct words are present but they are expressed with difficulty. In conditions such as a brainstem stroke where the muscles of articulation may be paralyzed, the sentences will sound garbled. In cerebellar lesions such as those of multiple sclerosis, "scanning speech" which is an interruption in the cadence of speech, may be the result. Words and phrases are expressed in hesitating groupings rather than in a smooth flow.

CRANIAL NERVE EXAMINATION

I: The Olfactory Nerve

Occlude the nostril on either side and ask the patient to identify the smell of coffee, tobacco, or mint. Irritants such as alcohol should be avoided. Local conditions such as rhinitis can also interfere with the sense of smell and should have been recorded as part of the ear-nose-throat examination.

II: The Optic Nerve

Visual acuity should be tested in each eye by having the patient read from a standardized vision card. If glasses are normally used for reading, then glasses should be worn for this test.

Visual fields should be tested in each eye. A simple method for confrontational testing is illustrated in Figure 8.1. The patient is asked to stare at the nose of the examiner and one or two fingers are held up in left and right visual fields. The patient is asked to report the sum of the number of fingers without looking away from the examiner's nose. For more precise testing, each eye can be tested independently in this matter. Furthermore, different areas of the visual field can be tested by holding fingers in the upper and lower quadrants. As an alternative to holding fingers in the various visual fields, a small red test object may be used. This may easily be done by placing a red mark 5 mm in diameter on one end of a tongue depressor. With the patient fixing his right eye on the examiner's left eye, a red test object is brought in from outside the visual fields until the patient states that he can see it. The other eye is tested in the same way. The examiner can compare his own visual fields with the patient's fields to estimate impairment. An alert, cooperative patient is needed for this kind of testing and, periodically, the side of the tongue blade without any red mark should also be used to verify that the patient is not reporting movement of the tongue blade alone.

The same red test object may also be used to test for color desaturation. The patient is asked to look at the red test object with one eye and then the other, and to report if the color is identical. In lesions of one optic nerve such as multiple sclerosis, the color seen by the affected eye will seem less bright and may be described as gray. This represents color desaturation and suggests optic nerve disease.

The head of the optic nerve may have been directly visualized by the use of the ophthalmoscope during the general physical examination. The appearance of the

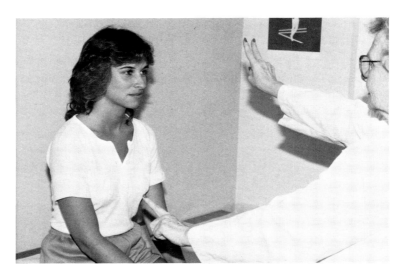

FIGURE 8.1   Examining the visual fields. The patient is asked to look at examiner's nose and to report the sum of the fingers being held up in both hands.

optic disc, particularly with regard to optic atrophy or papilledema, should be recorded here. **Papilledema** is caused by an increase in intracranial pressure such as might occur with an intracranial neoplasm. The physical signs commonly present include blurring of the margins of the optic disc and obscuration of small vessels. These vessels may be visualized on the surface of the optic disc and their course obscured by swelling that occurs at the disc margin; their course may be picked up again as they traverse the retina. Flame-shaped hemorrhages surrounding the disc may occur in more severe cases of papilledema. **Optic atrophy** appears as pallor of the normal color of the optic disc and can best be appreciated when there is asymmetry between the two eyes. Conditions such as multiple sclerosis or a tumor impinging upon the optic nerve can be present with optic atrophy.

III, IV, and VI: The Oculomotor, Trochlear, and Abducens Nerves

The nerves to the extraocular muscles are responsible for horizontal and vertical conjugate eye movements as well as innervation to the levator palpebrae muscles and the muscles for pupillary constriction. The eye should be observed with the patient looking straight ahead at a distant point to determine if the eyes are conjugate in the primary position of the gaze. The patient is then asked to look to the left and to the right. Paralysis of the sixth nerve will result in an inability of an eye to look laterally. The patient is then asked to look upward and downward with his eyes deviated first to the left and then to the right. A fourth nerve palsy will best be noted by the inability of the patient to look downward when his eye is directly laterally.

In lesions of the third nerve, **ptosis** is often present because of the involvement of the levator palpebrae muscle. The eye is deviated down and out because of weakness of the medial and superior rectus muscles. The third nerve also carries the parasympathetic fibers to the pupillary constrictor, and the affected pupil may therefore be dilated. The size of each pupil and its reaction to light stimulus should

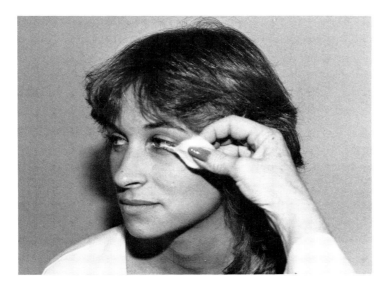

FIGURE 8.2   The corneal reflex. The end of a wisp of cotton is applied to the cornea. The patient's gaze is directed away from the field of the approaching stimulus.

therefore be observed. Lesions of either the third, fourth, or sixth nerves may result in disconjugate gaze and the symptom of diplopia. Diplopia as well as disconjugate gaze may also arise because of the intrinsic eye muscle imbalance rather than a primary cranial nerve abnormality. Ptosis is often present with myasthenia gravis, which is a disorder of the neuromuscular junction.

V: The Trigeminal Nerve

The trigeminal nerve carries sensory fibers from the face and motor innervation of the jaw muscles. The sensory division of the fifth nerve is divided into the first, second, and third divisions, which innervate the ophthalmic, maxillary, and mandibular portions of the face, respectively. These may be tested by touch or pinprick over the forehead, cheek, and jaw, respectively. The corneal reflex requires the normal function of both the ophthalmic division of the fifth nerve and the motor fibers to the orbicularis oculi, which is served by a motor branch of the seventh nerve. Testing for the corneal reflex is demonstrated in Figure 8.2. The patient's gaze is directed away from the incoming stimulus. The end of a wisp of cotton is lightly touched to the cornea, which normally evokes a brisk blink.

The motor division of the trigeminal nerve innervates the temporalis, masseter, and ptergoid muscles. Since the ptergoid muscles draw the mandible forward and medially, weakness in the trigeminal distribution will cause the chin to deviate toward the side of the lesion. Upper motor neuron lesions usually do not cause such changes since the trigeminal nerves receive bilateral upper motor neuron innervation.

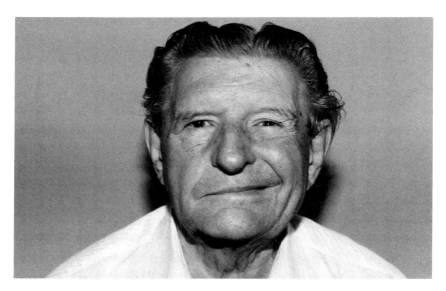

FIGURE 8.3   Right peripheral facial weakness due to Bell's palsy.

VII: The Facial Nerve

The facial nerve is primarily a motor nerve innervating the muscles of the upper and lower face. These functions are tested by asking the patient to grit his teeth, to close his eyes as tightly as possible, and to raise his eyebrows. Lesions of the peripheral seventh nerve will result in inability to close the eye tightly or retract the mouth in a position of smiling or grimace ipsilateral to the lesion. If the weakness of the muscles of the mouth are disproportionately affected compared with those around the eyes, the lesion is more likely to present a contralateral upper motor neuron lesion. Figure 8.3 shows a patient with a right-sided Bell's palsy—paralysis of the muscles innervated by the right seventh nerve.

The chorda tympani branch of the seventh nerve supplies taste to the anterior two-thirds of the tongue. The patient is asked to keep his tongue protruded while the examiner applies concentrated sugar or salt solutions on each side with a cotton swab. The patient is instructed to hold up one hand when he can identify the taste solution as being either sweet, sour, bitter, or salty. In Bell's palsy, which is an inflammatory lesion of the peripheral seventh nerve, taste is often lost ipsilateral to the facial weakness.

VIII: The Auditory Nerve

The auditory nerve is divided into the cochlear and vestibular branches. The auditory function of the cochlear branch is tested by various modalities of hearing. A vibrating tuning fork (256 cycles/s is standard) is held near the external auditory canal and the patient is asked to tell the examiner when the sound goes away. That threshold for sound is compared between each of the patient's ears. The ability to discriminate what the examiner whispers in each ear may also be recorded in Weber's test. A vibrating tuning fork is placed in the middle of the forehead and the patient is asked whether the sound can be heard in both ears, in one ear, or in neither ear. The sound is lateralized to the "normal ear" when unilateral nerve deafness is present, and is lateralized to the affected ear in cases of middle or external ear disease. In the Rinne test, a tuning fork is placed on the mastoid process and then next to the external auditory canal. When the sound carried by bone conduction can be clearly better heard than that carried by air conduction, disease of the middle or external ear is likely.

The vestibular branch of the auditory nerve carries afferent signals from the semicircular canals to the vestibular nuclei. Patients with lesions of the vestibular branch commonly complain of vertigo and may have nystagmus. **Nystagmus** is usually characterized by rapid conjugate involuntary eye movement, which may be horizontal, vertical, or rotatory. The rapid movement is preceded by a slower conjugate movement in the opposite direction. The nystagmus due to labyrinthine dysfunction does not change in direction as the direction of gaze changes, and the slow component of the nystagmus is toward the abnormal side in vestibular disease. Nystagmus may also be seen in lesions affecting the connections of the cerebellum; therefore, the presence of the nystagmus is not pathognomonic of vestibular disease.

The Hallpike maneuver is particularly useful in patients who complain of dizziness. The patient is seated on the examining table and his head is turned 45 degrees to the side and 45 degrees backward. The patient then lies down quickly and the examiner looks for the onset of nystagmus while the patient is asked to report any vertigo. Vestibular dysfunction is often associated with nystagmus that has a latency of several seconds and that fatigues, as opposed to nystagmus of cerebellar origin, which typically does not have a latency or fatigability.

IX and X: The Glossopharyngeal and Vagus Nerves

The glossopharyngeal and vagus nerves are tested together because they are closely related in anatomy and function. Unilateral lesions will produce deviation of the palate away from the affected side. This deviation is particularly noticeable when the patient is checked for gag reflex or asked to say "ahh." There is considerable variability in response when the gag reflex is tested, but it is rare for an awake patient to have no gag reflex. Asymmetry in sensation to stimulation of the two sides of the oropharynx suggests an ipsilateral lesion. Hoarseness may result from lesions of the recurrent laryngeal branch of the vagus nerve.

XI: The Spinal Accessory Nerve

The sternocleidomastoid muscle is tested by asking the patient to resist the examiner's attempt to turn his head. The trapezius muscles are tested by asking the patient to shrug his shoulders. Weakness of the trapezius results in the scapula being displaced downward and outward with sagging of the shoulder ipsilaterally. If both the trapezius and sternocleidomastoid are weak on the same side, the lesion is probably peripheral. If only the trapezius is weak, the lesion is probably central since the sternocleidomastoid muscle receives bilateral innervation.

XII: Hypoglossal Nerve

The hypoglossal nerve innervates the muscles of the tongue. The patient is asked to protrude the tongue. In lesions of the nerve, the tongue deviates toward the side of the lesion. In upper neuron lesions, the tongue deviates away from the lesion. Power may further be tested by instructing the patient to push out his cheek with the tongue against the resistance of the examiner. Peripheral weakness is manifest in difficulty pushing against the cheek contralateral to the affected nerve.

When hypoglossal dysfunction is chronic, fasciculations and atrophy may be present. Fasciculations are spontaneous contractions in individual motor units of a muscle. They are seen in lesions affecting the cell body of the motor neurons

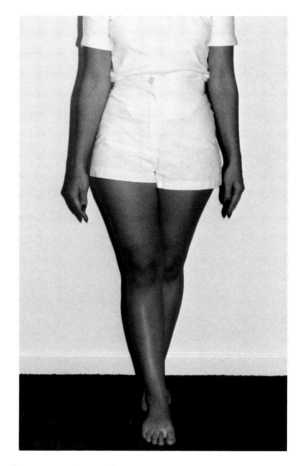

FIGURE 8.4   Tandem gait position.

and in some neuropathies. Since quivering of the muscles is common with the tongue protruded, observe the tongue resting on the floor of the mouth.

MOTOR EXAMINATION

Although observation of gait is an important part of the motor examination, the ability to walk normally requires integration with the sensory, visual, and vestibular systems as well. Posture, balance, symmetry of arm swing, and turning should be observed. The patient should then be asked to walk on his toes and then heels. A patient with weakness in the gastrocnemius muscles will be unable to walk on the toes. Next, the patient is asked to perform tandem gait (Figure 8.4). The heel of one foot is placed directly in front of the toes of the other foot in succession, walking as if on a tightrope. If this can be performed properly, then the patient is asked to repeat the maneuver walking backward.

Hopping up and down on each foot tests power and coordination in the legs. The hopping is often asymmetrical in quality, with the right leg performing better in right-handed people and vice versa. This should be tested prior to Romberg's test.

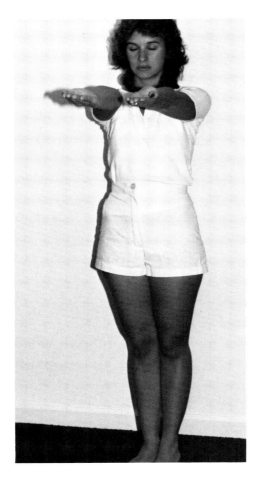

FIGURE 8.5   Romberg's test is a test of proprioception. If the patient is unable to maintain this position with the eyes open, then cerebellar dysfunction is suspect.

Romberg's Test

The patient stands with his feet shoulder length apart and his arms extended in front with eyes open. The patient is then asked to maintain this position with the eyes closed. Before asking the patient to close his eyes, the examiner stands next to the patient and extends his own arms so that the patient need not be afraid of falling. Romberg's sign, the inability to maintain balance with the eyes closed, indicates the loss of joint position sense. Normal balance is maintained by inputs from the visual, vestibular, and proprioceptive systems, as is demonstrated in Figure 8.5. Normal function of two of those three systems is adequate to maintain balance. When the patient with underlying loss of proprioception closes his eyes, only one of the three systems is left functioning, which is inadequate to maintain balance. A patient with cerebellar dysfunction and truncal ataxia may be unable to maintain balance even with the eyes open.

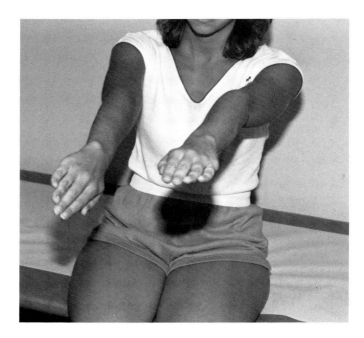

FIGURE 8.6   Pronator drift is often an early sign of a contralateral upper motor neuron lesion.

While performing Romberg's test, the presence of drift can also be observed. **Drift** is the slow downward displacement of one of the outstretched hands when the patient's eyes are closed (Figure 8.6). This is associated with upper motor neuron weakness from the contralateral hemisphere and is often associated with pronation of the hand as well as downward drift. Peripheral lesions affecting muscles of the shoulder girdle may also result in drift.

Tone/Bulk

Tone tests the passive resistance of muscles to flexion and extension. An increase in muscle tone is often associated with lesions of the upper motor neuron. In **spasticity,** there is a crescendo quality of passive resistance with a rapid decrescendo that has been characterized as "clasp-knife." **Clonus** is the rhythmic contraction and relaxation of a muscle that has been quickly stretched. It is usually associated with spasticity and hyperreflexia. To elicit ankle clonus, the examiner quickly dorsiflexes the foot, looking for the rhythmic contraction and relaxation of the gastrocnemius muscle associated with an upper motor neuron lesion. Although unsustained clonus may occur in some markedly anxious individuals, sustained clonus is almost always pathologic. With **rigidity** there is also an increase in tone; it is commonly associated with disorders of the extrapyramidal system, such as Parkinson's disease. In this condition, there is a persistent increase in tone with both flexion and extension at a joint that has been characterized as being like "lead pipe." When quick decreases in tone are superimposed on "lead pipe" rigidity, the term "cogwheeling" has been applied. Lesions of the central nervous system may less commonly result in **hypotonia.** In children this is often referred to as "floppiness" and has been compared to the resistance of a rag doll. This can best be evaluated by grasping the wrist of the patient and shaking the hand.

With experience in repetition of the neurologic examination, the examiner will soon recognize abnormalities of tone with these maneuvers. Musculature should be examined for evidence of atrophy or fasciculations. **Atrophy** is a loss of muscle bulk as a result of chronic denervation of a muscle or a group of muscles. Atrophy is usually preceded by the appearance of **fasciculations,** which are involuntary twitching of motor units due to denervation. Benign fasciculations often occur in nervous medical students who have learned about motor neuron disease. The key feature of benign fasciculations is that they are unassociated with weakness or atrophy.

Tremor

The presence of tremor is often noticed first during the history taking or while observing the gait. Tremors are characterized by their frequency, amplitude, and whether they are maximal at rest, posture, or action. The tremor of Parkinson's disease is maximal at rest with a frequency of 4 to 6 cycles/s that varies in amplitude. Essential tremor (which often is familial) or the tremor of hyperthyroidism is maximal with a sustained posture (standing with the hands outstretched). The frequency is approximately 10 cycles/s and the amplitude is small. Cerebellar tremors are characteristically described as action or intention tremors. The frequency and amplitude often increase as the patient reaches to pick up a coin or to touch his finger to his nose.

Power

Power in an individual muscle group is graded on a scale of 0 to 5:

0. No contraction.
1. There is a flicker of movement that is not functional.
2. There is movement of the body part but not sufficient to maintain it against gravity.
3. The body part can be maintained against gravity but not against resistance.
4. Some resistance against the examiner's effort is present but power is not normal.
5. Normal muscle power.

Pluses and minuses may be added for gradations of power. The following technique of recording (as recorded in a patient with a right ulnar nerve injury) is recommended:

	R	L
Wrist extensors	5/5	5.5
Opponens pollicis	5/5	5/5
First dorsal interosseus	3/5	5/5
Abductor digiti quinti	3/5	5/5
Extensor pollicis longus	5/5	5.5

CEREBELLAR EXAMINATION

Tests of cerebellar function are intimately related to other parts of normal motor function. These tests are often segregated, however, to better define lesions of the cerebellum and its connections with those of the motor cortex and its connections.

Patients with cerebellar dysfunction affecting balance will have been unable to perform tandem gait, which was tested earlier. They tend to fall to either side and often cannot stand with their feet together even if their eyes are open. In addition, lesions of the vermis of the cerebellum often produce nystagmus. Dysarthria (which was tested earlier) is manifest as difficulty in the articulation of speech. While lying on his back, the patient is instructed to put the right heel on the left knee and then run the heel down the shin. The same maneuver is then performed on the other side. In attempting to do this, patients with cerebellar dysfunction may have an action tremor ipsilateral to the side of the lesion.

While sitting, the patient is asked to extend his right arm and then touch the right index finger to his nose and alternately to the examiner's finger placed in front of him. This finger-to-nose movement is repeated several times with each arm. **Dysmetria** and past pointing occur when the patient has difficulty in anticipating the destination of his motor act and therefore cannot smoothly change the velocity and direction of the index finger. In such a case, he may jab himself in the cheek or completely miss the examiner's finger or push it backward. Ocular dysmetria can be observed by having the patient alternate his direction of gaze between a pencil placed directly in front of him and a light placed on either side. Normally an individual only requires one or two corrective moves to fix his gaze when changing directions, but the patient with cerebellar dysfunction may require multiple corrective movements. **Dysdiadochokinesia** is an impairment of the ability to make rapid alternating movements. This is typically tested by asking a patient to rapidly pronate and supinate each hand while lightly tapping the palmar and dorsal surfaces of the hand on the patient's leg. The same type of maneuver can be tested by asking the patient to tap the floor with his foot as quickly as possible. In these tests of rapid alternating movements the dominant extremity usually performs better, as was the case with hopping.

THE REFLEXES

The Muscle Stretch Reflexes

The muscle stretch reflexes (deep tendon reflexes) are obtained by striking the muscle tendon with a reflex hammer, thereby eliciting a reflex contraction of a muscle. When feasible, the examiner should be able to observe the muscle being tested and also feel the muscle for a contraction when its tendon is struck. The patient should be positioned so that the muscle is relaxed. Examples are illustrated in Figures 8.7 through 8.11.

Reflex hammers vary in size and shape. Because of its flexibility and length, the "Queen Square" hammer is preferred by many neurologists because it allows for greater "feel." This type of reflex hammer is illustrated in Figures 8.7 through 8.11.

Reflexes are graded from 0 to 4+, with 2+ representing the average and normal response.

0.   Absent.
1+.   Present but diminished.
2+.   Normal.
3+.   Brisk but not clearly pathologic.
4+.   Hyperactive and usually associated with clonus.

There is substantial variability between individuals, and anxiety often will make reflexes brisker in the individual. Comparison of responses between sides is important, however, because asymmetry of reflexes is virtually always pathologic.

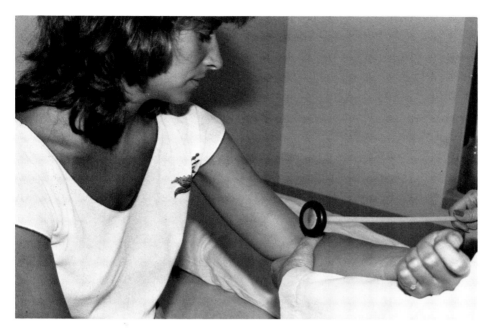

FIGURE 8.7   Biceps tendon reflex. The examiner's thumb is placed on the tendon; the thumb is then struck with the reflex hammer.

FIGURE 8.8   The brachioradialis reflex. The patient's arms are supported by the thumbs prior to percussion of the tendon.

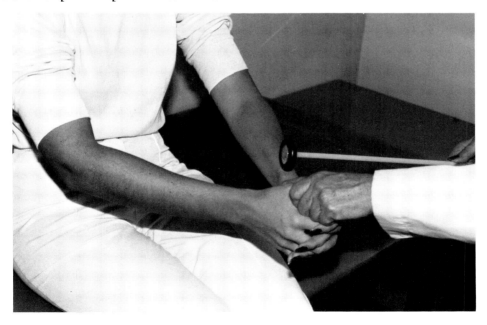

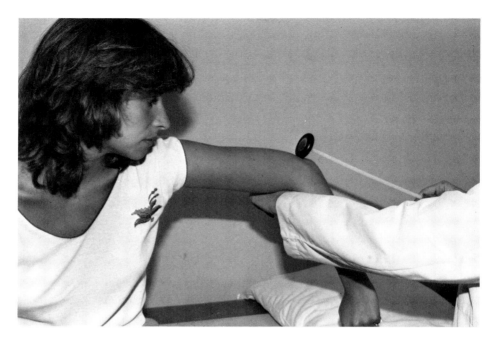

FIGURE 8.9   The triceps reflex. The relaxed arm of the patient is supported by the examiner as the tendon is percussed.

Recording of the reflexes in the clinical work-up is shown in the following example of a patient with a right sciatic nerve injury:

	R	L
Biceps	2+	2+
Brachioradialis	2+	2+
Triceps	2+	2+
Knee-jerk (quadriceps)	2+	2+
Ankle (gastrocnemius)	0	2+

If reflexes cannot be obtained with conventional technique of examination, reinforcement is employed. This is done by asking the patient to grit his teeth or clench his fists tightly while the reflex is tested. This maneuver increases the outflow from the γ-efferent system to the muscle spindles. By stimulating the muscle spindles in this way, reflexes may become elicitable when absent under normal circumstances. A reflex should therefore not be graded 0 unless it is not elicitable even with reinforcement.

The Superficial Reflexes

Unlike the muscle stretch reflex, which requires the percussion of a muscle tendon, superficial reflexes are motor responses elicited by touch stimulation. Examples of these include the corneal reflex and gag reflex discussed in the section on the cranial nerve examination. The abdominal, cremasteric, and plantar reflexes will now be described.

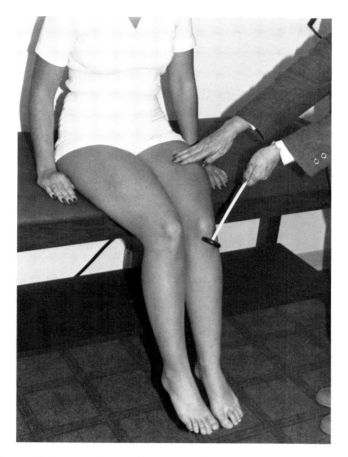

FIGURE 8.10   **The quadriceps (knee-jerk) reflex. The muscle is palpated as the patellar tendon is struck.**

The **abdominal reflexes** are tested by stroking the skin of the four quadrants of the abdominal wall with a blunt object. The handle of a reflex hammer or the stick end of a cotton applicator can be used effectively. In each of the four quadrants, a brisk muscle contraction should follow stimulation, thereby causing displacement of the umbilicus toward the stimulation. Since obese individuals, multiparous women, or persons with abdominal surgical scars may lose all of their abdominal reflexes, asymmetry between the two sides is particularly significant.

The **cremasteric reflex** is obtained in males by stroking the skin on the medial surface of the upper thigh and watching for ipsilateral elevation of the testicle secondary to contraction of the cremasteric muscle. The segmental innervation necessary for this reflex includes the L-1 and L-2 nerve roots. Unilateral loss of the cremasteric reflex suggests contralateral upper motor neuron lesion. Bilateral absence of the reflex may be present in elderly men as well as those with diseases of the scrotum.

The **plantar reflex** is obtained by stroking the lateral aspect of the plantar surface of the foot. A key is typically used to elicit the plantar reflex as it is drawn upward from the heel along the lateral aspect to the ball of the foot.

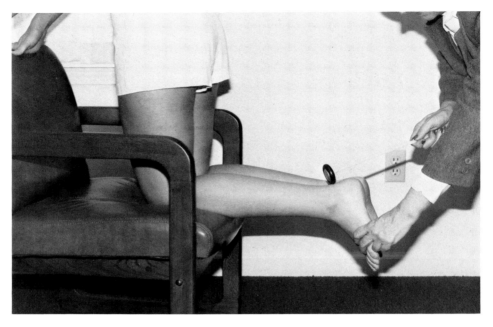

FIGURE 8.11   The gastrocnemius (ankle) reflex. The foot should be slightly dorsiflexed before striking the tendon.

Anxious or ticklish individuals may quickly withdraw their foot and, in such cases, the stimulus should be applied more softly. The examiner's finger may be substituted for a key in hyperreactors. The normal plantar response after early childhood is for plantar flexion of the toes to occur. The pathologic response is extension of the great toe, known as Babinski's sign, which is present with contralateral upper motor neuron lesions and is often associated with fanning of the other four toes. Patients with loss of sensation on the plantar surface of the foot may have no response to plantar stimulation and patients with paralysis of the extensor of the great toe are unable to produce Babinski's sign when tested.

THE SENSORY EXAMINATION

Of the various parts of the neurologic examination, the sensory examination is the most subjective. The examiner relies on the patient's interpretation of stimuli rather than the observation of involuntary responses. The examiner attempts to produce symmetrical stimuli between the two sides, but the patient may over-interpret insignificant differences. To help avoid these "false-positives" the stimuli are presented multiple times on each side. If the patient reproducibly observes an asymmetry in sensation between two sides, then it is significant. When an area of decreased sensory appreciation is reported, the examiner must then persist in testing to determine whether the area of the deficit is in the distribution of a peripheral nerve, dermatome, central lesion, or none of these. In lesions of peripheral nerves, the deficit is characteristically distal in the distribution of a glove or stocking. In central lesions a hemisensory deficit affecting face, arm, and leg is often present.

Light Touch

A cotton applicator is lightly stroked on the skin. Corresponding segments (such as the skin of the dorsum of the hand bilaterally) are touched and the patient is asked to compare the sensation. A variation is to ask the patient to close his eyes and report when a light touch is felt and where he feels it. For this part of the test, corresponding sides should not be tested sequentially because the patient may anticipate the next stimulus. In addition to numbness, when sensation is impaired patients may report dysesthesias to light touch. Such a response may typically occur after a traumatic peripheral nerve injury.

Superficial Pain

The skin is stimulated with a common pin to test for superficial pain. The patient is asked to compare the sensation of each side. In another variation, the patient is asked to close his eyes and identify the sensation as sharp or dull as the pointed or blunt end of the pin is applied to the skin. The latter approach allows for some objectivity in interpreting the patient's responses. The stimulus with the pin should be sufficient such that pain can be appreciated but should not be severe enough to draw blood. In instances where blood has been drawn by the stimulus, or in patients with known communicable diseases, the pin should be properly discarded. By using his own skin for practice, the examiner will quickly appreciate the appropriate pressure that needs to be applied.

Temperature

Testing for temperature appreciation is frequently omitted since it is redundant after testing for pain. Both sensory modalities are carried in the spinothalamic tract. Comparison of different areas to temperature can easily be tested, however, by applying the side of a metallic object like a tuning fork to the skin. The patient is asked if it feels warm or cool and is asked to compare corresponding body sides.

Vibration Sensation

A decrease in the appreciation of vibration when applied to the toes is often an early sign of peripheral neuropathy. Some decrease in vibratory appreciation normally occurs with aging, but it is usually very mild and symmetrical. The standard tuning fork has 128 vibrations/s and is applied over the bones of the great toes and the fingers. First, the patient is asked to compare the feeling between corresponding sides when the vibrating tuning fork is placed on each side. Next, the tuning fork is struck and placed on the left great toe and the patient is asked to report when he/she can no longer feel the vibration. This is then repeated on the right great toe and on the index fingers of each hand. If there is a decrease in vibratory appreciation in any extremity, the same procedure of testing is repeated in more proximal sites such as the medial malleolus and the patella.

Proprioception

The ability to identify the position of a joint in space is critical to motor control. The loss of such proprioception may result in "sensory ataxia" wherein the patient may be staggering, not because of a loss of coordination, but because he does not know precisely where his toes and feet are in space.

The great toe or the index finger is held distally on its sides. The digit is moved up and down in front of the patient in order to demonstrate what will be done and then the patient is asked to close his eyes. With each excursion upward

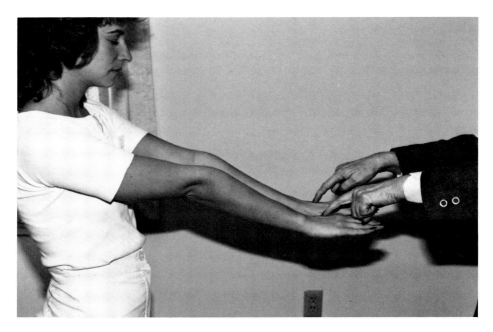

FIGURE 8.12   Extinction of one side to a double simultaneous stimulus indicates a lesion of the contralateral sensory cortex.

or downward, the patient is asked to identify the direction of motion. Excursions as small as 3 degrees of arc in the fingers and 5 degrees of arc in the great toe can be identified by normal subjects.

Stereognosis

The recognition of objects placed in the hands requires touch and position sense to be intact as well as central integration such that recognition of the object can occur. Loss of this ability is known as astereognosis. When the patient manipulates the object, such as a small key or small safety pin, coordination and the fine motor control of the fingers can also be observed. A penny may also be placed in the hand and the patient asked to identify both the denomination of the coin and the side that is "heads."

Extinction

Sensory inattention or extinction is tested by having the patient close his eyes and simultaneously tapping the dorsum of both hands as in Figure 8.12. With lesions of the parietal lobe, the contralateral hand may "extinct" the stimulation even when routine sensory examination of that extremity is normal. A similar extinction of the visual system may occur when the examiner's index fingers are simultaneously wiggled during the confrontational testing of visual fields. Extinction of one visual field may occur despite normal results when that field is tested individually.

AUTONOMIC FUNCTION

The presence of autonomic dysfunction can be observed in differences in color and texture of the skin. The skin may attain a shiny appearance, hair loss may be present, and swelling may be present because of altered vasomotor responses. The patient with autonomic neuropathy may complain that the affected part feels hot or cold and the examiner can feel for objective changes in temperature. Another test of the autonomic innervation of the skin is the scratch test or axon reflex. When the skin is scratched by the sharp end of a pin, a thin welt follows because of histamine release and vasodilation. In patients with impaired autonomic innervation, the lack of such a reaction may be noted.

Orthostatic hypotension may occur in autonomic neuropathy and can be observed by obtaining the patient's blood pressure initially in a supine position and then after the patient stands up. When there is a loss of autonomic control over the vasoconstrictor mechanism, the mean arterial blood pressure drops when the patient stands up. Dizziness and occasionally syncope occur when patients with orthostatic hypotension become symptomatic. Autonomic peripheral neuropathies are most commonly found in patients with diabetes mellitus; orthostatic hypotension on a central basis may be seen in Parkinson's disease.

THE TWO–MINUTE NEUROLOGIC EXAMINATION

This section is designed for the more experienced examiner who desires an efficient screening neurologic examination for the patient who has no apparent neurologic problem. This examination takes less than 2 minutes to perform and provides maximal screening for significant neurologic disease. It is certainly not intended to be a substitute for a more complete examination in the patient who has clinical evidence of a neurologic problem.

1. **Mental Status**—Level of alertness and speech should already have been observed while taking the history.
2. **Gait**—The patient is asked to walk several yards in a normal gait and then walk a few steps each on his toes, then heels, and then in a tandem position. Next, the patient stands in the position for Romberg's test and, while his eyes are closed, is tested for extinction. Any motor drift can simultaneously be observed in the outstretched arms.
3. While seated, the patient's fundi are examined and pupillary sizes are noted. The muscle stretch reflexes are next checked, and finally the plantar reflex is checked bilaterally.

Patients with lesions of the cerebral hemispheres often will have contralateral drift, extinction, and/or hyperreflexia and a Babinski sign. Patients with peripheral neuropathy often experience loss of reflexes early in the course of disease. The ankle reflexes are lost first in most systemic neuropathies, such as diabetic neuropathy.

CLINICAL CORRELATIONS

The purpose of this section is to correlate some of the characteristic physical findings in common neurologic disorders with underlying mechanisms. These examples of findings on examination demonstrate the importance of careful observation and interpretation of physical findings in the localization of neurologic lesions.

Parkinson's Disease

The characteristic findings on physical examination include rigidity, bradykinesia, and tremor. The rigidity may either be of the lead pipe or cogwheeling variety described earlier and is usually apparent when testing tone at the wrists or elbow. This rigidity is often translated by the patient into the symptom of stiffness and a loss of dexterity. Bradykinesia (slowing down of motor acts) is observed when the patient is walking or putting on an article of clothing. The tremor of Parkinson's disease is maximal at rest and has a frequency of 4 to 6 cycles/s. It is most apparent while the patient is walking with his/her hands at the sides or is sitting in an armchair with his hands hanging free. The underlying mechanisms for these physical findings is the degeneration of neurons containing dopamine in the substantia nigra. These cells contribute to a series of neural loops in the basal ganglia that modulate motor acts.

Multiple Sclerosis

Because of the multifocal lesions that may be present in the central nervous system in multiple sclerosis, the findings on examination are more variable than in most disorders. Motor, sensory, cerebellar, reflex, and even cranial nerve abnormalities may be present to different degrees in afflicted individuals. The physical findings have localizing values that may help to document the presence of multiple lesions. Such would be the case in a young adult with visual loss in one eye and ataxia. In examining such an individual, the visual loss may first be apparent when testing with the near vision card.

Other related findings may include optic atrophy and color desaturation. These findings are localizing to the ipsilateral optic nerve and cannot be explained by a lesion of the visual system posterior to the optic chiasm if the contralateral eye is normal. The finding of ataxia indicates a lesion of the cerebellum and its connections, particularly if proprioception is intact. This individual not only may have a positive Romberg's sign, but may also be unable to stand with his feet together even with eyes open. Gait is broad based, with a tendency to fall in any direction. A tremor of the head, nystagmus, and dysarthria may also be present in such an individual. Although a lesion of the cerebellar vermis is considered typical in such an individual, lesions of the afferent and efferent cerebellar fibers may produce similar findings.

In this example of a patient with both unilateral visual loss and cerebellar ataxia, one anatomic lesion cannot explain both physical findings. There is therefore evidence that at least two lesions are present, increasing the likelihood of the diagnosis of multiple sclerosis.

Stroke

An example of common findings in a stroke patient would be aphasia with a right hemiparesis, a right hemisensory disturbance, and a right visual field deficit. The presence of aphasia localizes the lesion to the left cerebral hemisphere in virtually all right-handed people and approximately 50% of left-handed people. The hemiparesis may include a droop of the right corner of the mouth as well as weakness of the right arm and leg. Hyperreflexia, spasticity, and Babinski's sign are usually present in this setting. The hemisensory disturbance may include numbness when tested with touch or pinprick, loss of joint position sense, diminished appreciation of vibration, and extinction to double simultaneous stimulation. The lesions responsible for the motor and sensory deficits may be cortical, subcortical, or both. The visual field disturbance commonly results from interruption of optic radiations as they pass near the internal capsule, where many infarctions occur. It is in this setting that a relatively small lesion can interrupt motor, sensory, and visual pathways in one area.

Cranial nerve abnormalities in a stroke patient indicate that the lesion is in the brainstem rather than in the cerebral hemispheres. An infarction of the left midbrain for example, may produce a left third nerve palsy and right hemiparesis (Weber's syndrome). The injury to the third nerve is manifest by ptosis, dilated pupil, and deviation of the left eye down and out. The hemiparesis is due to interruption of the pyramidal fibers in the cerebral peduncle. Since the interruption occurs rostral to the decussation of the pyramids at the lower medulla, the hemiparesis is contralateral to the lesion and the third nerve paralysis.

REFERENCES

1. Delp MH, Manning RT: *Physical Diagnosis.* Philadelphia, W.B. Saunders Co., 1981.

2. Bates B: *A Guide to Physical Examination,* ed 3. Philadelphia, JB Lippincott Co., 1983.

3. Stern TN: *Clinical Examination.* Chicago, Year Book Medical Publishers, Inc., 1964.

9
The Gynecologic Examination

Peter Grannum, M.D.

Dr. Grannum has been teaching students how to perform gynecologic examinations for more than 10 years. His clinic provides a scholarly, yet compassionate setting. Students at Yale University generally regard his course as one of the highlights of their medical training.

In the following pages, he has outlined in simple step-by-step terms how to conduct a gynecologic examination. His approach will help students retain this information throughout their careers.

The gynecologic examination is one of the most challenging examinations that the student will encounter during training. Learning to perform a comforting and thorough pelvic examination is truly an art. It is important to realize that most patients will demonstrate some anxiety for two reasons: (a) the fear of being told there is something wrong or that they may experience pain during the examination, and (b) exposure of one's genitals to an "unknown" person, which represents an element of body intrusion. This may be true in other examinations but is particularly so of the pelvic and rectal examinations.

A thorough knowledge of the pelvic anatomy is essential. The uterus was represented in Egyptian hieroglyphics as far back as 2900 BC (Figure 9.1). Leonardo da Vinci published detailed studies of the female anatomy in the 16th century. Several other notable physicians and researchers, such as Caspar Bartholin (1655-1738), Gabriele Fallopius (1523-1562), and Reijnier (Regner) de Graaf (1641-1673), have made considerable contributions to the knowledge of the female reproductive organs.

The pelvic examination should consist of four stages: (a) communication, (b) external examination, (c) speculum examination, and (d) bimanual examination.

COMMUNICATION

This is the one examination where communication with your patient is of the utmost importance. The patient should be greeted fully clothed and seated, in the office, preferably in a chair and not on the examination table. Having interviewed

Egyptian hieroglyphs
representing the uterus
are often seen on
representations of Tuart,
a hippopotamus-headed
goddess associated with
childbirth.

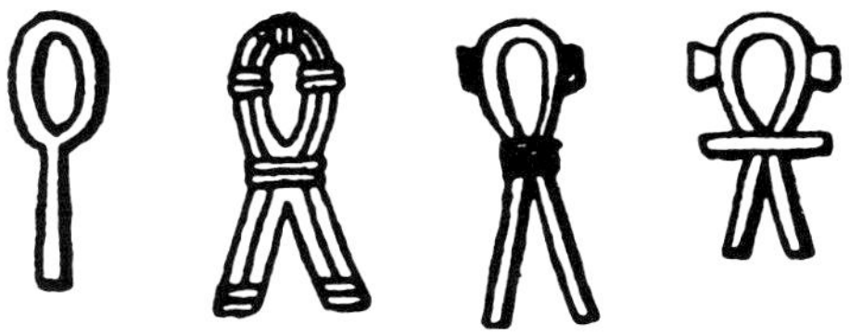

FIGURE 9.1   Egyptian hieroglyphs representing a uterus. Reprinted by permission from Knight B: *Discovering the Human Body*. New York, Lippincott and
Crowell Publishers, 1980, p 141.

the patient, she should then be asked to empty her bladder in preparation for the
examination, and be asked to change into a gown. Your attendant may prepare
the patient for you. You may discover that in some busy clinics, patients may have
already been asked by your attendant to empty their bladder and have already
changed. Most patients understand the reason for this. However, if
there is apprehension concerning this policy the recommended method mentioned
first should be adopted. The patient should be sitting on a chair on your entrance
into the examining room.

  Throughout the examination, you should always maintain eye contact and verbal
and tactile communication, and avoid the use of inappropriate terminology.

Eye Contact

Subtle changes in facial expressions may indicate either discomfort related to
the way in which the exam is being performed or pain from abnormalities of the
pelvic organs. You should respond by modifying the position or movements of your
hands, or by explaining to the patient that she may experience some discomfort
from this part of the examination because of an abnormality (eg, pelvic inflammatory disease, endometriosis, or an ovarian cyst). It may sometimes be necessary
to re-examine the abnormal area for a longer time in order to gain more information. This should be explained to the patient.

Verbal and Tactile Communication

Communicate with your patient verbally throughout the exam. Explain what is
going to be done. Inform her of your first body contact. This should be on her thigh,
preferably toward the anterior medial aspect. Indicate the beginning and end of
each part of the examination. At the end of the examination, explain all the results, after she has been able to sit up and cover herself. If the discussion is going

TABLE 9.1   Recommended Terms to Use and to Avoid During the Pelvic Examination

Do Not Use	Use
Move your bottom down	Slide down until you touch my hand (use the back of your hand)
Tumor	Mass
Bed	Examining table
Stirrups	Foot supports
Feel	Examine, palpate
Blades	Bills of speculum
Scraping	Collection of cells/samples (for Pap smear)
Spread your legs	Relax or move your knees apart
Stick finger(s)	Insert finger(s)
Pain	Discomfort

to be long, ask the patient to dress after you leave the office, and return when she is finished. Do not allow the door of the examining room to be opened for any reason during the exam, because this represents a breach of privacy.

Terminology

Avoid using terminology that could be construed as threatening or insulting (Table 9.1). Since the patient refers to you as Dr. X (using your surname), you should express the same respect unless she communicates otherwise.

Presence of Attendants

There should always be an attendant or chaperone accompanying you during the examination, preferably a woman. For the adolescent or elderly patient, or the very anxious, an accompanying friend or relative may be invited to be in the examining room. However, the adolescent patient should be asked about this privately, to prevent parents from intruding. In fact, important information may be withheld by the patient under those circumstances. If the patient desires to have her support person with her, it should be encouraged.

EXTERNAL EXAMINATION

Before proceeding with the speculum exam, the external female genitalia should be inspected. This includes the mons pubis, inguinal region, clitoris, labia majora and minora, and perineal area (Figure 9.2). An abdominal examination should always precede the pelvic examination (see Chapter 6). The patient should be in the lithotomy position with the head of the examining table slightly raised. This

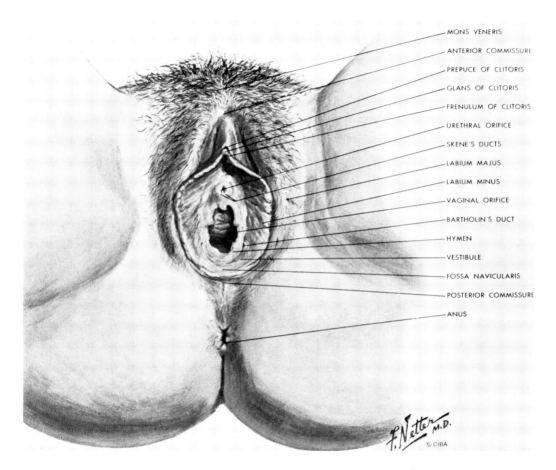

MONS VENERIS
ANTERIOR COMMISSURE
PREPUCE OF CLITORIS
GLANS OF CLITORIS
FRENULUM OF CLITORIS
URETHRAL ORIFICE
SKENE'S DUCTS
LABIUM MAJUS
LABIUM MINUS
VAGINAL ORIFICE
BARTHOLIN'S DUCT
HYMEN
VESTIBULE
FOSSA NAVICULARIS
POSTERIOR COMMISSURE
ANUS

FIGURE 9.2   External genitalia. Reprinted by permission from Netter F: *Vol II. A Compilation of Paintings on the Normal and Pathologic Anatomy of the Reproductive System.* **Summit, NJ, CIBA Pharmaceutical Products, Inc., 1954.**

allows continuing eye contact between physician and patient throughout the examination. The feet should be placed in the foot supports. The buttocks should be positioned at the edge of the table. Drapes should be placed between the patient's knees, but depressed enough to allow eye contact between patient and physician. Sterile gloves are not required for this part of the examination.

I. **External Genitalia Examination** (Figures 9.2 and 9.3)
   A. Inspect the inguinal region for lymph nodes and evidence of hernias (see Chapter 6)
   B. Inspect the clitoris, labia majora, and labia minora
   C. Palpate Bartholin's glands
   D. Inspect the urethral meatus and Skene's glands
   E. Inspect the perianal area

184

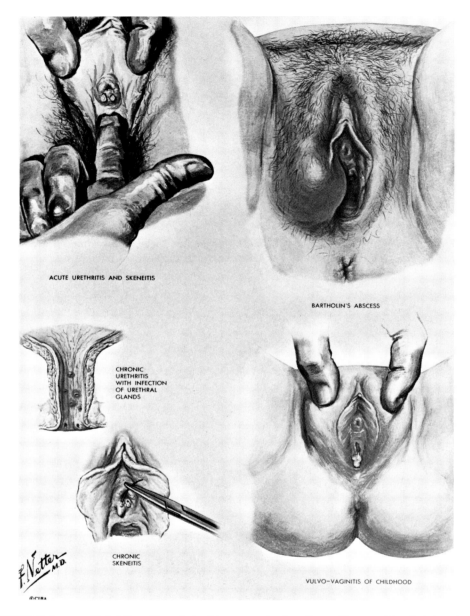

ACUTE URETHRITIS AND SKENEITIS

BARTHOLIN'S ABSCESS

CHRONIC
URETHRITIS
WITH INFECTION
OF URETHRAL
GLANDS

CHRONIC
SKENEITIS

VULVO-VAGINITIS OF CHILDHOOD

FIGURE 9.3   Vulvitis. Reprinted by permission from Netter F: *Vol II. A Compilation of Paintings on the Normal and Pathologic Anatomy of the Reproductive System.* Summit, NJ, CIBA Pharmaceutical Products, Inc., 1954.

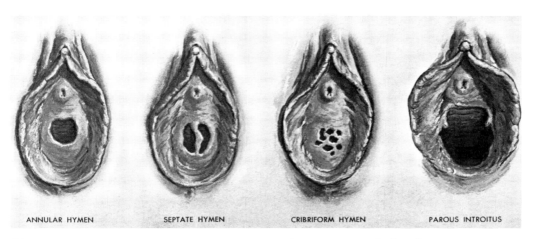

ANNULAR HYMEN   SEPTATE HYMEN   CRIBRIFORM HYMEN   PAROUS INTROITUS

FIGURE 9.4   Hymen and introitus. Reprinted by permission from Netter F: *Vol II. A Compilation of Paintings on the Normal and Pathologic Anatomy of the Reproductive System.* Summit, NJ, CIBA Pharmaceutical Products, Inc., 1954.

II. Examination of hymen and introitus

A. Check the hymen and introitus (Figures 9.2 and 9.4) (use index finger)
B. Palpate the cervix (use index finger)
C. Check for **pelvic relaxation** (Figures 9.5 and 9.6). Ask the patient to bear down, as if making a bowel movement. If there is pelvic relaxation, one of the following may be seen:
    1. Urethrocele—urethral area will descend; usually associated with cystocele
    2. Cystocele—anterior vaginal wall in area of bladder will descend
    3. Enterocele—posterior aspect of vaginal fornix will descend
    4. Rectocele—posterior vaginal wall will descend
D. Check for stress incontinence (involuntary loss of urine). Ask the patient to cough and/or bear down. Stress incontinence results from a change in the posterior urethral vesical angle, or change in the axis of the urethra. Reassure the patient that she should not be embarrassed by the loss during the examination. The examiner should be positioned to the side of the patient to avoid contact with the urine.
E. Check for uterine prolapse (Figure 9.7). Weakening of the supports of the uterus may allow this organ to descend through the vagina. Three types of uterine prolapse may occur: first-degree prolapse (the uterus and cervix descend into the vagina but not through the introitus); second-degree prolapse (the cervix descends through the introitus); and third-degree prolapse (the uterus lays outside the vaginal introitus). Second- and third-degree prolapses are easily seen. First-degree prolapse can be appreciated by placing the index finger into the vagina and at the same time asking the patient to bear down.

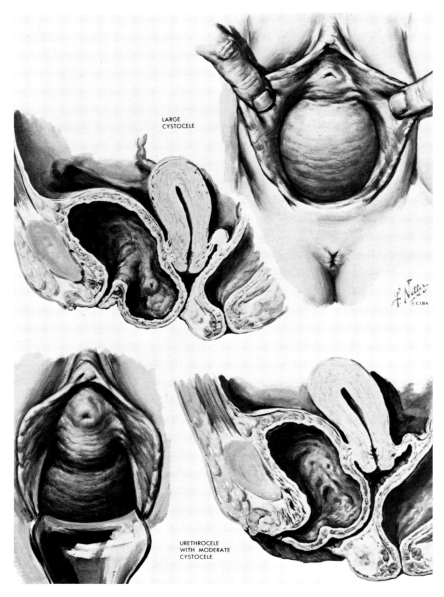

LARGE
CYSTOCELE

URETHROCELE
WITH MODERATE
CYSTOCELE

FIGURE 9.5   Cystocele and urethrocele. Reprinted by permission from
Netter F: *Vol II. A Compilation of Paintings on the Normal and Pathologic
Anatomy of the Reproductive System.* Summit, NJ, CIBA Pharmaceutical
Products, Inc., 1954.

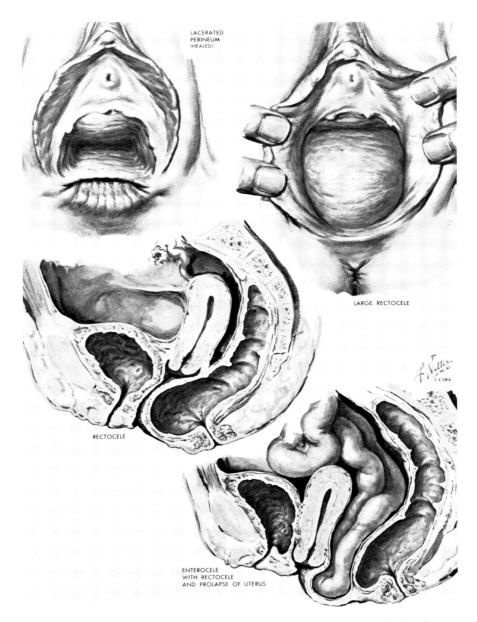

FIGURE 9.6 Rectocele and enterocele. Reprinted by permission from Netter F: *Vol II. A Compilation of Paintings on the Normal and Pathologic Anatomy of the Reproductive System.* Summit, NJ, CIBA Pharmaceutical Products, Inc., 1954.

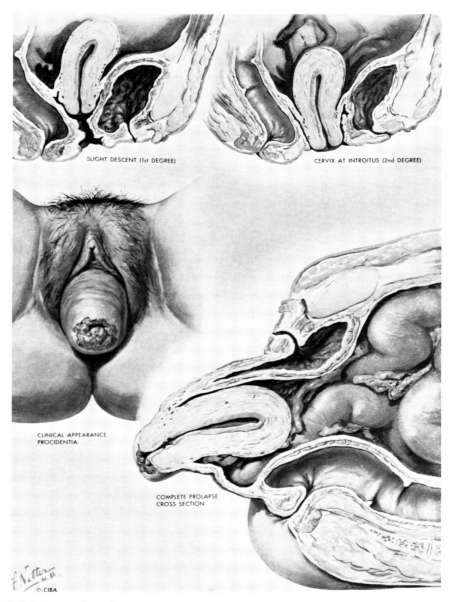

FIGURE 9.7 Uterine prolapse. Reprinted by permission from Netter F: *Vol II. A Compilation of Paintings on the Normal and Pathologic Anatomy of the Reproductive System.* Summit, NJ, CIBA Pharmaceutical Products, Inc., 1954.

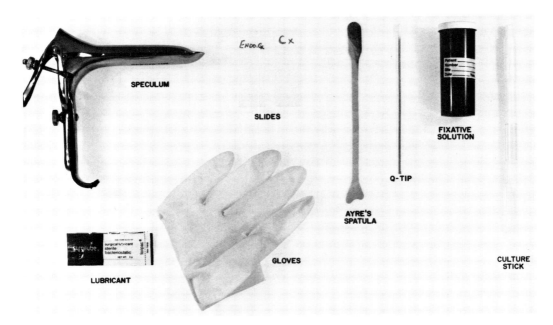

FIGURE 9.8   **Equipment used in a routine pelvic examination.**

SPECULUM EXAMINATION

The equipment used for the routine pelvic examination should include (a) warm speculum, (b) Ayre's spatula, (c) sponge forceps with swabs, (d) gloves, (e) culture sticks, and (f) slides for wet mounts (Figure 9.8). A sterilized speculum should be used. The speculum should be kept warm; a heating pad is useful, or it may be placed under warm running water just prior to the insertion. Allow the patient to touch the speculum to check the temperature before proceeding with the examination. This allows familiarization with the instrument and may reduce anxiety. If cultures are to be taken, or there is premature rupture of the membranes in the pregnant woman, strict sterile precautions should be adhered to, and a sterile speculum used.

Selection of Speculum

There are two basic types of specula, the Pederson (Figure 9.9) and the Graves (Figure 9.10). The Pederson has flat and narrow bills and comes in three sizes: standard (medium), narrow, and pediatric (Figure 9.11). The standard model is comfortable for the nulliparous woman, and should be the first choice for the first pelvic examination on a new patient. The narrow model may be more suited for the adolescent patient. The Graves speculum has wider bills that are more curved on the sides, and is also available in three sizes: large, medium, and pediatric (Figure 9.12). The medium and large sizes are useful for the multiparous woman. The pediatric specula (Pederson and Graves) are reserved for young children and may also be useful for the elderly and for the woman who has received

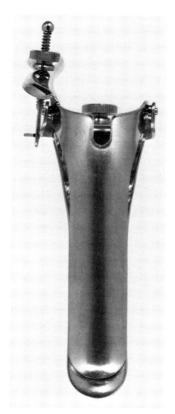

FIGURE 9.9   Medium Pederson speculum.

radiation therapy to the vagina. A wider bill speculum (eg, the Graves) is preferable if minor operative procedures are going to be performed (eg, endometrial or cervical biopsies [Figure 9.13]).

Speculum Insertion

The patient is asked to relax. A finger can be placed at the vaginal introitus depressing the posterior fourchette, allowing the transverse perineal muscles to relax. Two fingers may then be used to separate the labia. The speculum should be inserted obliquely to avoid pressure on the urethra (Figure 9.14). The instrument is inserted dorsally in a vector between the horizontal and vertical planes (approximately 45 degrees), and as it is advanced is simultaneously turned to a horizontal position (Figure 9.14). The bills should then be gently opened until the cervix is clearly visualized. The speculum can be locked to allow cervical inspection, collection of cells for the Pap smear, performing biopsies (Figure 9.13), or taking cervical cultures (eg, for gonorrhea, herpes, or Group B streptococcus).

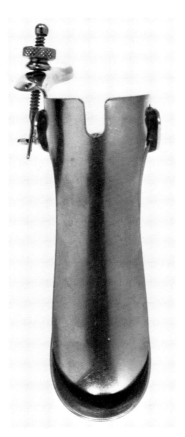

FIGURE 9.10   **Medium Graves speculum.**

Cervical Inspection

The Os

A pinhole os is usually an indication of nulliparity. If the woman has delivered by caesarean section without having dilated her cervix or had an early first trimester abortion, it may also appear nulliparous. The parous os has a transverse slit. Cervical lacerations can occur at the time of delivery and are seen at 3 and 9 o'clock. Large lacerations that are left unsutured will heal so as to give the cervix an almost "fish mouth" appearance (Figure 9.15).

Appearance

The normal cervix has pink, smooth, squamous epithelium. When there is active cervicitis, it appears red and will easily bleed when touched (friable). Old or chronic cervicitis may be evident by the presence of swollen nabothian follicles or cysts (Figure 9.15). Cervical polyps may be seen as a growth either from the surface of the cervix or protruding from the os as an endocervical polyp. Carcinoma of the cervix may appear as an ulcerative or fungating exophytic lesion (Figure 9.16). When there is an abnormal Pap smear and whitish plaques on the surface of the cervix (leukoplakia), colposcopy-directed biopsies may be indicated, because this combination may be premalignant. In carcinoma, in situ abnormal vascular

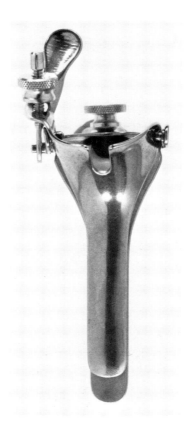

FIGURE 9.11   Pediatric Pederson speculum.

patterns seen on the colposcope, such as mosaic or punctation, would indicate the site for the biopsy (Figure 9.17). The colposcope allows direct vision of the cervix through the speculum at magnifications greater than 10 times.

In the pregnant state the cervix has a bluish hue because of congestion and cyanosis (Chadwick's sign). The cervix also has a softer consistency during pregnancy. In the pregnant woman routine tests include gonorrhea and Group B streptococcus. If there has been a history of herpes, or there is symptomatology or lesions, cultures from the appropriate sites should be taken. Scraping the herpes lesion to look for intracellular bodies (Tzanck preparation) is not as reliable as obtaining cultures. In the nonpregnant state, gonorrhea cultures are routine with herpes only taken if indicated.

Papanicolaou Smear and Cervical Cultures (Figures 9.13 and 9.18)

Collection of cells from the endocervical canal and squamocolumnar junction of the cervix can aid in the detection of early cervical cancer. Cultures should be done after the Pap smear has been performed. Since most early cancers exfoliate, collection and assessment of a sample of cells will improve early detection and improve the outcome of therapy. Cells from the endocervical canal are collected by placing a sterile cotton swab in the cervical os for 10 to 20 seconds. It should

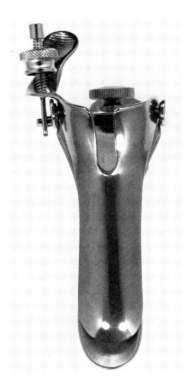

FIGURE 9.12   Pediatric Graves speculum.

be rotated in the os to improve the collection. The swab is wiped on a clean glass slide, which is then placed in a container of 95% ethanol for fixation. An Ayre's spatula (Figure 9.8) is used to collect the cells from the squamocolumnar junction. This junction or transformation zone is the starting point for carcinoma of the cervix. The long end of the spatula is placed in the os. The spatula is rotated 360 degrees to ensure a sample of the entire junction. The spatula is then wiped on a clean slide, which is also placed in the fixative. Cultures of the cervix are obtained by placing the culture swab in the cervical os for 10 to 20 seconds. The swab should then be placed in the appropriate medium for transport.

Vaginal Wall Inspection and Removal of Speculum

With the handles of the speculum in one hand and the thumb depressing the lever to gently separate the bills, withdraw the speculum until the bills have cleared the cervix. Allow the bills to slowly converge as the speculum is withdrawn, and at the same time rotate the speculum obliquely. The speculum should be at the oblique position when it reaches the introitus to avoid contact with the urethra. The vaginal walls should be inspected as the speculum is withdrawn. To visualize the posterior fornix, the speculum should be positioned under the cervix. The bills can be opened, elevating the cervix and allowing inspection of the posterior fornix. Visualization of the posterior fornix is useful in identifying an enterocele (Figure 9.6) or inspecting for a ruptured posterior fornix, often seen in the elderly rape victim.

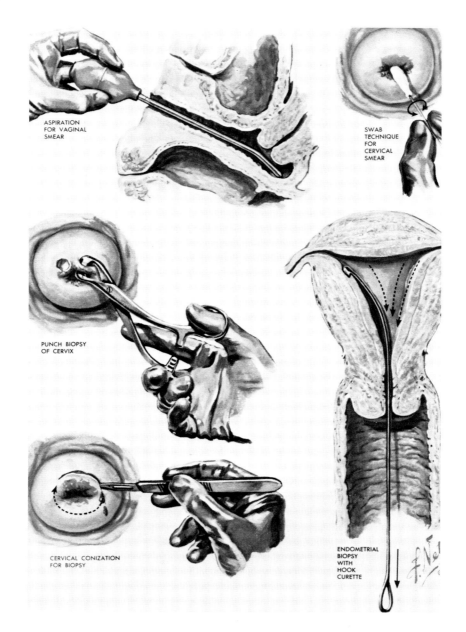

FIGURE 9.13 Diagnostic procedures: cervical smear and cervical and endo-metrial biopsies. Reprinted by permission from Netter F: *Vol II. A Compilation of Paintings on the Normal and Pathologic Anatomy of the Reproductive System.* Summit, NJ, CIBA Pharmaceutical Products, Inc., 1954.

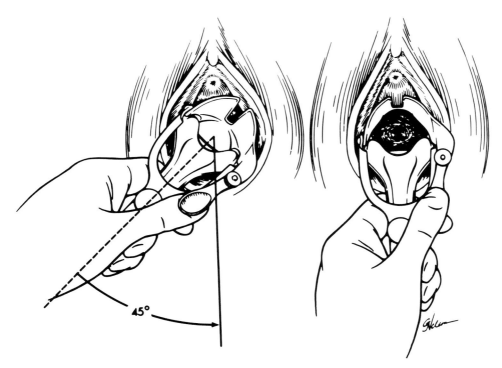

45°

**FIGURE 9.14   Insertion of speculum. Reprinted by permission from Maeck
JVS: Patient evaluation, in Mixter RW, Boynton SD, Leap B, Fitzpatrick JJ (eds):
Gynecology and Obstetrics, ed 2. New York, McGraw-Hill Book Company, 1981,
p 311.**

BIMANUAL AND RECTAL EXAMINATION

The rectal and rectovaginal exam should always be performed after the bimanual
examination.

Examination of the Uterus

The bimanual examination requires the use of a vaginal and an abdominal hand;
remove the glove from the abdominal one. Lubrication is necessary for this part
of the examination. Insert the index and second fingers of the vaginal hand into
the vagina in an oblique fashion, to avoid pressure in the urethral area. The index
finger is inserted first, ensuring relaxation of the transverse perineal muscles; then
the second finger is inserted. After both fingers have been inserted they are
directed posteriorly along the vaginal axis until the cervix is reached. With the
abdominal hand depressing the abdominal wall dorsally and the vaginal hand pushing
the cervix and body of uterus ventrally, the position, size, and consistency of the
uterus can be ascertained (Figure 9.19).

196

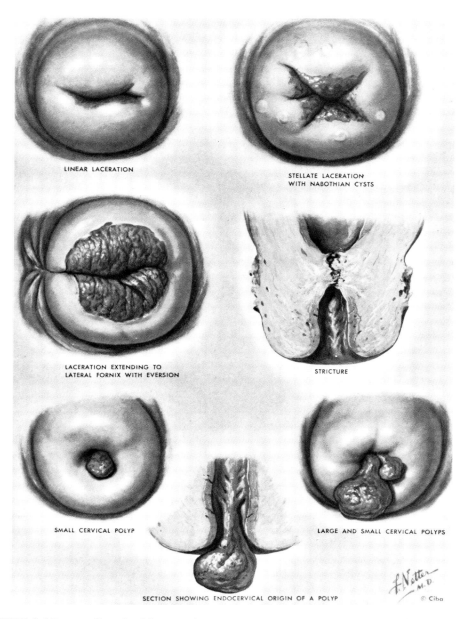

LINEAR LACERATION

STELLATE LACERATION
WITH NABOTHIAN CYSTS

LACERATION EXTENDING TO
LATERAL FORNIX WITH EVERSION

STRICTURE

SMALL CERVICAL POLYP

LARGE AND SMALL CERVICAL POLYPS

SECTION SHOWING ENDOCERVICAL ORIGIN OF A POLYP

FIGURE 9.15   Cervical lacerations, structures, and polyps. Reprinted by permission from Netter F: *Vol II. A Compilation of Paintings on the Normal and Pathologic Anatomy of the Reproductive System.* Summit, NJ, CIBA Pharmaceutical Products, Inc., 1954.

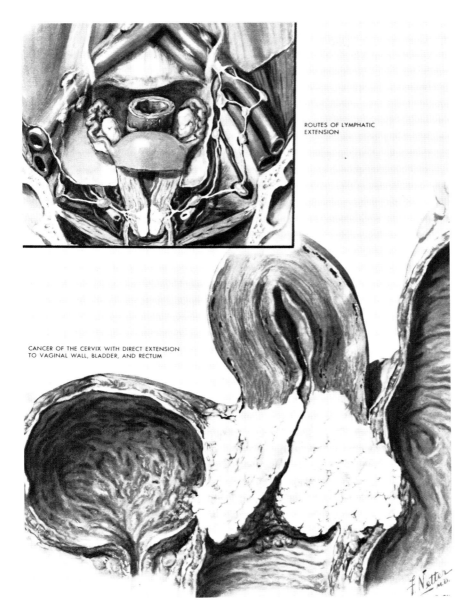

ROUTES OF LYMPHATIC EXTENSION

CANCER OF THE CERVIX WITH DIRECT EXTENSION TO VAGINAL WALL, BLADDER, AND RECTUM

FIGURE 9.16   Carcinoma of the cervix. Reprinted by permission from Netter F: *Vol II. A Compilation of Paintings on the Normal and Pathologic Anatomy of the Reproductive System.* Summit, NJ, CIBA Pharmaceutical Products, Inc., 1954.

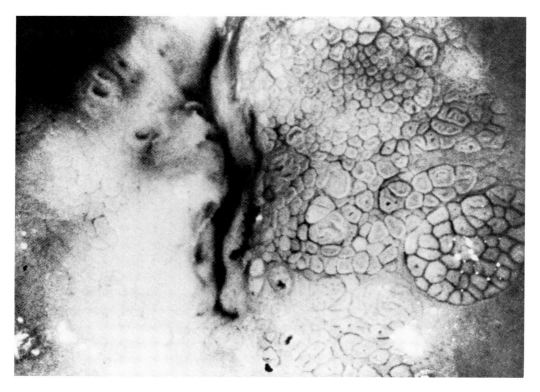

FIGURE 9.17   **Abnormal vascular patterns on colposcopy.**

Position

The uterus is supported by a number of ligaments (eg, round, cardinal, and uterosacral ligaments [Figure 9.20]). In addition, the levator ani sling forms part of the support mechanism. The uterus may assume different positions, determined by its attitude to the vaginal axis and the degree of flexion of the body of the uterus to the cervical axis (Figure 9.21). **Antiflexion** refers to an anteriorly positioned fundus, where the cervix remains in the vaginal axis plane. When the cervical axis changes either ventrally or dorsally from the vaginal axis, the uterus is said to be **verted** (anteverted or retroverted, respectively). Most often version and flexion are present simultaneously. The retroflexed and/or retroverted uterus may be difficult or impossible to palpate using the abdominal hand; in these cases rectovaginal examination (see below) should be performed. Knowledge of the position of the uterus is mandatory if the uterine cavity needs to be sampled (Figure 9.13) (eg, endocervical or endometrial biopsies) or for the placement of an intrauterine device.

Consistency

The consistency of the pregnant uterus is soft and globular. The nonpregnant uterus has a firm feel to it. The uterus containing multiple fibroids is usually enlarged, with a firm, irregular consistency. The nonpregnant cervix also feels firm, becoming softened during the gestational period.

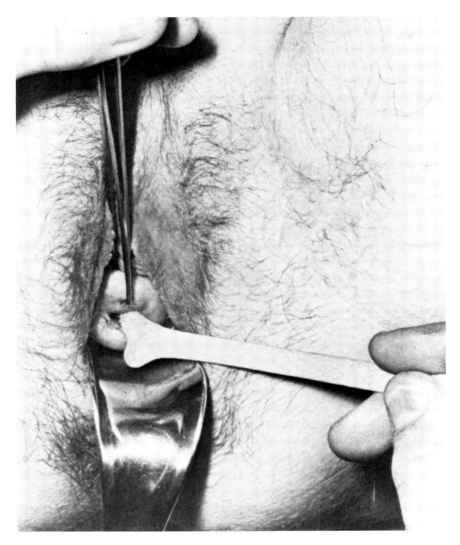

FIGURE 9.18   Collection of cells and cervical cultures.

Size

Knowledge of a normal-sized uterus comes only by experience. The size of the uterus, whether enlarged due to pregnancy or to a tumor, is described relative to the size of the pregnant uterus. At 12 weeks of pregnancy the uterus becomes an "abdominal organ" and is at the level of the pubic symphysis. At 20 weeks the uterus reaches the umbilicus, and at 36 weeks the xiphoid. As the fetus descends into the true pelvis, the fundus may recede from the xiphoid.

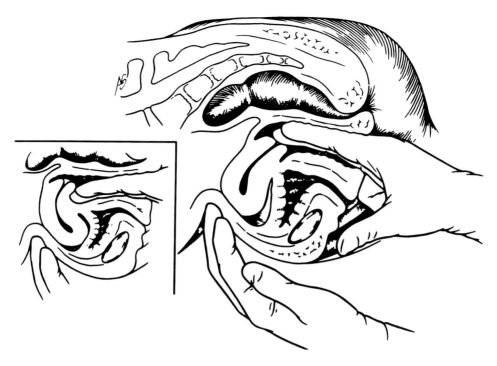

FIGURE 9.19   Bimanual examination for examination of the cervix and uterus.
Reprinted by permission from Maeck JVS: Patient evaluation, in Mixter RW,
Boynton SD, Leap B, Fitzpatrick JJ (eds): *Gynecology and Obstetrics,* **ed 2. New**
York, McGraw-Hill Book Company, 1981, p 312.

Tenderness

Gentle palpation of the uterus during the pelvic examination is important in
order to assess the presence of an inflammatory process (eg, pelvic inflammatory
disease or postpartum endometritis). The uterus and adnexae will be found to be
tender in these conditions, because the surfaces are usually involved in the
process.

Mobility of the Uterus and Cervix

In pelvic inflammatory disease, movement of the cervix to the left or right
will put tension on the inflamed serosa of the tubes and broad ligament. This will
elicit pain, and is referred to as "bilateral cervical excitation." Unilateral "cervical
excitation" refers to pain elicited with movement of the cervix to only one side,
commonly seen in tubal ectopic pregnancy. Inability to move the cervix or uterus
may represent cervical or uterine carcinoma that has spread to the pelvic side
walls, causing the uterus to become immobile.

Examination of the Adnexae

The fallopian tubes are generally not palpable. If they are inflamed (eg, pelvic
inflammatory disease), pain will be elicited. If the infection is long standing the
tubes may be indurated and palpable. The finding of a unilateral boggy mass in
the adnexal area is consistent with a tubal or ovarian ectopic pregnancy.

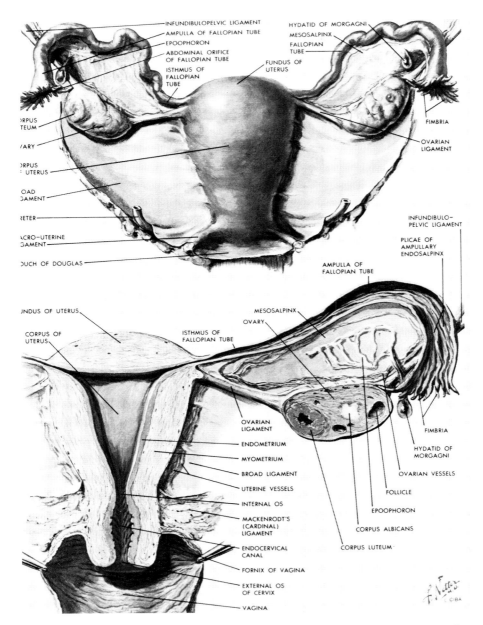

FIGURE 9.20   Internal pelvic organs and surrounding structures. Reprinted by permission from Netter F: *Vol II. A Compilation of Paintings on the Normal and Pathologic Anatomy of the Reproductive System.* Summit, NJ, CIBA Pharmaceutical Products, Inc., 1954.

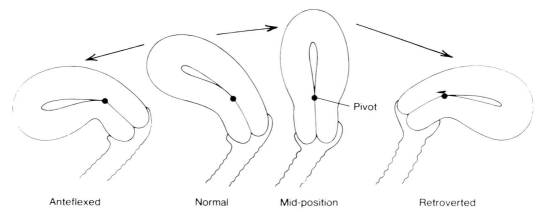

Anteflexed Normal Mid-position Retroverted

FIGURE 9.21   **Flexion and version of the uterus.**

FIGURE 9.22   **Bimanual technique for the examination of the adnexae. Re-
printed by permission from Maeck JVS: Patient evaluation, in Mixter RW, Boynton
SD, Leap B, Fitzpatrick JJ (eds):** *Gynecology and Obstetrics,* **ed 2. New York,
McGraw–Hill Book Company, 1981, p 313.**

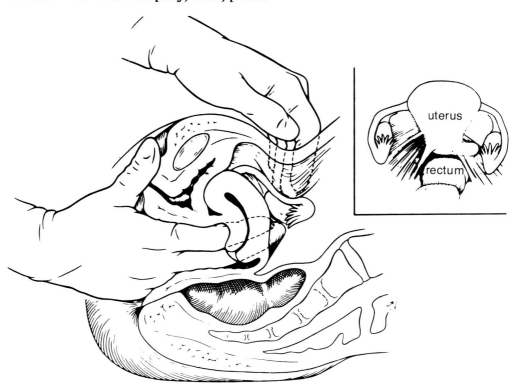

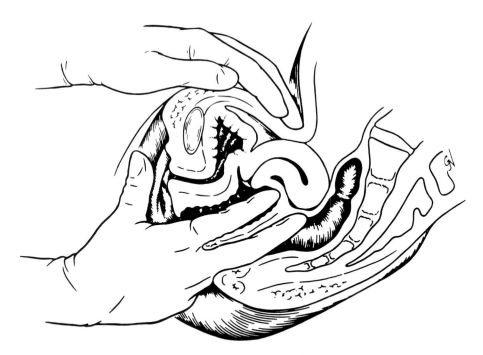

FIGURE 9.23   Bimanual rectovaginal examination.

Each adnexa should be palpated separately (Figure 9.22). The two fingers of the internal hand are placed in the fornix (lateral superior aspect). The external hand is placed on the right lower quadrant area of the abdomen. The aim is to palpate the adnexa between the hands. The external hand is pressed downward and medially, and the internal hand is moved ventrally. The two movements should be performed simultaneously. Normal ovaries should be palpable. Ovarian masses are easily palpable and should be described in terms of consistency, mobility, size, and degree of tenderness. Masses in the left adnexal area need to be distinguished from stool in the sigmoid colon. In that event the examination should be performed after evacuation.

Rectovaginal Examination

This part of the examination allows the study of the rectovaginal area, uterosacral ligaments, and the fundus of the retroverted and/or retroflexed uterus. Endometriosis can be detected by examining the uterosacral ligaments (Figure 9.23), where "beading" and tenderness can be appreciated. In Stage III carcinoma of the cervix, spread of the disease to the rectovaginal wall and rectum (Figure 9.16) can be palpated. The rectovaginal exam is useful in the differentiation between an ovarian cyst and stool in the sigmoid colon.

Use a fresh pair of gloves. With lubricant on the gloves, the index finger and the second finger are simultaneously placed in the vagina and rectum. Figure 9.23 illustrates how the retroverted uterus and the rectovaginal septum can be easily palpated. The abdominal hand may continue to be useful by depressing the uterus and cervix dorsally to aid in the palpation.

CONCLUSIONS

If care and sensitivity are used while performing the pelvic examination, most patients will continue to have their routine yearly check. An undignified, careless, and painful examination will reduce visits to the gynecologic office.

In addition, women should be taught the art of self-examination for inspection of the vulva, vagina, and cervix. Self-inspection and speculum examination can be taught to most women. Plastic specula are available for the self-examination. Education and counseling are important for increasing the woman's awareness of the pelvic organs. One excellent way to increase awareness is to have the patient participate during the pelvic examination. Most gynecologists have not encouraged patient participation, and so women are curious about their pelvic organs and are afraid and sometimes embarrassed to ask their physician to allow them to participate. Verbal communication and offering a mirror to the woman are useful in overcoming this problem.

ACKNOWLEDGMENTS

I would like to thank Jennifer Ferrigno, Nancy Kellet, Joanne Mezger, Kathy Pinto, Lyn Lombardi, Lucy Stein, and Jean Vulte for their help in the preparation of this manuscript. The above-mentioned are lecturers in the Department of Obstetrics and Gynecology, Yale University School of Medicine. They are responsible for the superb way in which this examination is taught in this medical school.

REFERENCES

1.   Maeck JVS: Patient evaluation, in Mixter RW. Boynton SD, Leap B, Fitzpatrick JJ (eds): *Gynecology and Obstetrics: The Health Care of Women,* ed 2. New York, McGraw-Hill Book Company, 1981, pp 305–317.

2.   Papanicolaou GN, Traut HF, Marchetti AA: *The Epithelia of Women's Reproductive Organs,* New York, Commonwealth Fund, 1948.

3.   Arey LB: *Developmental Anatomy.* Philadelphia, W.B. Saunders Co., 1954.

4.   Bryan AL, Nigro JO, Counsellor VS: One hundred cases of congenital absence of the vagina. *Surg Gynecol Obstet* 1949;88:79.

5.   Gardner HL, Kaufman RH: *Benign Diseases of the Vulva and Vagina.* Boston, GK Hall, 1981.

6.   Buscema J, Woodruff JD, Parmley TH, Genadry R: Carcinoma in situ of the vulva. *Obstet Gynecol* 1980;55:225.

7.   Burch TA, Rees CW, Reardon L: Diagnosis of *Trichomonas vaginalis* vaginitis. *Am J Obstet Gynecol* 1959;77:903.

8.   Gardner HL: *Haemophilus vaginalis* vaginitis after twenty-five years. *Am J Obstet Gynecol* 1980;137:385.

9.   Green TH Jr: Development of a plan for the diagnosis and treatment of urinary stress incontinence. *Am J Obstet Gynecol* 1962;83:632.

10. Marshall VF, Marchetti AA, Krantz KE: Correction of stress incontinence by simple vesicourethral suspension. *Surg Gynecol Obstet* 1949;88:509.

11. Monif GRG: *Infectious Disease in Obstetrics and Gynecology,* ed 1. New York, Harper & Row, 1974.

12.   DiSaia PJ, Creasman WT: *Clinical Gynecologic Oncology.* St. Louis, CV Mosby, 1980.

13.   Kistner RW: Conservative treatment of endometriosis. *Postgrad Med* 1958;25:505.

14.   Barber HRK: Ovarian tumors. *Clin Obstet Gynecol* 1969;12:929.

15.   Meigs JV: Fibroma of the ovary with ascites and hydrothorax—Meig's syndrome. *Am J Obstet Gynecol* 1954;67:962.

16.   Novak ER, Woodruff JD: *Novak's Gynecologic and Obstetric Pathology.* Philadelphia, WB Saunders Co., 1979.

10
Examination of the Eyes

Caleb Gonzalez, M.D.

INTRODUCTION

"The eyes are the mirrors of the soul." The eyes also can be an important source of information on the general physical condition of the patient. A thorough eye examination is essential for a complete diagnostic evaluation, especially in patients who present with symptoms whose origins are difficult to find.

During his or her career, the physician will identify many multisystem illnesses by the eye examinations, including tumors of the choroid, sarcoidosis, rheumatoid arthritis, diabetes, endocarditis, liver diseases, and congenital metabolic disturbances. The eyes give us a direct visualization of the fingerprints of arteriosclerosis by allowing us to perform a thorough examination of the retina vascular system under high magnification.

This chapter will be useful for the medical student during the time he or she is learning to examine the eyes either as part of the physical diagnosis course or during the rotations through medicine, pediatrics, neurology, the emergency room, and ophthalmology.

Besides the history, physical examination, and special examinations, this chapter is organized around those patient area problems seen most frequently by medical students. In each of the sections, the student is given relevant facts, examining procedures, illustrations, and interpretive information. The objectives for the student are:

This work was supported in part by Research to Prevent Blindness Inc. and the Connecticut Lions Eye Research Foundation.

1. To become familiar with history taking and ocular examination as performed by the ophthalmologist.
2. To be able to measure and record visual acuity and determine, if there is a decrease in vision, whether it is due to refractive error or ocular pathology.
3. To understand the different refractive problems of the eye.
4. To be able to perform an adequate ophthalmoscopic examination and differentiate a normal from an abnormal fundus.
5. To be able to recognize amblyopia and strabismus and be able to initiate the appropriate referrals.
6. To become familiar with the different types of glaucoma and be able to measure the intraocular pressure with the Schiotz tonometer.
7. To become familiar with the ophthalmoscopic signs of neurologic disorders, abnormal pupillary reactions, restriction of eye movements, optic nerve pathology, and gross visual field defects.
8. To be able to recognize common ocular injuries and determine the degree of emergency and whether it can be handled by a primary physician or needs referral to an ophthalmologist.
9. To be able to perform the necessary steps to evaluate a red eye and be able to decide whether the patient needs a referral to an ophthalmologist.

This chapter is not all-inclusive, and further resources will be needed for the complete preparation of the medical student in this field. He or she should buy at least one of the newest editions of any textbooks listed in the Additional Resources list at the end of the chapter, and, while a student, should try to come in contact with some of the self-instructional material that may be available in the medical school library or in the ophthalmology department, and if not available then a list of this material can be obtained by writing to the addresses given in the Additional Resources list.

ANATOMY OF THE GLOBE AND ADNEXAE OCULI

The Eyelids, Lacrimal System, and Orbits

The anatomy and structure of the ocular adnexae are depicted in Figures 10.1 through 10.5.

The Globe

The globe is a resilient sphere that is mildly inflated by internal fluids and turned by its own muscles. It rests in the bony orbit below the eyebrows, which keeps it protected against frontal blows. The orbital fat gives cushioning support to the eye and allows it to move freely. The eye muscles not only rotate the eyes in different positions of gaze, but they also hold both eyes straight.

The eyeball consists of three concentric layers: (a) an outer fibrous tunic composed of the cornea and sclera; (b) a medial vascular tunic composed of the iris, ciliary body, and choroid; and (c) the inner sensory tunic, the retina. The optical media is inside these tunics: from front to back, the aqueous humor, the lens, and the vitreous body. The globe has a volume of 6.5 cm^3, weighs about 7 g, and has a specific gravity of 1.077. Its average measurements are 24 mm anteroposteriorly and slightly less transversely and vertically.

The **cornea** forms the anterior one fifth of the eye, is completely transparent, measures about 12 mm in diameter, and has a radius curvature of 7.8 mm. The **sclera** forms the posterior four fifths of the outer covering of the eye. It is visible

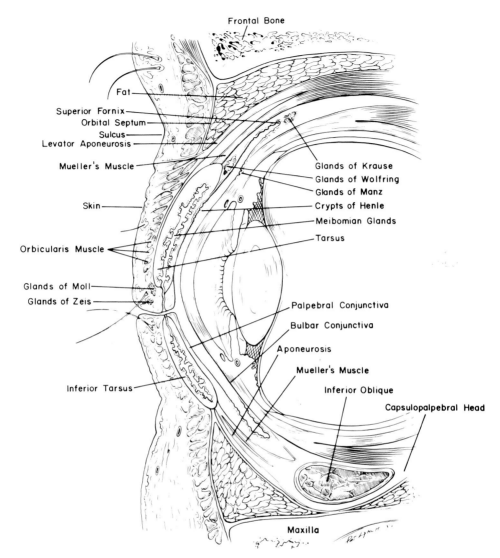

FIGURE 10.1   The eyelids.

as the white of the eye. It is thickest next to the optic nerve (1 mm) and thinnest just behind the insertion of the rectus tendons (0.3 mm). It is perforated by the optic nerve 1 mm above and 4 mm nasal to the posterior pole of the eye. In this area the sclera is thin and sievelike and forms the **lamina cribrosa,** through which the axons of the retina ganglion cells exit the eye. This is the weakest spot in the sclera and in glaucoma allows for the cupping of the disc.

The sclera is pierced by the posterior ciliary vessels (10 to 12 short ones and 2 long ones) and the ciliary nerves (6 to 10 short ones and 1 long one). The four to seven vortex veins exit 4 mm behind the equator. Between the limbus and the muscle insertions, the sclera is perforated by the anterior ciliary vessels, which come from the muscular branches to the rectus muscles.

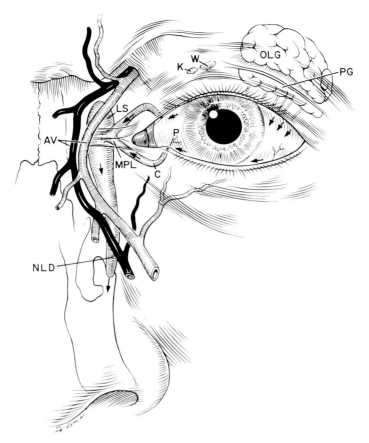

FIGURE 10.2   Lacrimal secretory system: OLG, orbital lacrimal gland; PG, palpebral gland; W and K, glands of Wolfring and Krause. Lacrimal excretory system: P, punctum; C, canaliculus; LS, lacrimal sac; NLD, nasolacrimal duct; MPL, medial palpebral ligament; AV, angular artery and vein.

The **choroid** extends from the optic nerve to the ora serrata and is the posterior part of the uveal tract. The **ciliary body** is the middle portion of the uveal tract and extends from the ora serrata to the corneal-scleral junction. It consists of the **pars plicata,** which contains the ciliary processes, anteriorly and the **pars plana** posteriorly. The whole ciliary body forms an anterior ring around the eye with a width of about 6 to 6.5 mm. The pars plicata is 2 to 3 mm wide and the pars plana 4 to 5 mm wide. The **iris** is the most anterior part of the uvea. It is 11 mm in diameter and 0.4 mm in thickness. Its central aperture is called the **pupil.** It floats in the aqueous humor and divides the anterior segment into anterior and posterior chambers, which communicate through the pupillary aperture. It slides freely on the anterior surface of the lens when dilating and constricting. The anterior chamber is 3.5 to 4 mm deep and the lens 3.5 to 4 mm thick.

The functional **retina** extends to within 7 mm of the ora serrata, and the nasal part of the retina reaches about 1 mm further forward than the temporal part, which is mainly responsible for the monocular temporal crescents in the visual field in each eye. With direct ophthalmoscopy, the peripheral retina can be seen to about 4 mm from the ora, which is about 8 mm from the limbus.

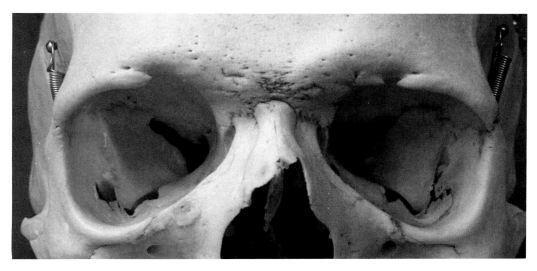

FIGURE 10.3   The bony orbits. Medial walls are parallel to each other. Each lateral wall is at a 45 degree angle from its medial wall. Lateral wall: zygomatic bone and greater wing of sphenoid bone. Floor: zygomatic bone, maxilla, and palatine bones. Medial wall: maxilla, lacrimal, ethmoid, and sphenoid bones. Roof: frontal bone and lesser wing of sphenoid bone.

FIGURE 10.4   Superior orbital fissure, annulus of Zinn, left orbital apex. O.N., optic nerve; SO, superior oblique muscle; LP, levator palpebrae muscle; SR, superior rectus muscle; LR, lateral rectus muscle; IR, inferior rectus muscle.

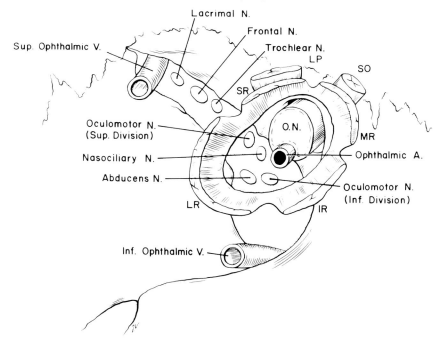

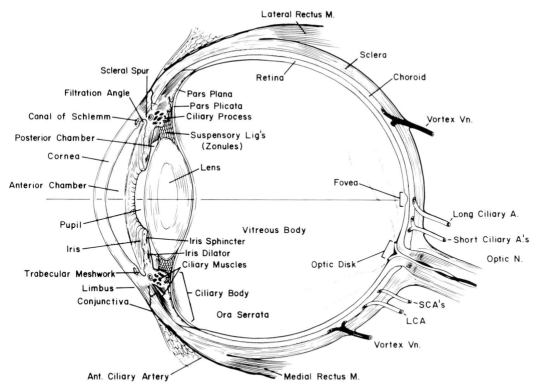

FIGURE 10.5   **Horizontal section of the globe, through the disc and fovea.**

The eyeball gets its blood supply from the ophthalmic artery through the posterior and anterior ciliary arteries and the central retinal artery. The central retinal artery is the first branch of the ophthalmic artery and enters the optic nerve 12 to 15 mm behind the sclera, running inside the nerve to the nervehead, where it branches to supply the inner layers of the retina. The posterior ciliary arteries start with two trunks from the ophthalmic artery, which divide into: (a) 10 to 20 short posterior ciliary arteries, which perforate the sclera around the optic nerve and supply the choroid and the nervehead; and (b) two large branches, the long posterior ciliary arteries, which perforate the sclera on either side of the disc and run forward in the suprachoroidal space to supply the ciliary body. Here they anastomose with the anterior ciliary arteries to form the major arterial circle and supply the iris. Muscular branches of the ophthalmic artery give rise to the anterior ciliary arteries. There are two for each muscle except the lateral rectus, which has only one. They continue with the tendons toward the limbus, where they perforate the sclera to end at the major arterial circle in the ciliary body.

HISTORY

Chief Complaint and Present Illness

The patient may have a minor or major complaint, but a good historian will elicit information that will shorten the time he or she has to spend with the patient. At times, the patient will describe physical signs as symptoms, such as "a red eye."

The three most common ophthalmologic complaints are disturbances of vision, pain (or discomfort), and abnormal secretions (or tearing).

If the patient reports loss of vision, careful evaluation and documentation should be performed to determine if it was limited to part of the field of vision or involved the whole field; if it was present only in one eye or both eyes; if the loss of vision was gradual or the onset was rapid; if it lasted a few seconds, a few minutes, less than one-half hour, or more than one-half hour; and if it is still present when the patient arrives for examination.

The most common cause of disturbances of vision is a refractive error (myopia, hypermetropia, astigmatism, or presbyopia). This type of nonpainful visual loss is gradual and of long duration as opposed to a nonpainful loss of vision secondary to organic causes, which is usually sudden. A sudden loss of vision without pain due to retina or optic nerve pathology is commonly due to occlusion of the central retinal artery or obstruction of the central retinal vein (secondary to pressure by an arteriosclerotic retinal artery). Both of these conditions have typical ophthalmologic findings. In the former the fundus is blanched, whereas in the latter the fundus will have multiple hemorrhages in the internal retinal layers around the course of the affected vessel(s). In elderly patients, a sudden loss of vision may be due to ischemic optic neuropathy, which could be due to hypertension superimposed on arteriosclerotic vessels supplying the optic nerve or to an autoimmune condition called giant cell arteritis (cranial arteritis, temporal arteritis). This latter type of acute, painless visual loss is often accompanied by fever, general malaise, and an elevated sedimentation rate and is diagnosed by temporal artery biopsy. It is important to distinguish the above two conditions because in cranial arteritis loss of vision may ultimately become bilateral and the vision in the second eye can be saved by starting the patient on high doses of steroids as soon as the diagnosis is made. Sudden visual loss with a normal fundus may also point to lesions between the optic disc and the optic chiasm, such as optic nerve tumor or inflammation (multiple sclerosis), pituitary tumors, parasellar lesions, carotid (or branches) arterial thrombosis, and anterior skull fractures or tumors. Sudden vision loss in a diabetic is usually due to vitreous hemorrhage. A sudden bilateral blindness is rare and, when present, is usually due to hysteria. Peripheral field disorders are usually not noticed until they are far advanced. They correspond to lesions in the visual pathways within the central nervous system.

Another common visual complaint is floaters (entopsia), which are shadowy specks or threads of different shapes and sizes that pass across the visual field, especially when the patient looks at a white wall. Large floaters of sudden appearance are more significant than small ones present for a long period of time. Almost all floaters are related to vitreous degeneration or vitreous pathology. When accompanied with lightning flashes (photopsias) they may herald the presence of retinal detachment. Photopsias are visual phenomena seen with the eyes closed. When monocular, they are usually due to retinal stimulation and when bilateral to occipital stimulation, as demonstrated by migraine phenomena. Migraine phenomena and migraine headaches may also be associated with hemianopsias. Distortion (metamorphosia), minification (micropsia), or magnification (macropsia) of a perceived image is usually secondary to macular disease. Double vision (diplopia) that is present when both eyes are open and disappears when one eye is closed is characteristic of paralytic strabismus.

Pain sensation in or around the eye must come from the lid, conjunctiva, cornea, iris, or ciliary body because they are the only ocular structures innervated by the trigeminal nerve. Nevertheless, intracranial pathology can refer pain to the orbital area. Reduced vision together with pain when moving the eyes is characteristic of optic neuritis. Localized eye fatigue after prolonged use of the eyes, as with reading, is called asthenopia and is a common symptom of refractive errors. Inflammation of the conjunctiva will give a gritty kind of sensation rather than an actual sensation of pain. In complaints of itching and burning, attention must be given to an allergic history or contact with irritants. Pain sensation from the eyelid, conjunctiva, and cornea is referred to the outer part of the upper lid. Herpes zoster and internal or external styes are also causes of pain in the lid areas. Questions regarding exposure to wind, hammering steel on metal, and time of the onset of pain are helpful. Pain associated with decreased vision and sensitivity to light (photophobia) directs the questioner to pathology of the cornea, iris, and ciliary body and possibly to acute angle closure glaucoma. Inflammation of these structures will also give rise to tenderness upon pressing on the globe. Severe, incapacitating headaches are usually not eye related.

The complaint of increased tearing must be classified as one of the following:

1. Intermittent tearing secondary to "dry eye" stimulating reflex tearing, such as seen in Vitamin A deficiency, trachoma, chemical burns, erythema multiforme, and keratoconjunctivitis sicca.
2. An overflow of a normal amount of tears (epiphora) due to an obstruction in the lacrimal secretory system. In infants this is usually due to an imperforated lower end of the nasolacrimal duct, whereas in adults it is due to infection of the lacrimal sac.
3. Production of excessive tears (lacrimation) due to foreign bodies, trauma, exposure to irritants, infections, or pathology of the anterior segment of the eye.

Following the exploration of the chief complaint, the history of the present illness is pursued in its entirety concentrating on the onset, duration, intermittency, disability, precipitating factors, and any associated signs.

Past History

In the past history are included the past ocular history, eye medications in use, and a general medical and surgical history. If the patient wears glasses, he is asked when he started wearing them and when they were last changed. History of previous eye trauma or eye surgery should be pursued in detail, including dates, hospitals, and physicians involved in the treatment. Previous eye problems such as lazy eye in childhood may eliminate an extensive work-up in evaluating poor vision in an adult after trauma.

Allergy to drugs or medications, especially to local eye medications, is obtained prior to instillation of any eye drops in the patient's eye. The patient should be questioned as to the use in the past or present of systemic medications, because these have been associated with eye pathology, for example, oral contraceptives (refractive disturbances), corticosteroids (cataracts and glaucoma), phenothiazines (retinopathy and cataracts), ethambutol (optic neuritis), chloroquine (central retinopathy), and chloromycetin (optic neuritis). Family history for eye conditions that have a hereditary basis, such as glaucoma, cataracts, macular degeneration, strabismus, retinoblastoma, and nystagmus, is also obtained.

PHYSICAL EXAMINATION

The inspection of each eye and the comparison of one eye with the other is the starting point of the objective examination of the eye. The anterior segment of the eye is better examined with lateral illumination in a slightly darkened room. In the "slit lamp" there is a magnifying lens that focuses the light on the conjunctiva,

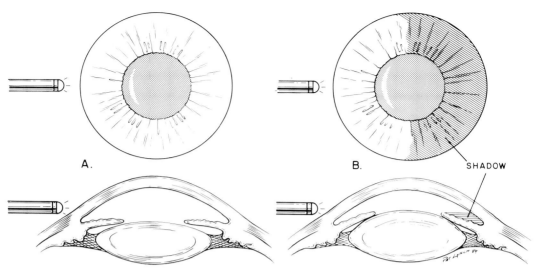

FIGURE 10.6   Anterior chamber depth evaluation. Penlight is placed at the limbus and contralateral iris area is observed for the presence of a shadow. Above: front view. Below: cross–section. A, deep anterior chamber. B, shallow chamber.

sclera, cornea, anterior chamber, or crystalline lens of the eye by moving the instrument forward. This could be simulated by using a plus condensing lens of between 10 and 20 diopters (10D to 20D) and placing it in the light path at a distance from the part to be examined that is equivalent to the focal length of the lens. The examiner can then use his naked eye or magnifying loupes to examine the tissue. The focal illumination distance for a 10D lens will be 10 cm and for a 20D lens will be 5 cm.

On examining the eyes, the examiner proceeds with the external eye examination in a systematic fashion. First, the status of the upper and lower lids is determined. It is noted if there is ptosis, swelling, or fat protruding into the lids; if the lids have a natural sulcus; if the lid borders are in contact with the globe with no ectropion or entropion; if there are any tumors or lesions around the lids; and if there is any swelling or redness. Then, attention is directed to the visual axes of the eyes. The patient is asked to look at a light or an attractive object, and the visual axes are compared to see whether they are straight on the object of regard or there is strabismus. If strabismus is present, then it is noted which way the deviated eye is turned. The object of regard is moved from one side to the other and up and down to see if both eyes follow together in a conjugate normal movement. Then, each eye is tested for mobility in all quadrants to be sure there are no limitations. During this part of the examination, the eyes are observed for the presence of rhythmic oscillatory back–and–forth movement, called nystagmus. Exaggerated outward position of the globe in the orbit (exophthalmos) or inward position (enophthalmos) eliminating or accentuating the sulcus is noted if present. Then, using the penlight, the cornea is illuminated laterally to see if it is shiny and if there are any foreign body opacities or corneal lesions, and to estimate the depth of the anterior chamber prior to pupil dilation for fundus examination (Figure 10.6). The peripheral visual fields are examined by fingers, hand, and red color confrontation in each eye while fixing straight ahead.

The conjunctiva is then examined for injection of the blood vessels, generalized redness, or papillary allergic reaction. After the bulbar conjunctiva, which is the part attached to the eyeball, is examined, the upper and lower lids are everted for examination of the palpebral conjunctiva, which is the conjunctiva lining the upper and lower lids. Rarely the sclera under the bulbar conjunctiva can be involved in a disease process, such as rheumatoid arthritis, or may be ruptured or lacerated during trauma. Foreign bodies in the eye are usually located either on the cornea or the palpebral conjunctiva under the upper lid close to the lid margin. Meibomian gland infections (internal stye) or chronic granuloma (chalazia) may protrude anteriorly through the skin or posteriorly through the conjunctiva. External styes (hordeolum) are caused by infections of the skin glands of Moll and Zeis.

Next, with good illumination, the pupils are checked for size, shape, equality, and reaction to light directly and consensually. The reaction of the pupil to direct light depends on the integrity of the visual apparatus (afferent limb), and on the integrity of the nerves to the iris constrictor musculature (efferent limb).

The rest of the examination is performed with the ophthalmoscope. First, transillumination of the ocular media is performed starting 2 or 3 feet away from the patient. Then the patient is slowly approached, with a focused image being maintained by appropriate rotation of the lens wheel of the ophthalmoscope. The disc or nervehead is evaluated first. Then the blood vessels are examined in the following order: first the nasal ones, superiorly and inferiorly, then the temporal ones, superiorly and inferiorly, as far into the periphery as can be seen. The central foveal area is then examined.

VISUAL ACUITY TESTING

Eye Chart

The first part of any ophthalmologic eye examination is the recording of the patient's visual acuity. This is important for legal purposes especially when the patient has had trauma to the eye. Distance vision is determined with the Snellen chart, on which each symbol is built in such a manner that the optotype (letter, number) as a whole subtends an angle of five minutes of arc, and each unit within the symbol subtends an angle of one minute of arc at a predetermined distance. One minute of arc at a distance of 20 feet is equivalent to about 1.8 mm, so the size of a full optotype will be five times that, or about 9 mm at 20 feet.

Astronomers years ago recognized that the eye is capable of perceiving two stars if the angle of separation between them is at least one minute of arc. This visual angle is called the minimal separable angle. The eye chart has lines of letters of different sizes. At the end of each line of letters is encoded the distance at which the letters in that particular line subtend an angle of five minutes of arc.

Testing Technique

The person to be examined is placed 20 feet (6 m) from the chart. (The distance of 20 feet was decided upon because rays of light originating from that distance are considered to be parallel for all practical purposes.) At that distance the person should be able to read the line of letters that subtends an angle of five minutes at that distance. If the person does so, his vision is recorded as 20/20 or 6/6. If the person cannot read this line of letters but can read those subtending an angle of five minutes at 40 feet while standing 20 feet from the chart, the vision is recorded as 20/40, or 6/12 in meters. An individual has normal visual acuity when each eye is best corrected to 20/20 and has abnormal visual acuity when the best corrected vision is worse than 20/20. Having a refractive error correctable with

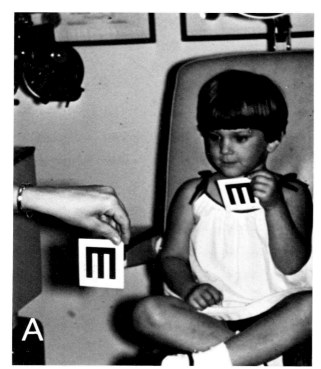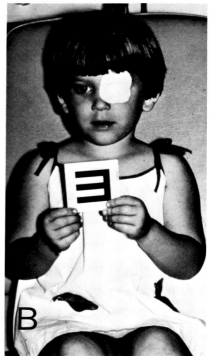

FIGURE 10.7   A: Four-year-old patient is being taught the "E" game. B: Non-tested eye patched with Elastoplast occlusor. Patient ready to be tested with full "E" chart.

glasses to 20/20 is not considered an abnormality of the visual system but simply a refractive error as opposed to organic pathology. In cases of organic pathology the vision cannot be improved even with the use of glasses. A legally blind person is an individual who has a best corrected vision of 20/200 or worse in his better eye or out of a possible 150 degrees of visual field in each eye has 20 degrees or less in the better eye.

Testing Children

Visual acuity reported by children depends on the age, intelligence, and attention span. By age 3 1/2 years, most children can report vision taken with the "E" chart. Before that age, the visual acuity in patients with strabismus is estimated by the ophthalmologist by the mode and preference of fixation in each eye. In testing children, the nontested eye must be covered with micropore adhesive tape or Elastoplast to prevent cheating and to give the child freedom to place his head in any position he/she desires (Figure 10.7). The patient practices the matching of different positions of the "E" on the chart with a big letter "E", which he holds in his hands. In the "E" game, the only task requested from the child is to match one of four positions: up, down, right, or left. As the test progresses and the "E's" become smaller in size and more letters are placed on each line, the patient still performs the same task because the optotype at which he is looking is always the same. A whole chart or an entire line is used rather than single letters, because patients with functional amblyopia may be able to read one or two extra lines when individual letters are used instead of a row of letters, giving a false visual acuity report.

Testing the Visually Handicapped

When a patient reports a vision worse than 20/200, the patient's nontested eye should be patched with an opaque tape or covered with the heel of the hand. The Snellen chart at distance will test the visual acuity from 20/20 to 20/200. If the patient cannot see a 20/200 line, the chart is brought closer to the patient. The distance at which the patient first can read a line of letters is recorded. For example, if he reads the 20/200 line at 10 feet, it is recorded as 10/200. The top of the fraction is the distance from the patient to the chart and the bottom of the fraction is the distance at which the specific letters subtend an angle of five minutes.

If the patient cannot see the top letter at a distance of five feet, then finger counting is used to approximate acuity. The vision is recorded as the farthest distance at which the patient can count fingers (CF). If within a few inches of his face the patient still cannot count any fingers, then he is tested for perception of hand motion. The vision is then reported as hand movement (HM) at the farthest distance he can see such movement. If the patient cannot see the movement of the hand, then a light is projected into the eye and the patient is asked if he can see it. The light is projected from each of the four quadrants, and the patient is asked to try to report the area from which the light is coming. If he does this accurately, then colored lenses can be interposed between the light and the patient, and the patient asked to report the color of the light. If he does this accurately, the vision is recorded as "light perception (LP) with projection and color discrimination." If he cannot discriminate the color, it is reported as "LP with projection but no color discrimination." If the projection is poor, then it is written only as "LP" or "LP with no projection." Finally, if the patient cannot see the light anywhere, it is written as "no light perception (NLP)."

Pinhole Vision

If the patient has glasses, the vision is always evaluated with the glasses on. If the patient cannot see well with his own glasses, it means one of two things: either the glasses need to be changed or there is some pathology causing the decrease in visual acuity. If the patient reports that he could see well with the glasses until recently, an organic disease process must be ruled out.

Looking through a pinhole of between 1 and 1.5 mm in diameter will have the effect of balancing up to about 5D of refractive error, helping to differentiate refractive error from organic pathology in diminished visual acuity. A pinhole can be placed in front of the patient's glasses if he/she wears glasses or in front of the eye if he does not wear glasses to determine grossly if the decreased visual acuity is due to a refractive error or to an organic disease. A pinhole can be made by perforating a piece of paper with an open paper clip.

Near Vision and Accommodation

The ability of the eye to change its refractive power by adding plus power in order to focus a close object on the retina is called accommodation. This is made possible by the contraction of the circular ciliary muscle causing a relaxation of the zonular fibers, increasing the curvature of the lens. The amplitude of this change depends upon the elasticity of the lens capsule and the lens fibers, which

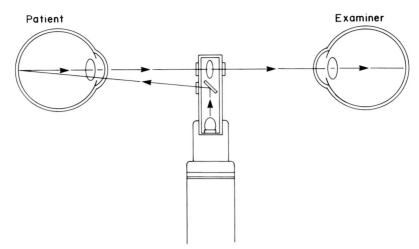

FIGURE 10.8   Optical principle of direct ophthalmoscopy.

decreases with age. The physiologic decrease of elasticity of the lens with age is called presbyopia and it begins in an emmetrope at about 45 years of age in cold climates and earlier in the tropics.

To read at a distance of one third of a meter, 3D of accommodation are needed, and for a distance of 16 inches, 2.5D of accommodation are needed in an emmetrope. To read comfortably at 16 inches for a long period of time without glasses, the patient will need at least 5D of accommodation. At age 45, the average emmetrope has 3.5D of accommodation. This may be enough to read for short periods of time in good illumination, but symptoms of fatigue may occur after prolonged reading. For near visual acuity testing, a commercially available near card can be used at 14 inches. Size 20/25 print is equivalent to the print of small bibles, 20/30 print is that of want ads, 20/40 is that of the telephone directory, 20/50 is that of newspaper text, 20/65 is that of magazines, 20/70 is that of adult textbooks, and 20/80 is that of children's books.

OPHTHALMOSCOPY

Direct Ophthalmoscopy

Within less than 10 years of the discovery of the ophthalmoscope by Helmholtz in 1850, optic nerve damage by glaucoma, detachment of the retina, and retinitis pigmentosa were all described. This instrument has made the field of ophthalmology possible. Helmholtz discovered that light falling into the eye is reflected through the same pathway as the incoming light source. He placed his eye directly into the pathway of the returning light (Figure 10.8) by using a mirror with a hole in the center to reflect light into the eye while he looked through the center hole directly into the path of light. Today, all ophthalmoscopes are self-illuminating, and they have a rotating disc with lenses that enable the physician to balance a refractive error, either in the patient or in himself, so that the fundus image will be seen in focus.

The examination is better performed if eye drops are used to dilate the pupil. Two types of drops can be used. Parasympatholytic drops, such as Mydriacil 1% and Cyclogyl 1%, paralyze the sphincter of the pupil and the ciliary muscle, producing both mydriasis (dilatation) and cycloplegia (paralysis of accommodation).

Sympathomimetic drops (Neo-Synephrine 2.5% or 10%) stimulate the dilator muscle of the pupil, causing mydriasis without cycloplegia. Combinations of these two types of drugs are commonly used by the ophthalmologist.

To examine the right eye, the patient looks straight ahead. The instrument is held with the right hand in front of the examiner's right eye. The index finger should be placed on the rotating disc that moves the lenses inside the instrument. Now, the examiner looks through the hole in the center at a distance of about 3 feet from the patient and observes whether the pupil being examined appears totally illuminated with an even red reflex. If there is no illumination or only part of the pupil is illuminated while some areas appear dark, it means that there is an opacity either in the cornea, anterior chamber, lens, or vitreous humor (all these structures together are called "the media") that interferes with the course of the returning light beam.

If there is a small foreign body in the cornea or a small opacity in the lens, it appears as a small, circumscribed, dark dot in a diffusely red-colored background. By having the patient move the eye up and down, we can use parallax to identify the location of the opacity. Any opacity in the cornea, the anterior chamber, or the anterior surface of the lens will move in the direction of the movement of the eye. Those opacities in the posterior surface of the lens or in the vitreous humor will move in the opposite direction. A naturally occurring opacity of the lens is called a cataract. It is named according to the location as anterior cortical, nuclear, and posterior subcapsular. The larger and more posterior the opacity in the lens, the greater the visual impairment will be.

The vitreous body is attached to the periphery of the retina and to the optic nervehead. Degenerative changes occur in the vitreous humor with age and in myopia causing it to liquify. Vitreous changes may be caused by hemorrhage and vascular changes such as those seen in diabetes and in trauma. Exudation of cells into the vitreous humor can be caused by inflammation of the iris, ciliary body, and choroid. All vitreous degenerations will cause opacities of the vitreous humor that will be seen by the patient in the form of dots or threads or large flakes. When there is a large exudative reaction of the vitreous humor or a large hemorrhage, the pupil on transillumination will appear dark instead of red. In asteroid hyalitis there are white glistening deposits suspended in the vitreous humor that resemble snowflakes and consist mainly of calcium soaps and lipids. This occurs in older patients, and causes no visual disturbances but makes it difficult to examine the retina with the direct ophthalmoscope.

The examination of the fundus proper should always begin with the examination of the nervehead. The fovea (center of the macular area) of the eye is very sensitive to light. Its examination causes discomfort and it is therefore examined last. The pupil will become miotic if not well dilated with drugs when the fovea is examined. Next, as you move closer to the patient's eye with the index finger turning the lens wheel of the ophthalmoscope slowly, the fundus structures will come into focus. If the patient is emmetropic, parallel rays of light will be reflected from the fundus returning in a parallel fashion into the examiner's eye. If the examiner is also emmetropic the incoming parallel rays of light will be refracted to focus on his/her retina and a sharp 15x magnified image of the patient's fundus will be seen. If the patient's eye is myopic the refracted light will be converging, and if the patient's eye is hyperopic the refracted light will be diverging. The examiner can obtain sharp images in these eyes by rotating the lens wheel of the ophthalmoscope to neutralize the patient's refractive error. If the examiner is emmetropic (or is using his or her glasses to correct his or her refractive error) and is not using his accommodation, the lens used to balance the patient's error will give an indication of the patient's refractive condition. With the lenses in the direct ophthalmoscope, astigmatism cannot be neutralized and the patient's retinal image, if the astigmatic error is high, will always remain slightly fuzzy.

Because the nervehead is nasal to the macular area, if the patient, while his right eye is being examined, is asked to look in the direction of the right ear of the examiner, the right nervehead will move into a temporal position and will be in the direct path of the examiner's vision. When examining the left eye, the patient is asked to look toward the examiner's left ear. First, notice the color of the optic nerve; observe the margins to see if they are sharp, blurry, or elevated; and evaluate the central cup. The nervehead is an oval disc that is colored slightly lighter than the orange-red color of the retina. Then, follow the retina blood vessels: start at the disc, go out with the arteries and come back with the veins. The ophthalmoscope allows for the examination of the retinal blood vessels, and in a sense, allows us to evaluate the vascular status of the rest of the body. The vessels are evaluated as to their width, their vascular reflections ("reflexes"), thickness of their walls, their course, and the ratio between the calibers of the arteries and the veins. The retina is completely transparent, so damage to it will show as an opacity. Finally, ask the patient to look directly at the light and evaluate the fovea.

The high magnification of the direct ophthalmoscope makes possible the observation of details in a small segment of the fundus, such as the blood vessels, the nervehead, and the macular area. It can also be used for measurements of differences in elevation of the fundus. If there is an elevated structure, such as the nervehead in papilledema or a tumor from the choroid elevating the retina, its height can be estimated by first focusing the instrument on the normal flat retina and then refocusing the instrument (by adding plus lenses) on the surface of the elevated structure. The difference between the two lenses will be the elevation of the retina/structure as measured in diopters. Three diopters' difference is equivalent, more or less, to 1 mm of elevation.

Indirect Ophthalmoscopy

The fundus can also be examined with a self-illuminating binocular indirect ophthalmoscope, which is supported with a headband. The patient is usually examined while lying down so that the patient's head can be approached from either side or from behind. Indirect ophthalmoscopy enables us to view the fundus of the eye stereoscopically. The examiner holds a condensing lens with one hand and can use the other hand to depress the sclera in order to examine the periphery of the retina or to draw on paper what he sees. When the pupil of the patient lights up by transillumination from the indirect ophthalmoscope, the condensing lens is brought into the beam of light. The condensing lens is held between the thumb and forefinger of one hand, the fourth or fifth finger of which is lightly resting on the patient's face. The patient and the examiner are about one arm's length apart (approximately 50 cm), and the condensing lens is about 8 cm from the patient's eye. The ophthalmoscope light, the condensing lens, and the pupil of the patient have to be in the same axis. With a +20D condensing lens a virtual inverted image of the fundus approximately 13 cm from the patient's eye will be seen with 3x lateral magnification (+30D = 2x; +15D = 4x). The axial magnification is equal to the square root of the lateral magnification (2 = 1.4; 3 = 1.7; 4 = 2). Indirect ophthalmoscopy requires practice because the image in the air is inverted such that the part of the fundus lying below the nervehead appears above it and the part of the fundus temporal to the nervehead appears on the nasal side. Also, the physician has to learn to avoid the distracting reflexes from the cornea and from the condensing lens while focusing on the image in the air. The distracting cornea and lens reflexes can be avoided by tilting the lens slightly, displacing them toward the lens margin. Three adjustments must be made before the examination is started: (a) the ophthalmoscope headband is adjusted over the head of the examiner, (b) the interpupillary distance of the oculars is set, and (c) the light is directed into the eye. For the initial examination of the disc (just as with direct ophthalmoscopy) the patient is asked to look at the right ear of the examiner when the right eye is to be examined and vice versa.

Indirect ophthalmoscopy has several advantages over direct ophthalmoscopy. The image is stereoscopic, so the disc elevation in papilledema, the width and depth of the optic nerve cup in glaucoma, and the retinal elevation in a detached retina, and in a melanoma of the choroid can be seen in a three-dimensional way. Because the light source is brighter, the fundus can be seen more clearly even when there are some opacities of the cornea or the crystalline lens. The periphery of the retina can be seen where most of the retinal tears, which produce detached retinas, are usually located. Because the image magnification is much less, more of the retina can be seen at a glance than with a direct ophthalmoscope, giving a better perspective of lesions that encompass a large section of the retina, such as diabetic retinopathy, detached retinas, and tumors inside the eye. For this same reason, it is more suitable for examination of uncooperative patients and children. It also allows for a more accurate evaluation of the contrast between the color of the nervehead and its environment.

OCULAR EMERGENCIES AND "THE RED EYE"

Ocular Emergencies

Ocular emergencies are classified into: (a) those to be treated within minutes, (b) those that can wait one to two hours, and (c) those that can wait one or more days. Emergencies needing treatment within minutes are chemical (acid or alkaline) burns and central retinal artery occlusion. In the case of chemical burns, the first person who gets to the patient should start immediate irrigation with copious amounts of aqueous solution, such as saline, eye irrigating solution, or tap water. Irrigation should continue for a minimum of 30 minutes, especially in cases of alkaline (lye) burns. If pieces of chemicals are in the conjunctiva, they should be removed. During irrigation an ophthalmologist should be contacted to determine appropriate, continuing treatment.

In central retinal artery occlusion, immediate massage of the eye is performed in an attempt to dislodge the thrombus/embolus. The patient is then asked to breath into a paper bag until a 5% carbon dioxide/oxygen mixture is available. Intraocular pressure can be lowered sharply either by the use of mannitol intravenously (2 g/kg of a 20% solution over 30 minutes) or by an anterior chamber paracentesis in an attempt to dislodge the thrombus/embolus. The paracentesis is performed by an ophthalmologist.

Emergency conditions that should be treated within one to two hours are: sudden loss of vision secondary to giant cell arteritis, corneal foreign body, acute angle closure glaucoma, corneal ulcer, lid laceration, penetrating injury to the globe, hyphema, purulent conjunctivitis in newborn infants and conjunctivitis in a patient who recently underwent intraocular surgery, and a retrobulbar hemorrhage either after trauma or after lid and/or orbital surgery. A blowout fracture of the orbit with an otherwise normal globe is not an emergency.

The following equipment is needed in the emergency or consultation room: strong light source, magnifying loupes, direct ophthalmoscope, Schiotz tonometer, distance chart and near vision card, pinhole, +2.00 lens, fluorescein strips, cobalt blue light, Desmarres lid retractors or bent paper clips, cotton swabs, eye pads,

paper tape, and Fox shield. Drugs needed are: proparacaine hydrochloride 0.5%
(Ophthetic), phenylephrine 2.5% (Neo-Synephrine), tropicamide 1% (Mydriacyl),
and pilocarpine 2%. After a short, pertinent history, based on the chief complaint,
the eye examination in the emergency room is performed in an orderly fashion.
The visual acuity is measured, preferably with a distance chart (using a pinhole
and a +2.00 lens to correct refractive errors and presbyopia, respectively, if
needed). Then the condition of the lids, conjunctiva, sclera, cornea, anterior chamber, and pupil is evaluated with a good light. This is followed by motility evaluation,
evaluation of visual fields by confrontation, intraocular pressure testing, and
finally ophthalmoscopic examination. Radiographs are ordered if there is a question of a foreign body or fracture of any of the orbital bones. To sedate children,
chloral hydrate 20 to 50 mg/kg of body weight or a pediatric cocktail (1 mg/kg
Demerol, 0.5 mg/kg Phenergan, and 0.5 mg/kg Thorazine) can be used.

Things to remember in the emergency room eye care:

1. No local anesthetic medication should be given to the patient to take home.
2. No ointments should be applied to the cornea prior to an ophthalmologic
   examination.
3. No atropine should be instilled in an eye; short-acting cycloplegics
   (Mydriacyl 1% or Cyclogyl 1%) are as effective.
4. No steroid eye medication should be used, except by an ophthalmologist.
5. When penetrating injuries to the globe itself are suspected, avoid any
   pressure to the globe.
6. Lid lacerations should not be sutured until the patient is evaluated by an
   ophthalmologist when: (a) they are through and through, especially in the
   upper lid; (b) they involve the lid margin; or (c) the lacrimal canaliculus is
   lacerated.

"The Red Eye"

A "red eye" refers to patients with conjunctival hyperemia with or without "ciliary
flush." Conjunctival hyperemia is an engorgement of the larger and more superficial bulbar conjunctival blood vessels. "Ciliary flush" is an injection of the deep
conjunctival and episcleral vessels surrounding the cornea, most easily seen in daylight, and appears as a faint violet ring in which individual vessels are indiscernible
to the unaided eye. It is a danger sign often seen in eyes with corneal inflammations, iridocyclitis, or acute glaucoma.

The combination of a few signs and symptoms will help make a tentative diagnosis in the red eye. Pain with photophobia and decreased vision will separate
corneal foreign body or ulcer, acute iritis, and acute glaucoma from conjunctivitis.
In corneal pathology, the pain will disappear with topical anesthesia. In acute
iritis, the pupil will be small and the intraocular pressure will be low. In acute
glaucoma, the pupil will be fixed and semidilated and the intraocular pressure
will be very high. In a red eye secondary to conjunctivitis there will not be a
"ciliary flush," the vision is not affected, and the pupil will be of normal size, re-
acting briskly to light both directly and consensually.

Allergic conjunctivitis is associated with itching, whereas bacterial and viral
conjunctivitis are associated with a gritty discomfort. A discharge in bacterial
conjunctivitis is purulent, with crust on the lashes; in viral it is serous and in allergic
it is mucous. In iritis, acute glaucoma, and corneal abrasion (or foreign body) there
is increased lacrimation but not true conjunctival discharge.

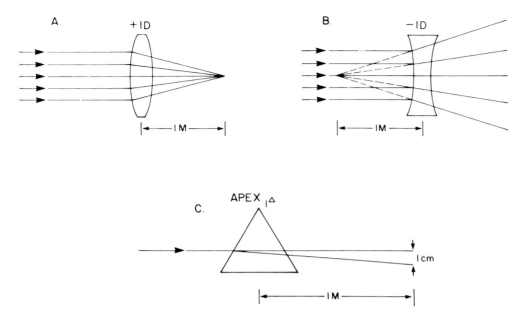

FIGURE 10.9   A: One positive lens diopter (+1.00D). B: One negative lens diopter (–1.00D). C: One prism diopter (1^Δ).

REFRACTIVE ERRORS AND REFRACTION

Optics

All anomalies of refraction can be explained in the lack of relationship between the refractive power of the eye (cornea and lens) and the length of the eyeball. The degree of refractive error, as well as the strength of the lenses needed for correction, is expressed in lens diopters (Figure 10.9). The focal length of a lens is the distance from the lens to the point where parallel rays of light going through the lens converge to a point that is called the focal point. One hundred divided by the focal length in centimeters will give the power in lens diopters. The stronger the lens is, the shorter will be the focal length. Lenses that converge parallel rays of light are called plus lenses. Some lenses diverge parallel rays of light as they emerge from the other side of the lens, and by tracing the rays backward to the left side of the lens an imaginary focal point will be reached. The distance between that point and the lens will be the focal length. These lenses are minus lenses because they have a negative focus. The power of this lens is found by dividing 100 by the negative focal length, being careful to keep the negative sign.

Emmetropia

In an emmetropic eye, parallel rays of light entering the eye will come to focus on the retina. This means that there is an optical agreement between the refracting powers (cornea and lens) and the length of the eyeball (Figure 10.10). The average adult eye is 24 mm in length; at birth the average eye is 19 mm in length. By age 3 years, the eye reaches its adult dimension and has a hypermetropia of about 2 lens diopters. As the eye enlarges from birth to age 3 years, the spherical lens

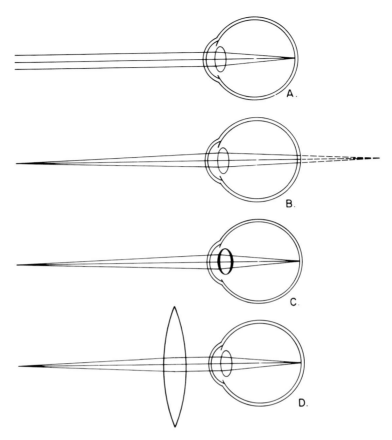

FIGURE 10.10   Emmetropia. A: Parallel rays of light focused on retina. B: Near vision rays of light focused behind retina. C: Near vision rays of light focused on retina with accommodation. D: Near vision rays of light focused on retina with a plus lens (in presbyopia).

becomes flatter, reducing its refractive power. If the refraction of the cornea and the lens is not changed and the length of the eyeball is changed by 1 mm, the effective refraction will be changed by 3D of myopia if it were lengthened, and by 3D of hyperopia if it were shortened. It follows that most refractive errors are due either to too short or too long an eyeball. After age 45 years, almost all emmetropes will need glasses for near vision.

Presbyopia

Near vision glasses are prescribed on the basis of the accommodation remaining. To test accommodation, a letter the size of a 20/30 in the near vision chart is placed close to the patient's eye and is moved slowly away until the patient can read it for the first time. One hundred divided by the distance in centimeters at which the patient can read the 20/30 line for the first time is the number of diopters of accommodation the patient has left. This amount of accommodation left determines the strength of the reading glasses given to the patient. When the amplitude of accommodation is less than 4 lens diopters, reading glasses are needed

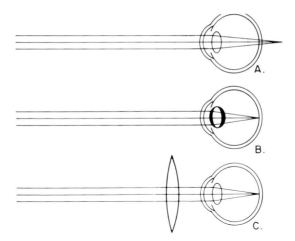

FIGURE 10.11   Hyperopia. A: Parallel rays of light focused behind retina. B: Parallel rays of light focused on retina with accommodation. C: Parallel rays of light focused on retina with a plus lens.

to be able to read comfortably for a long period of time and means that the patient has presbyopia.

Hyperopia or Farsightedness

Hyperopia, or farsightedness or hypermetropia, is usually due to a short axial length of the eye. Parallel rays of light will converge toward a focus behind the retina (Figure 10.11). In small degrees of hyperopia, young people can compensate for this refractive error by using accommodation, which increases the refractive curvature of the lens inside the eye. In moderate and large degrees of hyperopia, accommodation by itself will not be enough, and the patient will need convex plus lenses in front of the eye to focus the image on the retina. Natural emmetropes or persons made emmetropic by the use of glasses, when they look at a near object, will have to use their accommodation to converge the diverging rays of light. The use of accommodation at near point to keep the image clear will also bring convergence to keep the image single and miosis to improve the optical system of the eye. This triad is called the near reflex and occurs only in humans and higher primates.

In children with accommodative or refractive esotropia, the act of accommodation brings too much convergence, causing an ocular deviation that is corrected by the wearing of full hypermetropic correction lenses.

Myopia or Nearsightedness

Myopia is usually due to a long axial length of the eye and rarely due to too much refractive power of the cornea. Parallel rays of light are refracted by the myopic eye in such a manner that they focus in the vitreous body in front of the retina (Figure 10.12). Rays of light coming from the retina will leave the eye in a converging bundle, so that the far point of the myopia eye lies at a certain distance in front of the cornea. The greater the myopia, the closer the far point will be to the cornea. Myopic patients will have good vision without correction only in the area between the far point and the near point, and this is the reason that they hold

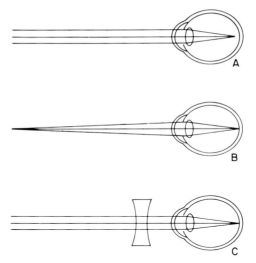

**FIGURE 10.12   Myopia. A: Parallel rays of light focused in front of retina.
B: Near vision rays of light focused on retina. C: Parallel rays of light focused
on retina with a minus lens.**

things close to the eyes when they are not wearing their glasses. The focusing
mechanism of the eye cannot compensate for myopia and the patient must wear
concave minus lenses.

The elongation of the eyeball in myopia causes stretching of all the structures
in the posterior part of the eye, which may bring secondary pathologic changes in
the vitreous humor, retina, choroid, and sclera. This causes a predisposition to
retinal tears and retinal detachments. In high myopia there is a bulging of the
sclera in the posterior pole called staphyloma. Around the area of the staphyloma
degenerative changes of the retina and vitreous can be observed with the ophthalmoscope in the form of pigmentary changes and atrophic areas. These changes
occur usually in the posterior pole, which is located temporal to the optic nervehead.

Astigmatism

Astigmatism is a refractive defect in which the refractive power of the eye is not
uniform in all meridians. Parallel rays of light entering the eye are bent unequally
in two principal meridians, and instead of a sharp point focus there are two focal
lines. Astigmatism is corrected by cylindrical (toric) lenses. Cylindrical lenses have
two meridians perpendicular to each other, with no refractive power in the axis
meridian and maximum refractive power in the other meridian. Astigmatism can
be *simple,* one focal line on the retina and the other in front (myopic) or behind
(hyperopic); *mixed,* one in front of the retina (myopic) and the other behind (hyperopic); or *compound,* both focal lines in front of the retina (myopic) or both behind
(hyperopic).

Refraction

A refraction is nothing more than the finding of the lens needed to balance the
patient's refractive error. In adult patients, after an objective refraction is done
using the retinoscope, trial lenses are placed in front of the patient's eyes to perform

the "acceptance." When cycloplegic medication is used it is called a cycloplegic refraction. It is called a manifest refraction when no cycloplegic medication is used. When only an acceptance is done without retinoscopy, it is called a subjective refraction. When only the retinoscopic findings under cycloplegia are used, as in children under the age of 7 years without an acceptance, it is called "Flash" retinoscopy, or objective refraction.

Retinoscopy is a form of transillumination (like ophthalmoscopy). The retinoscope has a perforated mirror with a central hole through which the examiner observes a streak of light projected from the instrument into the pupil and fundus of the eye. The pupils are dilated either with Mydriacyl 1% or Cyclogyl 1%. The examination is done in a darkened room and the examiner sits an arm's length away from the patient (two thirds of a meter). The light of the retinoscope is directed toward the patient's pupil and, by moving the light, a streak can be seen in the pupil moving either with or against the direction of motion of the instrument. If the emerging rays of light converge to a focus in the eyes of the physician, the pupil of the patient will appear evenly red and there will be no movement. In the case of hyperopia, the emerging rays of light will converge beyond the examiner's eye, and the streak of light in the patient's pupil will move in the same direction that the retinoscope is moved.

In myopia, the emerging rays of light will converge at the far point of the eye, which lies between the examiner and the patient. The crossing of the rays will produce a movement of the streak in a direction opposite to the motion of the retinoscope. To balance the refractive error, convex or concave lenses are placed in front of the patient's eye until his hyperopia or myopia is neutralized. There will be one combination of lenses that will abolish any movement of the streak, and at that moment the pupil will momentarily be evenly red. With this combination of lenses in front of the patient's eye, the far point of the eye lies on the retina of the physician, and, therefore, it corresponds to the degree of the refractive error. The retinoscopic examination is performed at a distance of two thirds of a meter, which corresponds to the focal length of a lens of 1.5D. This amount has to be deducted algebraically from the lens combination that neutralized the patient's refractive error. An emmetropic eye, therefore, will be neutralized with a +1.50 lens when the retinoscope is held at a distance of two thirds of a meter; at a distance of 1 meter, +1.00; and at a distance of one-half meter, +2.00. In a patient with astigmatism, one of the two principal meridians will be neutralized before the other. A cylindrical lens is added to the first lens in front of the patient's eye to neutralize the second meridian. When neutralization of the astigmatism is completed, the eye will be in a true spherical equivalent position free from any astigmatic influences.

Example of a refraction prescription:

+4.00	⌣	−2.25	x	180°
(sign and power of sphere)	(with)	(sign and power of cylinder)		(axis of cylinder)

Contact Lenses

When using contact lenses, the contact lens refracting surface substitutes for the refracting surface of the cornea. In the case of myopia, it weakens the converging power, and in the case of hyperopia it increases the converging power of the cornea. Soft lenses conform to the shape of the cornea, so they do not correct for corneal astigmatic errors. When hard contact lenses are fitted, the near surface of the lens will trap the tear film between itself and the cornea, filling out the area of more curvature, thus correcting corneal astigmatism. The hard and soft contact lenses stay in the eye by the surface tension of the tears between the lens and the cornea. The new "hard" contact lenses are made of a gas-permeable material and are tolerated better by the cornea. Soft contact lenses have a high water content and must be kept moist at all times to maintain their shape, either with the patient's tears while in the patient's eye or with sterilized salt solutions when they are stored. Overwearing of a contact lens causing a corneal abrasion may not be noticed until several hours after the lens has been removed. At this time, the eye will become reddened, the vision will become hazy, and there will be an increased sensitivity to light.

Fluorescein drops are used to help in the fitting of hard contact lenses and in the diagnosis of corneal abrasions. They should not be used with soft contact lenses because they will stain them. Hard and gas-permeable contact lenses are stored with wetting and cleaning solutions, which not only make the lenses cleaner but make them more comfortable when they are inserted into the eye. Contact lenses are indicated medically in patients who have had only one eye operated upon for cataract removal, without insertion of an intraocular lens. The contact lens will take over the converging power of the missing lens from the eye and the patient will be more comfortable without the magnification and the loss of side vision incurred with the use of aphakic spectacles. Soft contact lenses and gas-permeable lenses allow for more interchange of oxygen between the air and the cornea than the old hard lenses. Contact lenses will not stop the progression of myopia or keratoconus.

SPECIAL EXAMINATIONS

During the student's rotation through the ophthalmology service, he will be exposed to the following instruments and examination techniques.

Exophthalmometry

The cornea normally lies between 16 and 20 mm anterior to the lateral rim of the orbit. A difference of 2 mm between the anterior positions of the two corneas when compared to one another is considered abnormal. The orbit is a closed space, so any space-occupying lesion inside the orbit will push the eye forward, making it protrude. This is called proptosis or exophthalmos. Exophthalmos caused by tumors is usually unilateral, whereas that caused by thyroid orbitopathy may be bilateral. Exophthalmos can be measured by using a ruler placed on the anterior aspect of the lateral part of the orbit, parallel to the visual axis. By sighting across the ruler one can measure how far the cornea is anterior to the rim. An exophthalmometer (Hertel), which has a system of mirrors attached to each side, measures the protrusion of the eyes in a more accurate manner.

Tonometry

The intraocular pressure (IOP) can be measured either by indentation (Schiotz) tonometry or applanation (Goldmann) tonometry. In Schiotz tonometry a weight indents the cornea, displacing the fluid within the eye. The tonometer scale measures the amount of indentation, which is then converted to millimeters of mercury by the chart supplied with the tonometer (Figure 10.13). The instrument is placed directly on the center of the cornea of a reclining patient after the cornea has been anesthetized. In applanation tonometry an area with a diameter of 3.06 mm is flattened in the center of the cornea by the small, plastic Goldmann tonometer prism that is attached to the slit lamp. Besides topical anesthesia,

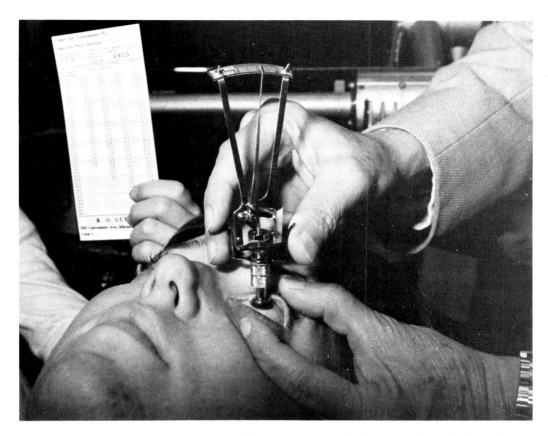

FIGURE 10.13   Schiotz indentation tonometer. Instrument is rested on top of the cornea after proparacaine 0.5% anesthesia. Chart to convert instrument's reading into millimeters of mercury is also shown.

fluorescein drops are instilled prior to "touching" the eye with this tonometer. The endpoint is reached by manipulating two opposing green half-circles (fluorescein stained), seen through the slit-lamp microscope while using blue light. The IOP is read in millimeters of mercury on the scale at the base of the instrument. Most ophthalmologists prefer applanation tonometry because it is not affected by the rigidity of the sclera. Normal average IOP is 16 mm Hg with a standard deviation of 2.5 mm Hg.

Slit-Lamp Examination

The slit lamp is an instrument that focuses a slit of light on the various structures of the eye while the same tissue is observed through a powerful microscope. The cornea, anterior chamber, lens, vitreous humor, and retina are all available for slit-lamp examination. To examine the vitreous humor and the retina with the slit-lamp microscope, a fundus contact lens is placed on the front surface of the eye. The slit lamp is extremely important for the ophthalmologist to be able to diagnose and treat diseases of the cornea and inflammations of the uvea. It is useful to differentiate types of cataracts and to categorize lesions in the macular area. It is an important tool used to evaluate progress after cornea and cataract surgery.

Gonioscopy

Gonioscopy is the examination of the angle of the anterior chamber of the eye. The gonioprism lens is placed on the cornea after topical anesthesia and the angle is observed through the slit-lamp microscope. Several zones can be differentiated by the amount of pigment they have. The most anterior zone is the end of the corneal endothelium (Schwalbe's line). The next one is the trabecular meshwork, which has some pigment. Then comes the nonpigmented scleral spur followed by the deeply pigmented ciliary body band. The main use of gonioscopy is to differentiate open-angle glaucoma, in which all the structures of the angle are clearly visible, from narrow-angle glaucoma, in which none or only some of the anterior structures of the angle are visible.

Keratometry

With the keratometer, the curvature of the cornea in two principal meridians can be measured, giving an indication whether corneal astigmatism is present or not. This instrument is indispensible in the prescription of contact lenses and in the prescription of glasses for patients with large corneal astigmatic errors. It is also valuable in the preoperative and postoperative evaluation of patients needing corneal transplant and cataract surgery.

Ophthalmodynamometry

The ophthalmodynamometer (ODM) is an instrument that has a spring gauge that indents the sclera while the examiner looks at the central retinal artery. Because the pressure from the instrument makes the pressure inside the eye increase to approximately the level of the systemic diastolic pressure, the central artery will start pulsating. This will be the ocular diastolic pressure. Then, as more pressure is applied, the central artery will stop pulsating. This will be the ocular systolic pressure. The normal ophthalmic artery pressure is about 78% of the systemic blood pressure. A pressure difference of 15% or more between both eyes may indicate occlusion of the internal carotid artery. The central retinal artery is a branch of the ophthalmic artery, which is the first branch of the internal carotid artery. For the test to be positive, there must be about 85% occlusion of the internal carotid.

Fluorescein

Fluorescein is a vegetable dye that is soluble in water, blood, and in connective tissue. It is nontoxic and can be injected intravenously. When illuminated with blue light it fluoresces a bright yellow-green color. Its four major uses in ophthalmology are: (a) to diagnose corneal pathology, (b) to diagnose patency of the lacrimal drainage system, (c) to evaluate the fit of hard contact lenses, and (d) intravenously to help in the diagnosis of disturbances of blood flow in the choroid and retina. Sterile 0.25% fluorescein solution (Fluress) or a fluorescein-impregnated strip (Fluor-I-Strip) is applied to the cornea. If an abrasion is present, the defect in the surface epithelium will appear green in white light and yellow under blue light. To test tear excretion, a small cotton-tipped applicator is placed in the nose under the inferior turbinate, then one drop of 2% fluorescein is placed in the conjunctival sac and the patient's head is bent forward. Within five minutes the fluorescein should appear in the nose if the lacrimal excretory system is patent (Jones' test).

Fluorescein Angiography

Five or 10% sterile fluorescein soluble solution is injected intravenously into the patient's arm, and the fundus of the eye is evaluated for disturbances of the pigment epithelial layer or permeability changes of the retinal vessels with the use of appropriate optical filters. The changes can be visualized (angioscopy) with a slit-lamp examination and a fundus contact lens or can be photographed (angiography) with a fundus camera. The injected dye first reaches the choroidal blood vessels in 8 to 10 seconds, producing a diffuse "flush" of the entire ocular fundus. Then, the dye appears at the disc 0.5 to 1 second later before entering the central retinal artery branches. The arterial phase is the initial stage in which the fluorescein is present only in the arterial vessels. The next phase is the capillary phase representing a fine, granular fluorescence of the whole retina. Beginning of flow of the dye through the venous channel indicates the venous phase. At the beginning of this stage, the dye coming from small vessels does not mix immediately with the blood already present in the other vessels. The fluorescein and the normal blood run parallel to each other in the larger veins in a laminar fashion. Later on, the veins are completely filled with the dye. The interval between the entrance of the dye and the beginning of the venous flow is the retinal arterial circulation time. This interval is the shortest for the vessels supplying the macula. "After phase" is the time after the fluorescein has left the retinal vessels. Normal retinal vessels are not permeable to fluorescein, so only in pathologic, inflammatory, or degenerative conditions of the retina, such as diabetic retinopathy and retinal vein obstructions, will fluorescein leak into the retina.

STRABISMUS AND AMBLYOPIA

Terminology

Strabismus terminology is specific to this subject, and some introductory definitions will be given. **Strabismus, cast, squint,** or **tropia** is a misalignment of the visual axis. **Amblyopia** is decreased vision in one eye with best correction glasses without observable organic disease. A difference of two lines or more in vision from one eye to the other is considered significant amblyopia. **Convergence** occurs when both eyes move toward each other and **divergence** refers to the eyes moving away from each other. In **esotropia,** one eye is turned toward the nose. In **exotropia** one eye turns out toward the temple. The tendency of one eye to turn in toward the nose when it is covered but straighten out when the cover is removed is **esophoria;** toward the temple, **exophoria. Intermittent exotropia** is a manifest exodeviation, which may be present intermittently either for distance fixation or only when the patient is tired. **Fusion** is the ability of the central nervous system to superimpose into a single image the images that it receives from both eyes simultaneously. **Stereopsis** is the ability to perceive objects in three dimensions using horizontal disparity as the only clue. Stereopsis is possible because of the horizontal separation of the eyes and the partial decussation of the optic nerves. **Ductions** are movements of one eye and **versions** are movements of both eyes together.

Hypertropia is a vertical divergent deviation in which one eye is up when the other one is fixating and, when the fixation switches to the higher eye, the lower eye goes down. **Dissociated vertical deviation** (DVD) is the upward deviation of one eye when the other eye is fixing and, when fixation is switched to the higher eye the lower one does not go down. DVD could be manifest deviation or could be a latent deviation present only when a cover is placed in front of the eye. An **overacting inferior oblique** muscle causes the elevation of the eye moving toward the nose when both eyes are moving together in a horizontal direction. **Nystagmus**

is the spontaneous, rhythmic movement of the eyes. **Latent nystagmus** is the rhythmic movement of both eyes present only when one eye is covered. **Near point of convergence** (NPC) is the closest that both eyes can move toward each other while maintaining the object of regard as single. **Near point of accommodation** (NPA) is the closest that one particular eye can see an object clearly. **Accommodative convergence** is the convergence brought in by the use of accommodation. The **accommodative convergence/accommodation ratio** (AC/A) is the amount of accommodative convergence brought in by each unit of accommodation. The first is expressed in prism diopters and the second in lens diopters.

Diagnosis

Strabismus is usually diagnosed by inspection, but at times the width of the nasal bridge and the shape and size of the epicanthal folds at each side of the nose may give the false impression of strabismus (pseudostrabismus). To diagnose strabismus an attractive object is placed in front of the patient's eyes, such as keys, toys, or small cartoon characters pasted on tongue blades. While the patient is looking at the object of regard, the examiner gently covers one eye, the one he thinks is the fixating eye, while maintaining his observation on the apparent misaligned eye. If the patient has strabismus, then a shift of the nonfixing eye will be made to assume fixation on the object of regard. This is called the cover test. Strabismus is classified into comitant and incomitant deviations.

Incomitant Deviations

Incomitant deviations occur when the degree of misalignment changes in different positions of gaze so that there is a limitation or restriction of the movement of one or both eyes. Incomitant deviations are divided into the congenital and acquired types. The congenital types include restrictive syndromes, such as Duane's syndrome, Brown's syndrome, Moebius' syndrome, and strabismus fixus. In all of these syndromes shortly after birth a restriction of the movement of one or both eyes is noticed because of innervational and/or mechanical factors (Figures 10.14 and 10.15). Included in acquired incomitant deviations are those caused by paralysis of the third, fourth, and sixth cranial nerves secondary either to tumors, diabetes, viral diseases, or trauma. Limitation of motion causing incomitant strabismus can also be secondary to entrapped orbital tissue in a fracture of the floor of the orbit, eye muscle changes in thyroid disease, or myoneural problems in myasthenia gravis. All the acquired incomitant deviations in patients above age 7 years are accompanied by double vision, and usually the patient has an abnormal position of the head in an attempt to compensate for the lack of movement of the affected eye.

Comitant Deviations

Comitant deviations are those in which the degree of misalignment of the visual axes is the same when the patient looks in different positions of gaze. There is no loss of the effective eye muscle power and each eye can move freely. As a rule, the terms "strabismus" and "comitant deviation" are used synonymously, and the patients suffering from this condition are primarily treated by their ophthalmologist. (Patients with incomitant deviations may be primarily treated by neurologists.) Although the etiology of comitant deviations is unknown, there is a higher familial incidence, and they are more common in patients with prematurity, developmental delay, cerebral palsy, Down's syndrome, and other conditions that affect the delicate development of the central nervous system. Strabismus is present in

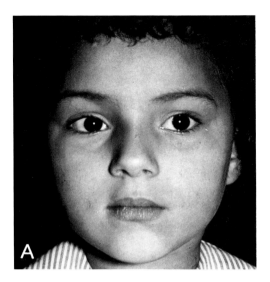 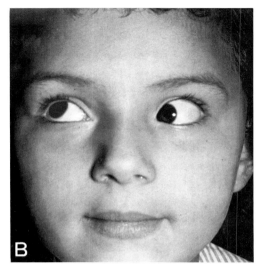

FIGURE 10.14   Brown's syndrome. A: Compensatory head position with no deviation in primary position, head turned to patient's right and chin elevated. B: Underelevation of affected left eye on adduction with widening of palpebral fissure.

2% to 3% of the population. Comitant strabismus encompasses more than 90% of all ocular deviations. Eighty percent of these will have esotropia and about 20% will have exotropia. About 70% of the esotropias start before the age of 1 year and about 85% of the exotropic patients have an intermittent deviation.

Accommodative Esotropia

Accommodative esotropia is an acquired deviation with usual onset between the ages of 1 1/2 and 4 years. The accommodative esotropes had a chance of having both eyes work together in a normal fashion and developing normal binocular reflexes prior to the onset of their ocular deviation, and as a result they have a better chance of getting a functional cure with adequate therapy. They are divided into three groups according to their response to their full cycloplegic hypermetropic correction (with atropine). Atropine 0.5% is used three times per day for three days in each eye prior to examination. If the patient's deviation is completely straightened out with the use of the full hypermetropic atropine refraction findings, the patient is called a full accommodative esotrope (Figure 10.16). If the eyes are straightened for distance fixation but not for near fixation, the patient is an accommodative esotrope with a high AC/A ratio and is treated with an addition of bifocals to his distance, hypermetropic prescription. If the patient's deviation is reduced markedly with the use of the atropine refraction findings but not corrected fully for distance or near vision, then the patient is called a partially accommodative esotrope, and, in addition to the use of glasses, the patient is a candidate for surgical correction for that part of the deviation not straightened out by the glasses.

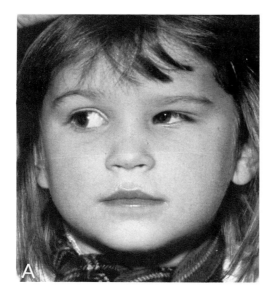
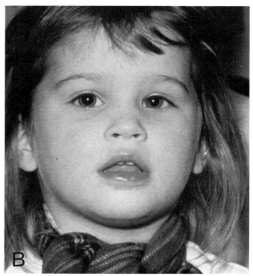
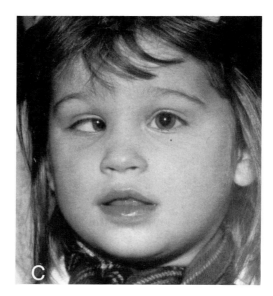

FIGURE 10.15   Duane's syndrome, type I. A: Narrowing palpebral fissure and retraction of left eye on gaze to patient's right. B: Compensatory head position with face turned to her left. C: Limitation of abduction of left eye with widening of palpebral fissure on gaze to her left.

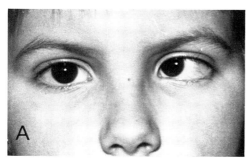
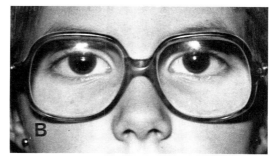

FIGURE 10.16   Accommodative esotropia. Atropine refraction: +4.50 sphere each eye. A: Left esotropia without glasses at distance and near. B: Deviation corrected with atropine refraction findings at distance and near fixation.

Congenital Esotropia

Patients with congenital esotropia are those in whom the onset of the deviation occurs prior to age 6 months. Glasses are rarely used as a form of therapy in patients with congenital esotropia. Almost 100% of them will need surgery in an attempt to straighten the eyes (Figure 10.17). It is believed that if the eyes are straightened out prior to age 2 years, there is a better chance of attaining a more permanent alignment of the visual axes and a better binocular cooperation than if they were operated on at a later age. During the first visit to the ophthalmologist, the congenital esotropes have a full eye examination, including a cycloplegic refraction with Mydriacyl 1% and/or Cyclogyl 1% and ocular media and fundus studies. Organic pathology, such as cataracts, retinoblastoma, colobomas, toxoplasma retinopathy, and retinopathy of prematurity, could be present together with the strabismus or could be the cause of the ocular deviation. Full retinoscopic findings are prescribed for a patient with myopia or with high astigmatic error. Minor or moderate degrees of hypermetropic corrections are not prescribed until after surgery and only if a residual esodeviation remains or if the esotropic deviation returns. High degrees of hypermetropic refractive error may be prescribed prior to surgery to evaluate its effect on the deviation. The horizontal deviations in congenital

FIGURE 10.17   Congenital esotropia. A: Esotropia prior to surgery. B: Six months after recession of the medial rectus in each eye.

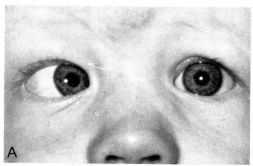
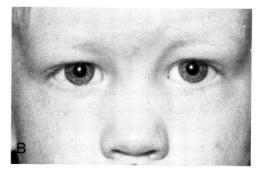

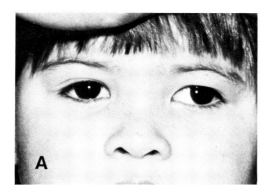 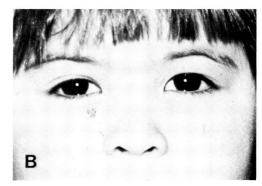

FIGURE 10.18   Intermittent Exotropia. A: Exotropia prior to surgery. B: Six months after recession of lateral rectus each eye.

esotropes may be complicated by the presence of dissociated vertical deviations, overacting inferior oblique muscles, and/or latent nystagmus. Any of these conditions may be present at the onset of the deviation or may show themselves after the surgery is performed.

Exotropia

Exotropias usually start around the age of 1 year and are divided into intermittent, in which the deviation is present occasionally, and constant, in which the deviation is present all the time. Constant or sensory exotropias are associated with poor vision in one eye, as in anisometropic amblyopia or monocular cataract. The treatment of esotropia, whether constant or intermittent, is surgical once the vision problem, if present, has been corrected (Figure 10.18).

Amblyopia

Amblyopia is a preventable type of blindness that occurs in 2% of the population. It must be treated before the age of 7 years and preferably before the age of 5 years to get a permanent cure. Visual acuity screening at the first grade level is almost too late if permanent results are to be expected with adequate therapy. Amblyopia occurs when the patient does not use one eye normally in the act of vision. Each eye must be used adequately until visual maturity arrives between ages 7 and 9 years in order to develop and maintain good vision in each eye for the rest of the patient's life. Patients with alternating or intermittent deviations rarely develop amblyopia. Only about 15% of exotropes are constant, and most congenital esotropes have some type of alternation in their deviations. As a rule, almost all accommodative esotropes have a constant deviation with amblyopia when first examined.

Amblyopia associated with strabismus is called strabismic amblyopia. In anisometropic amblyopia, there is a significant difference (at least 1.50D) between the refractive errors of each eye. This apparently is distasteful to the visual system, which ignores the image from one of the eyes, thus setting the stage for the development of amblyopia in that eye. Anisometropic amblyopia in a patient with strabismus is discovered during the first examination, whereas anisometropic amblyopia in a patient with the eyes straight is usually not discovered until it is too late because there is no outward evidence that it is present. The main purpose of visual acuity screening performed between the ages of 3 and 5 years at nursery, prekindergarten, and kindergarten levels is to discover patients with anisometropic amblyopia without strabismus. Patients with strabismus and amblyopia should have been under the care of an ophthalmologist already by this age.

Visual acuity is judged in the patient with strabismus and amblyopia by the mode of fixation before the age of 3 years. After this age, the "E" chart is used as described previously. When the child learns the alphabet, the regular Snellen chart at 20 feet is used to measure the vision in each eye. In testing vision in children, the nontested eye is always occluded with micropore tape or a piece of Elastoplast to prevent cheating.

Prior to the treatment of functional amblyopia, one must differentiate it from organic loss of vision secondary to congenital or acquired intraocular lesions. Interestingly enough, organic pathology with visual loss during infancy, as in retinoblastoma, can be the cause of strabismus. Amblyopia secondary to obstruction of the visual pathways in infancy, as in cataracts, is called deprivation or occlusion amblyopia. Dense, bilateral, congenital cataracts must be removed within the first few weeks of life in order to prevent permanent deprivation amblyopia.

NEURO–OPHTHALMOLOGY

Ocular Motility

The primary position of gaze is that in which the head is upright and the eyes are looking straight ahead toward the horizon. The action of individual eye muscles are as follows: medial rectus, adduction (toward the nose); lateral rectus, abduction (toward the temple); superior rectus, elevation, adduction, and intorsion (tilting of the 12 o'clock position of the cornea toward the nose); inferior rectus, depression, adduction, and extorsion (12 o'clock position of the cornea tilted toward the temple); superior oblique, depression, abduction, and intorsion; inferior oblique, elevation, abduction, and extorsion. In conjugate movements of both eyes (versions) in the six diagnostic positions of gaze, the prime movers of each eye are called yoke muscles and are identified in Figure 10.19. In the midline positions the following muscles are used: up, both elevators in each eye (right superior rectus, right inferior oblique and left superior rectus, left inferior oblique); and down, both depressors in each eye (right inferior rectus, right superior oblique and left inferior rectus, left superior oblique).

Innervation of the eye muscles by cranial nerves is as follows: Lateral rectus, by the abducens (VI) nerve; superior oblique, by the trochlear (IV) nerve; medial rectus, superior rectus, inferior rectus, and inferior oblique, by the oculomotor (III) nerve. This nerve also innervates the levator palpebrae superioris muscle of the lid.

Paralytic Strabismus

Damage to the cranial nerves innervating the eye muscles cause incomitant paralytic strabismus with characteristic findings as follows: (a) VIth nerve, involved eye in adduction (esotropia) with face turned to the same side; (b) IVth nerve, involved eye elevated (hypertropia), extorted with chin depressed and head tilted to opposite shoulder; and (c) IIIrd nerve, involved eye abducted (exotropia), and depressed (hypotropia) with face turned to opposite side plus ptosis in the same side. Spontaneous recovery in a few months is the rule in paralytic acquired strabismus especially when due to viral diseases, diabetes and hypertension. Aneurysm is suspected when there is also pupillary involvement.

THE YOKE MUSCLES

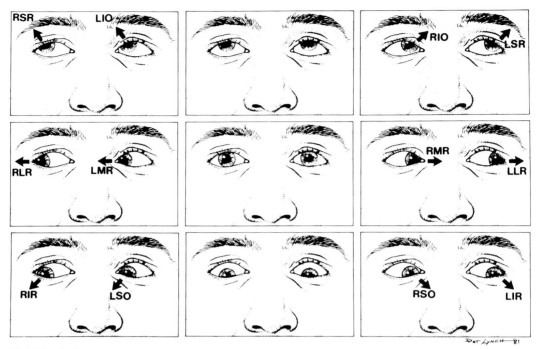

FIGURE 10.19   Yoke muscles. The six diagnostic positions with their yoke muscles, the straight ahead position, and the midline positions (up and down) are shown.

Red Lens Test

Diagnosis of individual muscle paralysis is done by the prism and cover test and also by subjective tests, such as Lancaster red/green test or the red lens test. The red lens test is easy to perform and can be done at the bedside. A red filter is placed over the patient's right eye and he/she is asked if his diplopia is side by side, up and down, or a combination of both. If it is only side by side the light is moved first to one side and then to the other and the patient is asked to report in which side the double images are more separated. Once this side is identified, we know that the farther away image belongs to the eye with the involved muscle which is lagging behind sending the image farther away. The color of the light identifies the eye. If the patient instead reports that the diplopia is vertical or a combination of horizontal and vertical, then the light is moved to the diagnostic positions of gaze described above (the four corners) looking for the area of greater vertical separation of the images. Again in this area the further away image will identify the involved eye and the muscle which is the prime mover in this position by the color of the image.

Graves' Disease

Graves' disease is an autoimmune disorder characterized by one or more of the following clinical findings: hyperthyroidism with diffuse hyperplasia of the thyroid gland, infiltrative ophthalmopathy, and pretibial myxedema. The ocular involvement

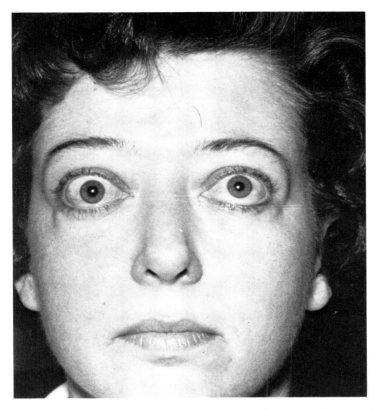

FIGURE 10.20   Graves' disease. Exophthalmos, lid retraction, conjunctival hyperemia, and left hypertropia secondary to "restricted" right inferior rectus muscle are shown.

may appear before or at the same time as the hyperthyroidism or after the patient is euthyroid with treatment. In other patients, it may appear with hypothyroidism secondary to treatment for hyperthyroidism with either radioactive iodine or surgery. In other patients with typical thyroid ophthalmopathy some endocrinologic tests are negative. Lid retraction, lid lag, conjunctival injection over the areas corresponding to the horizontal rectus muscles, proptosis, and limitation of movement of the eye muscles (inferior and medial rectus) are the most common ophthalmologic findings. Graves' disease is the most common cause of unilateral and bilateral exophthalmos in adults (Figure 10.20).

Dreaded complications of Graves' are corneal exposure with ulceration and visual loss secondary to optic nerve compression by engorged extraocular muscles in the apex of the orbit. Treatment consists of tarsorrhaphy to protect the cornea, decompression of the orbit to increase its volume and release the pressure on the optic nerve, and eye muscle surgery to increase ocular motility. NO SPECS is a mnemonic to remember the classification of thyroid ophthalmopathy: "N" for no physical signs or symptoms, "O" for only signs, "S" for soft tissue involvement with signs and symptoms, "P" for proptosis, "E" for extraocular muscle involvement, "C" for corneal involvement, and "S" for sight loss.

240   **Physical Diagnosis**

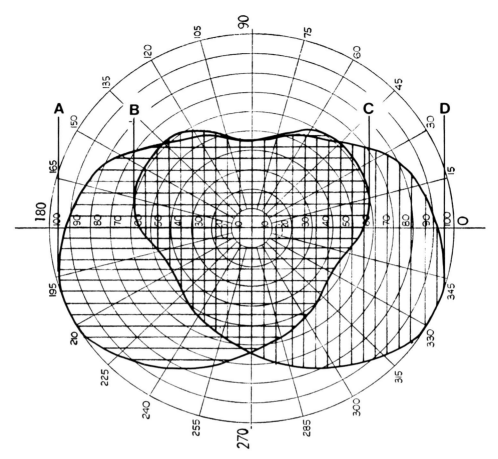

FIGURE 10.21   Visual fields. A–C: Left monocular field. B–D: Right monocular field. A–D: Total binocular field. B–C: Superimposed binocular field. A–B: Left monocular temporal crescent. C–D: Right monocular temporal crescent.

Visual Fields

The total field of one individual, steadily fixating eye is about 150 degrees (Figure 10.21). The total field of both eyes fixating on one spot (including the temporal crescents in each eye, which come from the most distal nasal retinas and do not participate in fused binocular vision) is about 180 degrees. The superimposed binocular field, which is the field seen by both eyes at the same time, is 120 degrees. Visual fields, as tested in ophthalmology and neurology, are determined with only one eye open while it holds fixation steadily straight ahead; the nontested eye is occluded. The central field of one eye is the innermost 30 degrees of vision and it is charted at a distance of 1 m on a black screen using white circular objects varying from 2 to 9 mm in diameter with the patient wearing his/her best correcting glasses. The central field is damaged in diseases of the ganglion cell axons (nerve fiber layer), especially at the disc and fovea, and of axons in the optic nerve up to the chiasm. The additional 120 degrees of the peripheral field are charted in a device called a perimeter.

The peripheral field is damaged in glaucoma and by tumors or vascular lesions involving the visual fibers from the chiasm to the occipital cortex. A scotoma is an island of decreased visual function surrounded by normal function. The best example of a scotoma is the blind spot. Hemianopsia occurs whenever there is a visual defect in the right or the left half of the visual field. In homonymous hemianopsia, the same side of the visual space of a single eye is affected in each eye, for example, the nasal half in one eye and the temporal half in the other. In heteronymous hemianopsia, opposite sides of the visual space are affected, as occurs in bitemporal or binasal hemianopsia.

Visual Field Defects

Visual field pathology anterior to the chiasm will produce monocular visual field defects without respect for the midline. Central scotomas correspond to lesions affecting the central field of vision in one eye, usually secondary to inflammation, compression, or ischemia of the optic nerve. Lesions affecting the superior and inferior arcuate nerve fiber layers will give characteristic arcuate scotomas, most commonly seen in glaucoma (Figure 10.22). Bitemporal hemianopias are caused by lesions involving the chiasm. Lesions posterior to the chiasm will produce homonymous field defects without compromising vision unless the occipital cortex is involved. The most common cause of homonymous hemianopsia is a vascular lesion. Temporal lobe lesions cause visual field defects that are denser above, whereas parietal lobe lesions yield visual field defects that are denser below.

Two tests help differentiate macular from optic nerve pathology: photostress recovery time test and color vision test. Each eye is tested individually. In the photostress test, the patient looks at the smallest line he can read on an eye chart or in a newspaper. Then he looks directly into a penlight held 2 to 3 cm from the eye to be tested for 10 seconds. The penlight is then removed and the time elapsed until the patient is able to read the same line again is recorded. Within one minute is normal, past two to three minutes is diagnostic of macular disease, since recovery time is not prolonged in optic nerve disease. Congenital color vision defects affect both eyes equally in 8% of males and 0.5% of females. They are constant through life and are not associated with retinal or optic nerve pathology. The perception of red color is affected early in optic nerve pathology (neuritis, ischemia) but not in macular disease. Ishihara color plates can be used to test each eye individually, or simple comparisons between each eye with a red-topped medicine bottle may suffice.

Optic Nerve

The optic nerve contains one million nerve fibers and is divided into four portions:

1. Intraocular, which is 1 mm long and 1.5 mm in diameter.
2. Orbital, which runs from the globe to the optic canal and is 25 to 30 mm long and 3 to 4 mm wide. In this area, the nerve fibers become myelinated and pia, arachnoid, and dura coverings are added.
3. Intracanalicular optic nerve, which is 4 to 9 mm long, runs posteriorly and medially (in this area it is accompanied by the ophthalmic artery).
4. Intracranial, which is between 10 and 16 mm in length, runs posteriorly, medially, and cephalad and "ends" at the optic chiasm.

All the fibers from the ganglion cells in the temporal retina go through the chiasm and the optic tract to the lateral geniculate body on the same side and those from the nasal ganglion cells cross to the lateral geniculate body of the opposite side.

242

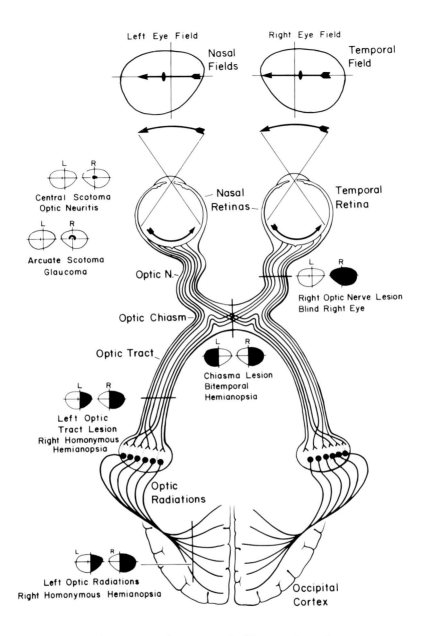

FIGURE 10.22   Diagrammatic anatomic illustration of common visual defects, as seen from above.

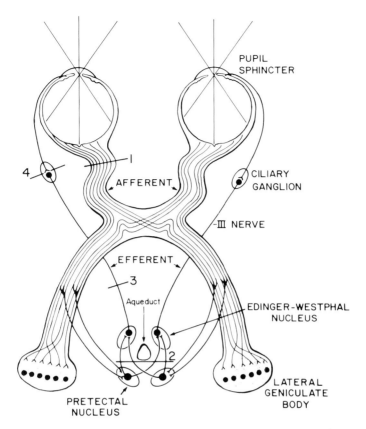

FIGURE 10.23   Pupillomotor pathways. Lesions at the locations marked will cause the following pupillary defects: 1) If complete, amaurotic; if partial, afferent pupil; 2) Argyll Robertson pupil and Parinaud's syndrome; 3) Paralytic pupil; 4) Adie's pupil.

All of these fibers, which originated in the ganglion cells in the retina, will synapse at the lateral geniculate body with "visual" fibers that then terminate in the visual occipital cortex via the geniculocalcarine optic radiations.

The pupillomotor fibers leave the optic tracts prior to the lateral geniculate body and enter the brainstem. They synapse in the pretectal nuclei, from where they are distributed to the ipsilateral and contralateral Edinger-Westphal nucleus via an intercalated neuron. The efferent parasympathetic pupillary fibers leave the midbrain with the third nerve and synapse at the ciliary ganglion (short root). The postganglionic fibers reach the sphincter and the ciliary body through the short ciliary nerves (Figure 10.23).

Afferent Pupillary Defects

One of the most important signs in neuro-ophthalmology is the afferent pupillary defect. It is an objective sign of anterior visual pathway disease and is abnormal specifically in pathology of the papillomacular bundle or optic nerve and in chiasmal syndromes. No pupillary defect is noted in cataracts, strabismic amblyopia, papilledema, or refractive errors. Whereas the efferent limb of the pupillary reflex must be tested with drugs, all that is needed to test the afferent limb is a strong light. Because of the partial decussation of the retinal fibers in the chiasm and the crossover of the pupillary afferent fibers in the midbrain through the intercalated nucleus, light stimulus to one eye (direct) will bring an identical response (consensual) through the efferent motor limb to each pupil.

During the examination, the patient is placed in a semi-darkened room, and while he fixates at distance, a strong light source is shone into one eye. This will bring a direct response to that pupil and a consensual response to the fellow eye's pupil. The light is then shone into the other eye and both pupils are observed again for direct and consensual responses. If the pupils constrict normally to direct light, the near reflex need not be examined. In all light-near dissociated syndromes (see below), the response to direct light is the one that is absent, not the response to near accommodation; however, if the direct light response is absent, then the near response must be tested.

In an amaurotic pupil (blind eye), the involved pupil does not react directly but reacts consensually. In "pupillary escape" or Marcus Gunn pupil, there is an "afferent pupillary defect" secondary to optic nerve or papillomacular bundle damage. For example, by abruptly swinging the penlight alternately from eye to eye in the case of a subtle optic nerve lesion in the left eye, although both pupils may constrict briskly to direct light testing, when the light is moved from the right eye to the left eye, the left pupil will dilate slightly. In other words, the "consensual" response in the affected eye is slightly better than its "direct" response.

Sympathetic Pupillary Defects

The sympathetic innervation to the dilator muscle of the pupil and to the smooth muscle of the lids starts in the hypothalamus with sympathetic fibers descending in the spinal tract as the first-order neurons. The second-order neuron leaves the spinal cord at the level of C-8-T-2, coursing through the posterosuperior chest area and ending at the superior cervical ganglion in the neck near the carotid artery bifurcation. From there, postganglionic fibers go to the sweat and vasoconstrictor fibers of the face via the external carotid, and other postganglionic fibers follow the internal carotid to join the ophthalmic division of the third nerve. Through the nasociliary and the long ciliary nerves, they reach the ciliary ganglion (sympathetic root) and the iris dilator muscle. Via the ophthalmic artery, they also reach the smooth muscle of the lids. Lesions of the sympathetic pathway will cause Horner's syndrome, which consists of miosis plus ipsilateral ptosis and diminished sweating (Figure 10.24). "Cluster headaches" with incomplete Horner's syndrome (no anhidrosis) occur in middle-aged men. In Horner's syndrome the pupils react normally to light and near, but the lack of dilatation of the miotic pupil to two drops of cocaine 10% in 30 minutes to one hour determines the diagnosis and differentiation of postganglionic from preganglionic Horner's syndrome is done by using 1% Paredrine. Cocaine works by blocking the presynaptic recovery of the neurotransmitter norepinephrine. Cocaine fails to dilate the pupil in a sympathetic lesion because there is less norepinephrine in the synaptic cleft.

Efferent Pupillary Defects

In physiologic anisocoria the pupils will react briskly to light and will dilate to 10% cocaine and the near reaction is intact. Pharmacologic anisocoria, in which the larger pupil does not react well to light secondary to inadvertent atropinization, is diagnosed when the larger pupil does not constrict to 1% pilocarpine. A patient with Adie's pupil or a dilated pupil secondary to third cranial nerve damage will constrict to this medication. Third nerve palsy will also be accompanied by eye

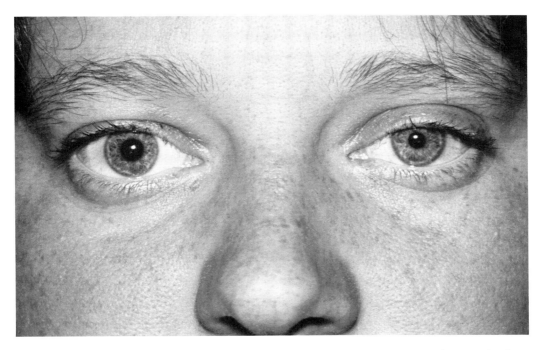

FIGURE 10.24   Horner's syndrome. Ptosis, miosis, and anhydrosis on left side. Note "upside down" ptosis, left lower lid.

muscle problems. A denervated, dilated, tonic pupil (Adie's) will even constrict with pilocarpine 1/8%.

Light–Near Dissociation

Three types of conditions have light-near dissociation: Parinaud's syndrome, Argyll Robertson pupils, and Adie's pupil. In Parinaud's syndrome the lesion is in the midbrain; the pupils are usually "dilated" and they do not react to light but react well to accommodation. In Argyll Robertson pupils the pupils are irregular, "miotic," and do not react to light but react to accommodation. This latter syndrome is caused by syphilis (tabes dorsalis). In Adie's pupil the pupil is "dilated," has poor or no reaction to light, and reacts to accommodation with a "tonic" constriction. The lesion is in the ciliary ganglion and may be idiopathic or secondary to inflammation or trauma of the area. The dilatation in Adie's pupil is a post-ganglionic denervation hypersensitivity. Pilocarpine 1/8% or Mecholyl 2.5% will produce miosis in the Adie's pupil but not in an atropinized, third nerve-damaged, or normal pupil. Adie's syndrome besides the tonic pupil includes partial or complete absence of knee and ankle tendon reflexes and occurs in young females.

CATARACTS AND GLAUCOMA

Cataracts

The opacification of the lens in cataracts is usually due to disorganization of the orderly arrangements of the lens fibers, increasing light scattering (Figure 10.25). The lens has no blood vessels and obtains its nutrition from the aqueous humor. It

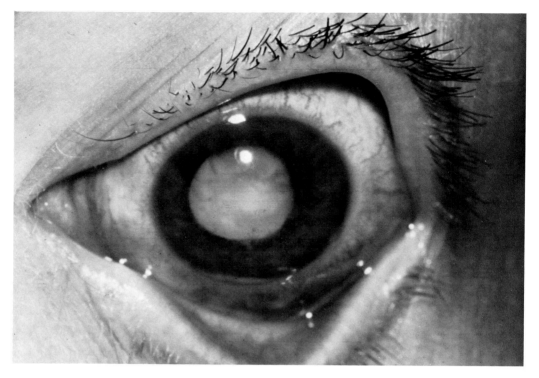

FIGURE 10.25   Advanced cataract.

keeps itself dry with the use of the sodium/potassium ATPase pump. The pump may be damaged by trauma or by the prolonged use of steroid medication (as in arthritis), allowing opacification in the lens. Cataracts may take a long time to develop, as in the case of senile cataracts, or may develop in a very short period of time, such as occurs when there is direct trauma to the lens capsule with a penetrating injury. Traumatic cataracts can also be caused by shock waves secondary to a blow to the eye or by gamma radiation. The opacity secondary to traumatic cataract is due to destruction of tissue and will not resolve with time. From age 14 to age 44, diabetes is the most common cause of the formation of cataracts. Cataracts are four to six times more common in diabetics than in nondiabetics.

Senile cataracts can be divided into three broad categories, depending on the location of the primary light scattering opacity:

1. Cortical cataracts, which have water-filled clefts between the lens fibers in the lens cortex.
2. Nuclear cataracts, which have dense aggregates of several proteins causing a yellowish-brown discoloration in the "center" of the lens.
3. Posterior subcapsular cataracts, which have opacity mainly at the level of the posterior capsule of the lens.

The cortical and nuclear cataracts may take years to decrease vision, whereas the posterior subcapsular cataracts reduce vision very rapidly in the patient.

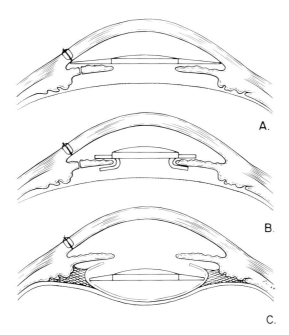

A.

B.

C.

FIGURE 10.26   Intraocular lenses. Intracapsular cataract extraction corrected with anterior chamber lens in A and with an iris plane lens in B. Extracapsular cataract extraction corrected with a posterior chamber lens in C.

Congenital cataracts are usually accompanied by other systemic problems such as mental retardation and hearing problems, except when they are due to a defective gene inherited as a dominant characteristic from one of the parents. Other causes of congenital cataracts are infections in the mother during the first 2 months of pregnancy by rubella, toxoplasmosis, or mumps; and enzyme deficiency, such as occurs in aminoaciduria. They are also found frequently in association with Down's syndrome and ectopic dermatitis.

There are presently three types of intraocular lenses used in the surgical treatment of cataracts: (a) an anterior chamber lens, which is placed in front of the iris in the anterior chamber; (b) an iris plane lens, which is placed in the pupillary space; and (c) a posterior chamber lens, which is placed behind the iris in the posterior chamber (Figure 10.26). It should be noted that an iris plane intraocular lens is supported by the iris and could dislocate if the pupil were dilated. Fortunately, these lenses are not in use anymore in this country; but as a rule, a non-ophthalmologist should not dilate the pupils of a patient with an intraocular lens in place unless he/she gets permission to do so from the surgeon who operated on the patient or from an ophthalmologist who has examined the patient.

Glaucoma

Glaucoma is a normally preventable form of blindness usually caused either by an insidious or an acute rise in intraocular pressure (IOP). This increase in IOP damages the nerve fiber layer throughout the retina, the nerve fibers at the optic nerve (neuroretinal rim), and the optic nerve itself, causing characteristic field changes as tested by perimetry. The glaucomas are divided into four groups:

(a) primary open-angle glaucoma, (b) primary angle closure glaucoma, (c) secondary glaucoma, and (d) low-tension glaucoma.

The aqueous humor is formed by the ciliary epithelium in the posterior chamber. It travels predominately through the pupillary space into the anterior chamber and escapes through the fine trabecular meshwork in the anterior chamber angle into collector channels and aqueous veins, which empty into the episcleral and conjunctival blood vessels. There is an equilibrium established between the inflow and the outflow of this fluid. In angle closure glaucoma, there is a relative pupillary block that makes it difficult for the aqueous humor formed in the posterior chamber to gain access to the anterior chamber. This causes the iris to bulge forward against the angle meshwork, blocking outflow. Since the ciliary body continues to produce aqueous humor, IOP increases. There seem to be anatomic and physiologic predispositions of eyes to develop angle closure glaucoma, such as: small anterior segments with shallow anterior chambers, size and position of the lens, and greater lens-iris apposition, as seen in the older population with increasing lens thickness.

In open-angle glaucoma, the most common of the glaucomas, there is no mechanical limitation in the flow of aqueous humor from the posterior to the anterior chamber, but there is a resistance to the outflow at the trabecular level, decreasing the outflow facility. Secondary glaucomas, which may be of open- or closed-angle mechanism, have an identifiable underlying primary problem. Some untreated eyes can develop typical glaucomatous changes although they may never register IOP higher than what is considered "normal." These eyes may show disc pallor as seen with the ophthalmoscope and typical glaucomatous field changes by perimetry. These patients have low-tension glaucoma. Their treatment is similar to that used for primary open-angle glaucoma. On the other side of the spectrum, occasionally IOP higher than "normal" will be recorded in patients with healthy eyes. These patients are followed at frequent intervals but not treated unless glaucomatous nerve damage or field changes can be corroborated.

Primary Open-Angle Glaucoma

Primary open-angle glaucoma is a disease of the elderly with onset usually after age 40; it affects about 2% of the population of this age group. It is characterized by increased intraocular pressure, open anterior chamber angle, cupping of the optic nerve, and characteristic visual field defects. It has a slow, painless progression and can take 5 to 10 years to produce the pathologic changes in the optic nervehead. Once the optic nerve fibers are damaged, the visual field loss is permanent, even if the IOP can be maintained within tolerable limits afterward. In treated or untreated eyes, tolerable levels of IOP are determined by the pathophysiology of each individual eye.

The average IOP for nonglaucomatous eyes is 16 mm Hg. Intraocular pressure readings of two standard deviations over average, that is, 22 mm Hg, should be considered suspicious, especially in any patient at risk. Patients at risk are those with a family history of glaucoma, with diabetes, with high myopia, or who respond to a trial of topical steroid drops for a period of 4 weeks with an increase in IOP. The damage to the retinal nerve fiber layer and ganglion cell layer in glaucoma is not visible with the ophthalmoscope unless it is advanced. Nevertheless, it can be seen in red-free fundus photos, and it is documentable with the perimeter. The damage to the optic nervehead can be observed and recorded because of the loss of the neuroretinal rim with enlargement of the physiologic cup and increased pallor of the optic disc.

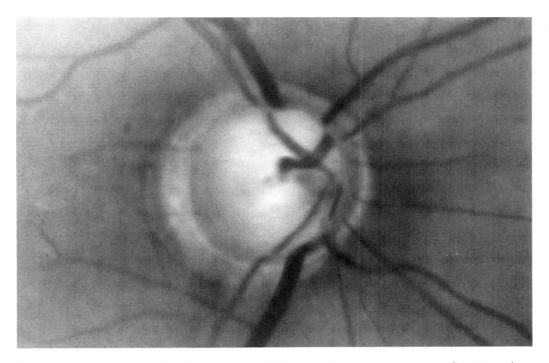

FIGURE 10.27   Optic disc cupping. Wide and deep optic disc cup (right eye) in advanced glaucoma. Blood vessels pushed nasally curling around the edge of the excavation.

Optic Cupping. The normal optic cup is a small, circular, white area in the center of the optic disc, which represents a "separation" of the nerve fibers as they leave the eye to form the optic nerve. The white area in the center of the depression is the lamina cribrosa, which is a finely perforated connective tissue membrane through which the nerve fibers pass when leaving the eye. The optic nerve at this level is composed of glial tissue, nerve fiber axons, and capillaries. The layer of nerve fiber tissue composing the optic disc around the physiologic cup is called the rim. When it is normal, it is pinkish in appearance as compared to the cup in the center. The ratio of optic cup diameter to that of the optic disc is estimated visually to the nearest tenth horizontally and vertically. This ratio is genetically determined and is equal in both eyes of the individual; it is considered physiologically when the ratio is less than 1:3 (0.3). The cup/disc ratio can be used either to make a presumptive diagnosis of glaucoma or to follow patients already known to be glaucomatous. Suspicious patients will be those with a cup/disc ratio greater than 0.4 or those with a difference in cup/disc ratios between the two eyes of greater than 0.2. As the glaucomatous process continues and the cup becomes larger, the retinal vessels will be pushed toward the nasal side and appear to curl tightly around the edge of the cup (Figure 10.27). Nevertheless, congenital variations from patient to patient regarding the cup/disc ratio can mislead an inexperienced observer in differentiating a physiologic cup from a glaucomatous cup, especially in patients with physiologic large cups. Glaucoma experts follow their patients with stereo-optic nervehead photos to document cup/disc ratio changes.

Results of visual field testing, demonstrating the characteristic visual field defects of glaucoma, are helpful in making the diagnosis and in following the progression of the disease while under treatment. The arcuate nerve fibers entering the optic disc from above and below the macula from the temporal retina are usually the first affected, giving the characteristic nasal field defects an arcuate shape. These defects usually are continuous with the blind spot and end at the nasal horizontal meridian. The central and temporal fields of vision are the most resistant to glaucomatous changes.

Primary Angle Closure Glaucoma

Primary angle closure glaucoma is also a disease of the elderly. The addition of new fibers to the lens with age increases its thickness, pushing the iris forward and making the anterior chamber dangerously shallower in those patients with an already anatomically predisposed shallow anterior chamber. If the pupil mid-dilates in darkness, the base of the iris will mechanically block the aqueous humor from getting into the filtration angle, precipitating an attack. At the same time, the iris slides upon the lens, blocking the passage of aqueous humor from the posterior to the anterior chamber. The aqueous humor continues to be produced by the ciliary body and the IOP rises. The more the pressure increases in the posterior chamber, the more the iris is pushed forward against the filtration angle. The acute glaucoma attack is characterized by intense ocular pain, blurred vision, haloes around lights, and nausea and vomiting. The examination reveals markedly diminished vision, hazy cornea, mid-dilated nonreactive pupil, injected scleral and conjunctival blood vessels, and a shallow anterior chamber. The ophthalmologist must look at the angle with a gonioprism. If the cornea is too edematous to see through, it can be temporarily cleared by dehydration with the use of topical glycerin. If glycerin is not available, the examiner can always look at the angle of the other eye because the anatomic configuration of both angles is about the same in most patients. Some patients may have had minor attacks through the years with the formation of peripheral, anterior synechiae, and present themselves with a chronic angle closure glaucoma.

Angle closure glaucoma can be precipitated in a predisposed narrow anterior chamber angle by dilation prior to a fundus examination. When the pupil is semidilated, the iris and lens can come into apposition, blocking the aqueous humor passage from the posterior chamber through the pupil into the anterior chamber and producing the acute attack. Because the treatment for this condition is an iridectomy in the affected eye and a prophylactic iridectomy in the fellow eye, the monitored precipitation of an attack can be rewarding for the patient. In patients with narrow angles, the ophthalmologist may use provocative tests to induce an attack. This is done either by putting the patient in a dark room (in which the pupils will mid-dilate) and then determining the IOP one hour later or by using drops of Mydriacyl 1%. The pressure is checked every 15 minutes and, if the pressure increases by at least 8 mm Hg or an attack is precipitated, the patient is treated medically to break the attack, and then surgery is performed to obtain a cure.

Other Glaucomas

Glaucomas can be associated with a swollen lens (phacomorphic glaucoma), causing a pupillary block with the same signs and symptoms as acute glaucoma. Glaucoma can also be caused by an inflammation (uveitides) by blocking the outflow. Neovascular glaucoma is associated with blood vessel proliferation in the iris and the angle secondary to retinal ischemia. This may occur in diabetes mellitus with proliferative retinopathy or following a retinal vein occlusion. There is a glaucoma associated with the prolonged use of systemic steroids, which is

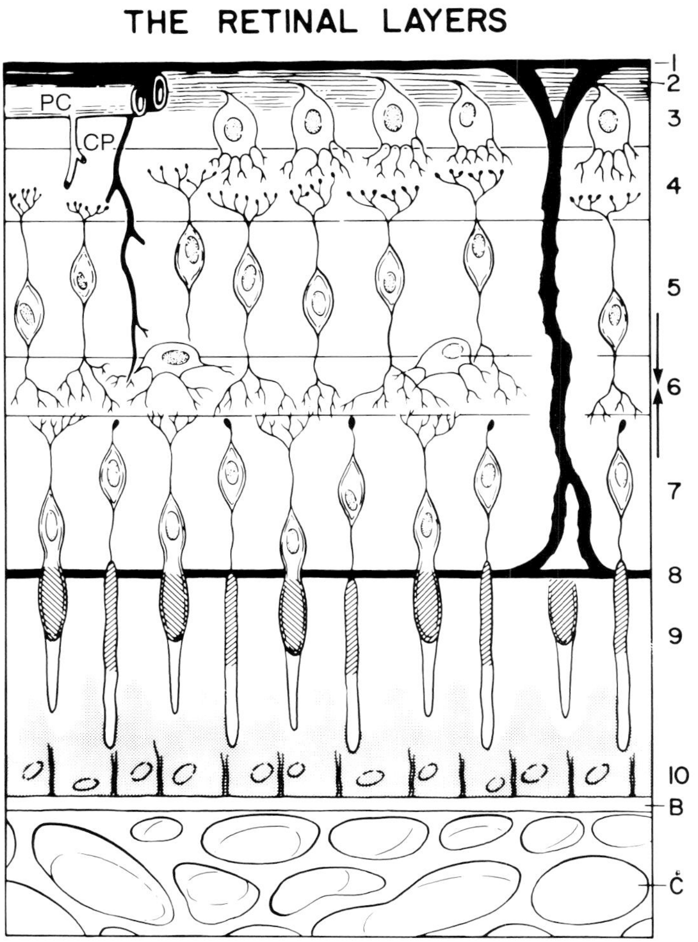

THE RETINAL LAYERS

FIGURE 10.28   Microscopic retinal layers. 1) Internal limiting membrane.
2) Nerve fiber layer. 3) Ganglion cell layer. 4) Inner plexiform layer. 5) Inner
nuclear layer. 6) Outer plexiform layer. 7) Outer nuclear layer. 8) External
limiting membrane. 9) Rod and cone layer. 10) Pigment epithelium layer.
B: Bruch's membrane. C: Choroid choriocapillaris. M: Mueller's cell. PC: Precapillary arterioles. CP: Capillaries. (Arrows: Layers 1 to 6 are supplied by
retinal circulation, and 6 to 10 by choroidal.)

indistinguishable from primary open-angle glaucoma except that the pressure decreases once the steroid medication is discontinued. Congenital glaucoma is characterized by marked photophobia, tearing, and blepharospasm. Diagnosis is made
by the presence of large hazy corneas, cupping of the optic disc, and high IOP.
Congenital glaucoma is sometimes associated with other congenital defects and
seems to have a genetic predisposition. Its treatment is surgical.

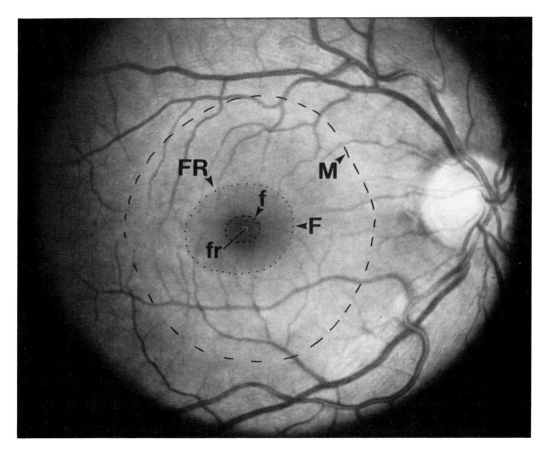

FIGURE 10.29   Retinal central area, right eye. M: Macular area. F: Foveal area. FR: Foveal reflex. f: Foveolar area. fr: Foveolar light reflex. Note: Disc and fovea are approximately 1.5 mm in diameter each.

THE RETINA

Retinal Layers

The retina records, processes and erases images automatically and regulates the size of the pupil by responding to changes in light levels. Its sensitivity is higher than any photographic film available. The retina is a multilayered, crystal clear membrane about 0.2 mm in thickness, lying between the vitreous body and the choroid. Embryologically it is composed of two parts: the sensory retina and the pigment epithelium (Figure 10.28). The microscopic structure of the retina is similar to that of the cerebral cortex and consists of 10 layers from the vitreous towards the choroid.

Macula, Fovea, Foveola, and Foveolar Avascular Zone

The retina has about 130 million photoreceptor cells, 7 million of which are cones and the rest are rods. They convey their impulses into one million optic nerve fibers. The cones are responsible for daylight and color vision and are located in

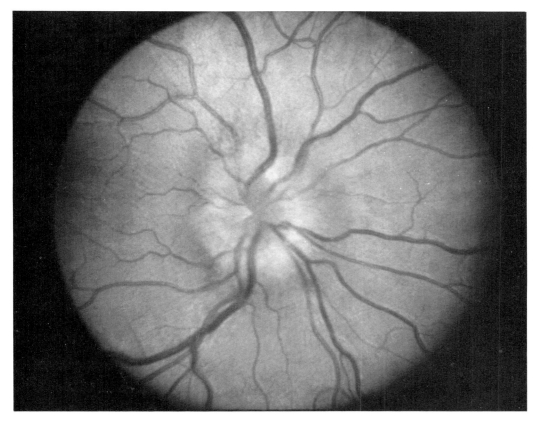

FIGURE 10.30   Papilledema. Hyperemic disc with blurred, elevated margins.

the posterior aspect of the retina with about 14% of them in the central macular area which encompasses 18 degrees of the central visual field. The center of the macula area is about 4 mm temporal to the center of the optic disc and its boundaries cannot be seen ophthalmologically. The foveal depression in the center of the macula can be appreciated in young subjects by a light reflex arising from the thickened internal limiting membrane just before its slope starts, and measures about 1.5 mm in diameter (Figure 10.29).

The foveola is the name given to the 0.3 mm diameter center of the fovea. In this area there are no rods and each cone connects with its own bipolar and ganglion cell. Their visual impulses run through the papillomacular bundle to enter the nervehead on the temporal side. The foveolar avascular zone (FAZ) is an area described by fundus fluorescein angiograms varying between 0.25 and 0.6 mm diameter in which capillaries cannot be identified. This is an important landmark for retinal surgeons.

Optic Disc

The optic nervehead (disc, papilla) lies nasally to the fovea and is composed of nerve fibers coming out of the ganglion cell layers of the retina on their way to the central nervous system. Only the internal limiting membrane and the nerve

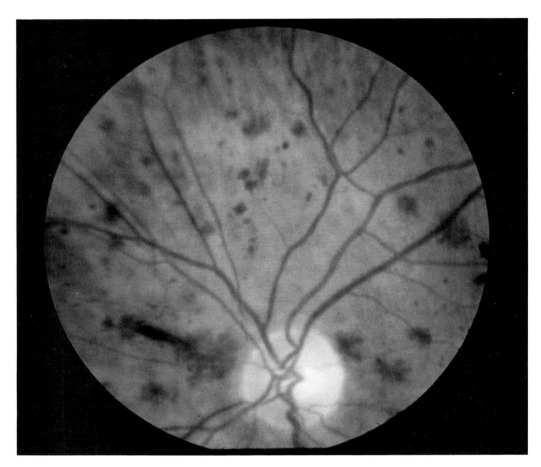

FIGURE 10.31   Diabetic retinopathy. Nonproliferative, "background."

fiber layer (the two innermost layers of the retina) are present in this area. The optic disc is not sensitive to light and corresponds to the physiologic blind spot in the visual field. Outside the eye, the optic nerve has the same sheath as the brain (pia, arachnoid and dura). The dura merges with the sclera and the pia with the choroid. The space between these two sheaths is filled with cerebrospinal fluid. An increase in the cerebrospinal fluid pressure will produce papilledema with blurred disc margins and elevation of the disc over the surrounding retina (Figure 10.30). Increased intraocular pressure on the optic nerve will cause atrophy of the optic disc axons and its capillaries, making the disc appear white with sharp borders by ophthalmoscopy. The nervehead, as seen by the ophthalmoscope, measures about 1.5 mm; this measurement is used as a yardstick for fundus lesions.

Retinal Detachment

In retinal detachments, the neurosensory retina is detached from the retinal pigment epithelium and the space between these tissues is filled with fluid. Detachments accompanied by a hole going through all the layers of the retina (retinal

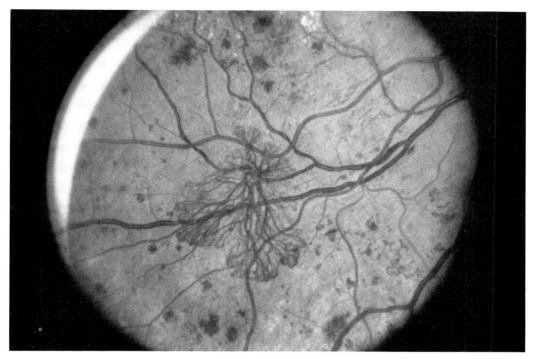

FIGURE 10.32   Diabetic retinopathy. NVE. Proliferative. Note: New blood vessels on the surface of the retina.

break) are called rhegmatogenous. Detachments secondary to traction of the vitreous or exudation from choroidal or retinal vessels, not accompanied by a hole, are called nonrhegmatogenous. Rhegmatogenous retinal detachments are more common than nonrhegmatogenous.

Diabetic Retinopathy

For the past 10 years, diabetic retinopathy has been the leading cause of blindness in the 20 to 64 year old age group in America. It takes about 10 to 20 years of the duration of diabetes before the retina is damaged. This retinopathy occurs in about one-third of all diabetics. The longer life span of diabetics with improvement in their treatment is causing a marked increase in diabetic retinopathy. Diabetes affects the retinal blood vessels and not the choriocapillaris and as such is primarily a disease of the internal layers of the retina. Diabetic retinopathy is divided into a nonproliferative (BDR-background diabetic retinopathy) phase and a proliferative (PDR-proliferative diabetic retinopathy) phase. The nonproliferative phase is produced by focal areas of retinal capillary obstruction and permeability changes, and areas of intraretinal ischemia. The capillaries are damaged both at the pericyte and endothelial levels (thickening of the basement membrane followed by platelet-RBC aggregations). The capillary obstructions and permeability changes are seen ophthalmoscopically and by fluorescein angiography as microaneurysms, intraretinal microvascular abnormalities (IRMA, interpreted as new blood vessels or old "shunt vessels), small, round hemorrhages, hard exudates and when advanced, macular edema (Figure 10.31). Damage to the precapillary arterioles will produce closure of

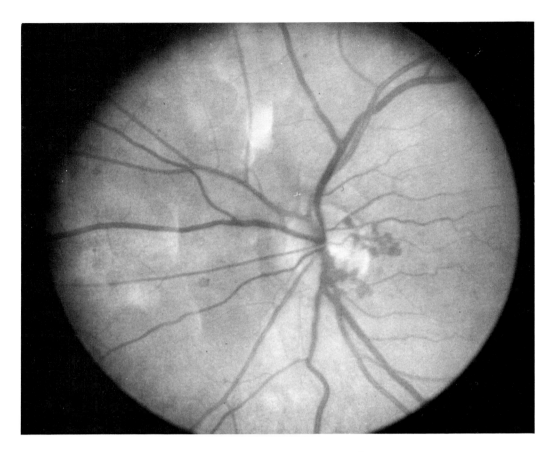

FIGURE 10.33   Diabetic retinopathy. NVD. Proliferative. Note: New blood vessels on the disc.

terminal arterioles with retinal infarction seen clinically as cotton wool exudates, white thread-like arterioles, venous beading and large blot hemorrhages. These changes may occur in both normotensive and hypertensive diabetics.

Proliferative diabetic retinopathy develops as a response to a presumed vaso-proliferative factor which is initiated by the retinal ischemia present in the pre-proliferative period. First, a few fine vessels appear on the surface of the retina (NVE-neovascularization elsewhere) (Figure 10.32) or at the optic disc (NVD-neovascularization at the disc) (Figure 10.33). Then, fibrous tissue develops with an increasing vessel size, followed by a regression and contraction of the fibro-vascular tissue, leaving a relatively avascular fibrous sheet. Vitreous detachment together with contraction of this new fibrovascular tissue will cause vitreous hemorrhages and tractional retinal detachments. As this fibrovascular proliferation is presumed to be a response to retinal ischemia, it is also seen in other ischemic-like retinal diseases, such as retrolental fibroplasia, retinal vein obstruction and sickle cell retinopathy.

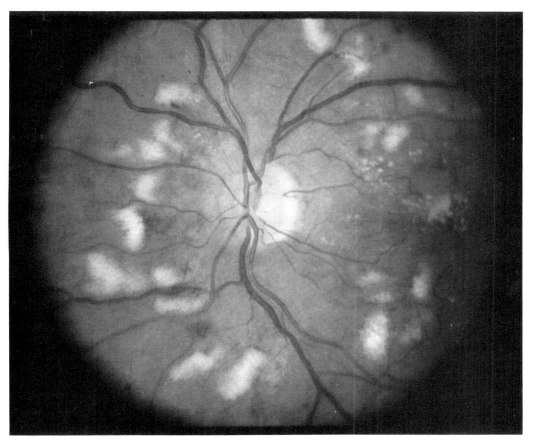

FIGURE 10.34   Hypertensive retinopathy. Stage III. Cotton-wool spots, arteriolar attenuation, hemorrhages, AV nicking, and hard exudates (in macular area).

Hypertensive Retinopathy

Hypertension causes sclerosis of the arterioles and as a result early changes in the ocular fundus can be observed with the ophthalmoscope. It has been classified in four stages: Stage I, slight general attenuation of retinal arterioles; Stage II, more pronounced general attenuation, focal attenuation, broadening of the arteriolar reflex and peripheral arteriovenous crossing changes (AV nicking); Stage III, severe, general and focal attenuation, thickened arteriolar walls (copper-wire and silver-wire), marked AV nicking, cotton-wool spots, splinter and large hemorrhages in the nerve fiber layer and hard exudates, especially around the macular area in the form of a star (Figure 10.34); Stage IV, Stage III plus papilledema. Stages I to II are characteristic of chronic essential hypertension and Stages III and IV are seen in acute increase of blood pressure, such as in malignant hypertension and toxemia of pregnancy. Cotton-wool spots are an ischemic response of the retina secondary

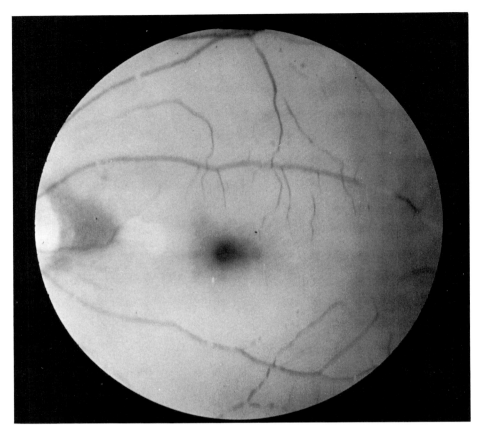

FIGURE 10.35   Central artery occlusion. Marked retinal edema with "cherry red spot."

to closure of end precapillary arterioles. Hard exudates and small, round hemor-rhages are secondary to retinal capillary endothelial permeability changes (break in the blood-retinal barrier).

Retinopathy of Prematurity (ROP)

Retinopathy of prematurity (RLF-retrolental fibroplasia) is a disorder of premature infants who have been exposed to a high concentration of oxygen. In these infants this seems to cause a retinal vasoconstriction with subsequent delay in vasculariza-tion of the peripheral retina. When the infant is later moved to a lesser concentra-tion of oxygen (as room air), there is a rapid proliferation of new blood vessels on the surface of the periphery of the retina. With time this fibrovascular tissue contracts, dragging the macula temporally. The process may "burn out" at any time, but if it continues, it will lead to a total retinal detachment with a mass of fibrous tissue behind the lens. Premature infants under birth weight of 1500 gm are at risk, especially those receiving high capillary oxygen tension for too long a time shortly after birth.

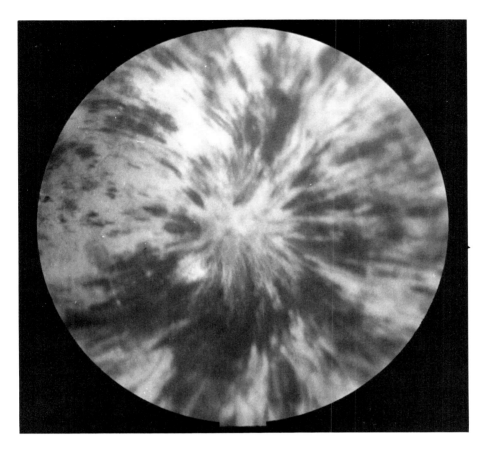

FIGURE 10.36   **Central vein obstruction. Multiple hemorrhages with marked retinal edema.**

Retinal Arterial Occlusions

An occlusion of a central retinal artery will cause the total sudden loss of vision in the affected eye. The retina will become edematous and thus will lose its transparency, appearing white especially in the perifoveal area where the ganglion cell layer is denser. Lack of blood supply will cause a starvation of all the inner layers of the retina including the inner nuclear layer. The pigment epithelium, the photoreceptors and the outer nuclear layer will not be involved since they are supplied by the choriocapillaris. The foveola will appear as a red spot (cherry red) surrounded by the whitish opaque retina, because it lacks the inner layers of the retina and because in this area the pigment epithelium is denser (Figure 10.35). Occlusion of any of the branches of the central retinal artery could also occur, producing an edematous white area in the area of infarction. Occlusion of a precapillary arteriole will produce a typical yellowish-white, cotton-wool spot. Ischemia of the central arterial system will cause a transient blindness (amaurosis fugax), and if prolonged, may even cause a permanent central artery or branch occlusion. Commonly the occlusion is due to embolization from a distant area, such as heart valves or atheromatous plaques from the internal carotid. Massage of the eye in an acute stage may make the thrombus/embolus move distally in the arterial tree causing less permanent damage.

Retinal Vein Obstruction

An obstruction of the central retinal vein or any of its branches is usually associated with hypertension and ophthalmoscopically will be seen as marked dilatation and tortuosity of the veins peripheral to the obstructed area with multiple hemorrhages and retinal edema (Figure 10.36). Obstruction may be caused by direct pressure of an arteriosclerotic central artery or one of its branches at an AV crossing. Further complications of retinal vein obstruction are macular edema and neovascularization of the retina and optic disc with secondary vitreous hemorrhage and/or neovascular glaucoma. Laser photocoagulation may be done to reduce the blood flow in the affected area, and in an attempt to reduce the leakage from vessels in the therapy of macular edema. Pan retinal photocoagulation (PRP) is at times used to destroy new blood vessels and also can be done to prevent neovascular glaucoma.

REFERENCES

1. Allen EW: *Essentials of Ophthalmic Optics.* Oxford, Oxford University Press, 1979.

2. American Academy of Ophthalmology: *Ophthalmology Study Guide for Students and Practitioners,* ed 4. San Francisco, American Academy of Ophthalmology 1982.

3. Anderson D: *Testing the Field of Vision.* St. Louis, CV Mosby Co, 1982.

4. Apple DJ: *Ocular Pathology.* St. Louis, CV Mosby Co, 1985.

5. Brown G, Tasman W: *Congenital Anomalies of the Optic Disc.* New York, Grune & Stratton, 1982.

6. Carr R, Siegel I: *Visual Electrodiagnostic Testing.* Baltimore, Williams & Wilkins, 1982.

7. Casey TA, Mayer DS: *Corneal Grafting.* Philadelphia, WB Saunders Co, 1984.

8. Coakes RL: *An Outline of Ophthalmology.* Bristol, Wright Co, 1985.

9. Collins J: *Handbook of Clinical Ophthalmology.* New York, Masson Publishing Co, 1982.

10. Darrell RW: *Viral Diseases of the Eye.* Philadelphia, Lea & Febiger, 1985.

11. Davson H: *The Eye,* ed 3. Orlando, Academic Press, 1984.

12. Deutscht FD: *Paton and Goldberg's Management of Ocular Injuries.* Philadelphia, WB Saunders Co, 1985.

13. Doxanas MT, Anderson RL: *Clinical Orbital Anatomy.* Baltimore, Williams & Wilkins, 1984.

14. Duane T: *Clinical Ophthalmology,* Vols. 1-5. Philadelphia, Harper & Row, 1985.

15. Epstein DL: *Chandler & Grant's Glaucoma.* Philadelphia, Lea & Febiger, 1986.

16. Fraunfelder FT, Roy FH, Mayer SM: *Current Ocular Therapy,* ed 2. Philadelphia, WB Saunders Co, 1985.

17. Gittinger JW Jr: *Ophthalmology: A Clinical Introduction.* Boston/Toronto, Little, Brown & Co, 1984.

18. Gonzalez C: *Strabismus and Ocular Motility.* Baltimore, Williams & Wilkins Co, 1983.

19. Grayson M: *Diseases of the Cornea,* ed 2. St. Louis, CV Mosby Co, 1983.

20. Hammerschlag SB: *Computed Tomography of the Eye and Orbit.* Norwalk, Appleton-Century-Crofts, 1983.

21. Harley RD: *Pediatric Ophthalmology,* ed 2. Philadelphia, WB Saunders Co, 1983.

22. Havener WH: *Synopsis of Ophthalmology: The Ophthalmology Book,* ed 6. St. Louis, CV Mosby Co, 1984.

23. Hollwich F: *Pocket Atlas of Ophthalmology.* Chicago, Year Book Medical Publishers, 1981.

24. Jackson CRS, Finlay RD: *The Eye in General Practice,* ed 8. Edinburgh, Churchill Livingstone, 1985.

25. Jaffe N: *Cataract Surgery and Complications.* St. Louis, CV Mosby Co, 1984.

26. Jones L, Reeh M, Wirtschafter J: *Ophthalmic Anatomy.* Rochester, American Academy of Ophthalmology, 1970.

27. Kanski JJ: *The Eye in Systemic Disease.* London, Butterworths, 1986.

28. Kanski JJ, Packard RB: *Cataract Surgery and Lens Implant Surgery.* London, Churchill Livingstone, 1985.

29. Kolker AE, Hetherington J: *Becker-Schaffer's Diagnosis and Therapy of The Glaucomas,* ed 5. St. Louis, CV Mosby Co, 1983.

30. Kritzinger E, Wright B: *The Eye and Systemic Disease.* Chicago, Year Book Medical Publishers, 1984.

31. Lee J: *Contact Lens Handbook.* Philadelphia, WB Saunders Co, 1986.

32. Leigh RJ: *Neurology of Eye Movements.* Philadelphia, FA Davis Co, 1983.

33. Leitman M, Gartner S, Henkind P: *Manual for Eye Examination and Diagnosis.* Oradell, Medical Economics Co, 1981.

34. McPherson A, Hittner H, Kretzer F: *Retinopathy of Prematurity.* Toronto, BC Decker Inc, 1986.

35. Michaels DD: *Visual Optics and Refraction.* St. Louis, CV Mosby Co, 1985.

36. Milder B, Rubin ML: *The Fine Art of Prescribing Glasses Without Making a Spectacle of Yourself.* Gainesville, Triad Scientific Publishers, 1978.

37. Miller N: *Walsh and Hoyt's Clinical Neuro-Ophthalmology.* Baltimore, Williams & Wilkins Co, 1984.

38. Moses RA: *Alder's Physiology of the Eye.* St. Louis, CV Mosby Co, 1981.

39. Newell FW: *Ophthalmology: Principles & Concepts,* ed 6. St. Louis, CV Mosby Co, 1986.

40.   Peyman GA et al (eds): *Principles & Practice of Ophthalmology,* Vols. 1-3. Philadelphia, WB Saunders Co, 1981.

41.   Reinecke R, Herm R: *Refraction.* Norwalk, Appleton-Century-Crofts, 1983.

42.   Renie WA (ed): *Goldberg's Genetic and Metabolic Eye Disease,* ed 2. Boston/Toronto, Little, Brown & Co, 1986.

43.   Rice TA, Michels RG, Stark WJ: *Ophthalmic Surgery.* St. Louis, CV Mosby Co, Toronto, Butterworths, 1984.

44.   Roy FH: *Ocular Differential Diagnosis,* ed 3. Philadelphia, Lea & Febiger, 1984.

45.   Schepens CL: *Retinal Detachment and Allied Diseases.* Philadelphia, WB Saunders Co, 1983.

46.   Sears ML, Tarkkanen A: *Surgical Pharmacology of the Eye.* New York, Raven Press, 1985.

47.   Shields JA: *Diagnosis and Management of Intraocular Tumors.* St. Louis, CV Mosby Co, 1983.

48.   Silverstone DE, Hirsch J: *Automated Visual Field Testing.* Norwalk, Appleton-Century-Crofts, 1986.

49.   Smolin G, O'Connor GR: *Ocular Immunology,* ed 2. Boston, Little, Brown & Co, 1986.

50.   Spalton DJ, Hitchigs RA, Hunter PA: *Atlas of Clinical Ophthalmology.* Philadelphia, JB Lippincott Co, 1984.

51.   Spencer WH: *Ophthalmic Pathology,* ed 3. Philadelphia, WB Saunders Co, 1986.

52.   Theodore F, Bloomfield S, Mondino B: *Clinical Allergy and Immunology of the Eye.* Baltimore, Williams & Wilkins, 1983.

53.   Vaughn D: *General Ophthalmology,* ed 11. Los Altos, Lange Medical Publications, 1986.

54.   Walsh TJ: *Neuro-ophthalmology: Clinical Signs and Symptoms.* Philadelphia, Lea & Febiger, 1985.

55.   Weinstein GW et al: *Key Facts in Ophthalmology.* London, Churchill Livingstone, 1984.

56.   Wilensky JT, Read JE: *Primary Ophthalmology.* New York, Grune & Stratton, 1984.

57.   Zide BM, Jelks GW: *Surgical Anatomy of the Orbit.* New York, Raven Press, 1985.

Self-instructional Material

A complete up-to-date list (with prices) of available self-instructional material in the form of tapes, slides and videocassettes with or without workbooks can be obtained by writing to the addresses given below. This material should be available for medical student use at the medical school ophthalmology department, the university hospital, and at the Veterans Administration Hospital libraries.

1. Health Sciences Consortium, 200 Eastowne Drive, Suite 213, Chapel Hill, NC 27514.

2. Media Library, University of Michigan Medical School, Ann Arbor, MI 48109.

3. National Medical Audio Visual Center (GSA), Order Section, Washington, D.C. 20409.

4. Ophthalmology Development Fund, Department of Ophthalmology, University of Kentucky Medical Center, Lexington, KY 40506.

11
The Head and Neck Examination

Keat-Jin Lee, M.D., and Thomas Vris, M.D.

Few areas of the body provide such a complex array of structures for the skillful and knowledgeable examiner as the head and neck regions, and few examinations are as diagnostically rewarding as the systematic head and neck examination. The examination consists of two basic parts: an inspection and palpation of the external features of the head and neck region and an internal examination using special illumination and instrumentation.

The examiner will need a source of coaxial illumination such as a head mirror or a headlight. The coaxial principle allows the examiner's line of vision to be in the same pathway as the line of illumination. The head mirror accomplishes this by having a hole centrally placed in the mirror. This again places the line of vision and the direction of the light beam on the same pathway. Certain headlights are so constructed to allow for this coaxial illumination.

The sensitive mucosal linings of the oral and nasal cavities will frequently require topical anesthesia before an adequate examination can be carried out. The most commonly used anesthetics are 2% Pontocaine spray, 1% Xylocaine spray, and Cetacaine. It is important to wait five to ten minutes after the application of the topical anesthetics before examining the patient. This will allow time for the local anesthetic to take effect. This is a very important step and one that is commonly missed by beginning students.

Mirrors are used in otolaryngology to reflect light into the larynx and the hypopharynx as well as up into the nasopharynx beyond the soft palate. A selection of mirror sizes should be available ranging from Number 00 to Number 6. A Number 4 mirror is usually very appropriate for indirect laryngoscopy examination. A Number 1 or 2 mirror would be appropriate for nasopharyngoscopy examination.

This chapter was reprinted from Lee KJ, Vris T: Otolaryngology-- head and neck physical diagnosis, in Lee KJ, Stewart CH (eds): *Ambulatory Surgery and Office Procedures in Head and Neck Surgery,* Orlando: Grune and Stratton, 1986, pp 1-17, by permission.

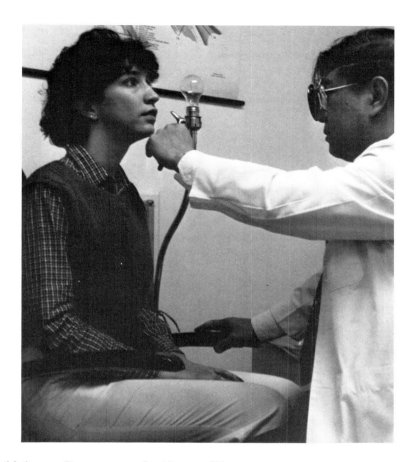

FIGURE 11.1   Proper examination position.

Fiberoptic nasopharyngoscopy and laryngoscopy have become an important contribution to the examination of the internal recesses of the head and neck region. They provide an unparalleled view of the laryngeal and nasopharyngeal structures. Adequate anesthesia is again very important before the fiberoptic nasopharyngoscope or laryngoscope is passed. The oropharynx and the nasal vestibules are carefully sprayed with topical anesthetic. Cotton pledgets soaked in vasoconstriction solution such as ephedrine or a topical anesthetic powder (cocaine) can be placed along the nasal mucosa to decongest the tissues. The lens of the fiberoptic nasopharyngoscope or laryngoscope should be covered with a thin film of liquid soap to prevent fogging, or may be slightly warmed by dipping it in warm water prior to insertion. A slight lubricant should be used to facilitate the passing of the scope. A detailed examination of the nasopharynx including the eustachian tube orifices and Rosenmueller's fossa can be made. Passing the fiber-optic scope further inferiorly, a view of the hypopharynx and the larynx can be achieved.

The head and neck examination is best performed with the patient sitting forward in front of the examiner. All instrumentation and the topical anesthetics as well as the light source should be readily available to the seated examiner. It is always wise to sit in the position illustrated in Figure 11.1 and not in the position illustrated in Figure 11.2.

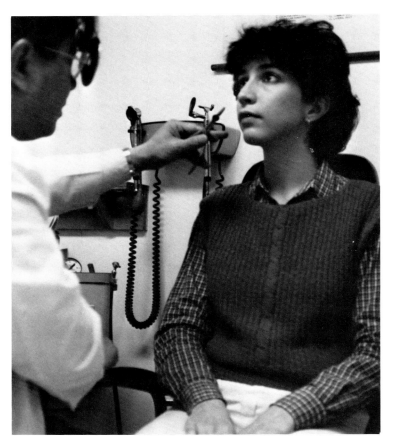

FIGURE 11.2   Improper examination position.

THE EXTERNAL HEAD AND NECK EXAMINATION

This aspect of the examination consists of inspection and palpation. However, before the clinician can appreciate the pathology of the neck region, he/she should have a mental picture of the anatomic structures within the neck. The hyoid bone, thyroid cartilage, cricoid cartilage, and trachea are midline structures. The mandible superiorly, the trapezius muscle posteriorly, and the clavicle inferiorly, together with the midline structures, form the confines of a rectangle. The sternocleidomastoid muscle, which is attached to the mastoid tip superiorly and to the clavicle inferiorly, dissects this rectangular space into an anterior triangle and a posterior triangle. The anterior triangle is bordered by the mandible, the anterior margin of the sternocleidomastoid muscle, and the midline structures. The posterior triangle is bordered by the trapezius muscle, the clavicle, and the posterior margin of the sternocleidomastoid muscle. The internal jugular veins span the triangles from an inferior to superior direction. Surrounding the internal jugular veins are located numerous lymph nodes. These nodes can be involved with inflammatory processes or with metastatic diseases. It is important to describe any lymph adenopathy as being in the low jugular nodes, midjugular nodes, or upper jugular nodes. It is also important to describe any neck masses in relation to the triangles mentioned above as well as in relation to the other anatomic structures. The posterior digastric muscle and the anterior digastric muscle form a digastric sling in the upper portion of the anterior triangle. The submandibular gland is located in the anterior aspect of the digastric triangle. The digastric triangle is bordered by the posterior digastric muscle, the anterior digastric muscle, and the mandible. The carotid bifurcation, or the carotid bulb, is slightly below the digastric triangle. It is essential for students to familiarize themselves with all of these structures by examining each other.

Inspection

Begin by noting the patient's head position. Is the head thrust forward in the sniffing position, signifying a possible upper airway obstruction (eg, an enlarged epiglottis, which is an anterior structure flapping posteriorly to compromise the upper airway)? Please note if the head is tilted to one side, possibly attributable to torticollis of the sternocleidomastoid muscle or an expanding neck mass.

An overall appraisal of the morphology and symmetry of the head and face should be made. Is there a flattening of the malar eminence, suggesting an undiagnosed facial fracture, or a fullness due to neoplasia in the maxillary antrum? The normal face is roughly divided into equal thirds by horizontal lines drawn through the eyes and through the mouth. Disharmony of the middle and lower thirds of the face resulting in relative prognathic or retrognathic configurations may reflect a malocclusion secondary to trauma or developmental malformation. Dental occlusion is generally categorized in three classes: Class I is normal, Class II is commonly referred to as an overbite, and in Class III the mandibular teeth are more anterior than the maxillary teeth as a result of relative mandibular overgrowth or prognathism. It is of interest to note that the mandible and certain parts of the ossicles in the middle ear are derived from the first branchial arch (mandibular arch). Hence, any malformation of the mandible may be associated with malformation of the middle ear ossicles, giving rise to a conductive hearing loss.

The skin of the head and neck region should be carefully inspected for lesions. Malignant and premalignant skin lesions are strongly correlated with sun exposure, which in most individuals is greatest to the head and neck region. Basal cell carcinoma frequently arises on the nasal dorsum, malar eminence, forehead, eyelid, and around the auricle. The usual basal cell carcinoma is a round elevated lesion with a rolled-up border and a central ulceration. A slight whitish discoloration may or may not be present. Squamous cell carcinoma is the next most common malignant lesion of the skin. Squamous cell carcinoma has a more flattened, scaly appearance than the basal cell carcinoma. It is also more ulcerative. It is important to note at this juncture that basal cell carcinoma is usually less aggressive than squamous cell carcinoma. However, basal cell carcinoma that exists in the auricle within a 1 cm radius of the external auditory canal is also very aggressive and should be treated more like a squamous cell carcinoma than a basal cell carcinoma.

Melanoma of the head and neck has a greatly improved prognosis when detected early. Hence, any pigmented nevus that has changed in recent months or has begun to ulcerate or bleed should be looked upon with great suspicion.

The examiner should also be aware of congenital benign nevi, strawberry and cavernous hemangiomata, neurofibromas, and café-au-lait spots. It is important to note that hemangiomas in the infant do usually regress to a greater or lesser extent by the age of 2. Hence, aggressive surgical treatment should not be applied under the age of 2 unless the hemangiomas are compromising vital structures. Patients with neurofibromas oftentimes develop acoustic neurinoma. Acoustic

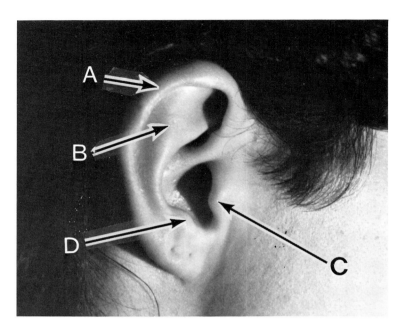

FIGURE 11.3   Normal auricle: A, helix; B, antihelix; C, tragus; D, antitragus.

neurinoma is a form of a cerebellopontine angle tumor giving rise to sensorineural
hearing loss, tinnitus, and vertigo.

The special features of the external head and neck that we normally unify
into one recognizable entity when we "learn a face" should each be inspected for
structural abnormalities. Thus the normal auricle has a natural curvature ending
in an attached lobule (Figure 11.3). The size of the concha and the presence of an
antihelix determine the angle at which the ear stands out from the head. The lack
of an antihelical fold gives rise to a "shell-shaped" ear, otherwise known as a lop
ear. Some mothers think that the child's ear is too large and hence request an
otoplasty. In most instances it is not that the ear is too large, but rather that the
lack of an antihelical fold causes the ear to appear to be too large.

The external nose has a bony dorsum made up of the nasal bones, the nasal
processes of the maxilla that form an angle with the frontal bone at the root of
the nose. Nasal gliomas or encephaloceles originating from the anterior cranial
fossa may exist at this junction. The lower portion of the nose is shaped by nasal
cartilages that form the tip and the alae nasi. The columella at the caudal end of
the nasal septum forms the nasal labial angle with the philtrim of the upper lip.
Each of these elements is of major importance in defining facial features. In the
inspection of the head and neck region, the presence of periorbital edema,
erythema, or chemosis should alert one to the possibility of infection in an adjacent
sinus. Exophthalmos may of course be a sign of thyroid disease but may also reflect disease of the facial bone such as histiocytosis or fibrous dysplasia. It is
important to check for the extraoccular musculature movements that are innervated by the third, fourth, and sixth cranial nerves. Injuries to the orbit from
surrounding sinuses may cause limitation of these movements. Impairment may also
be a result of facial bone fractures. Infection involving the cavernous sinus or a
pituitary tumor may also give rise to limitation of the extraoccular muscle movements.

Palpation

Routine palpation of the head and neck should begin with the sinuses. Pressure on the superior and inferior orbital rim will elicit tenderness in an infected ethmoid, frontal, or maxillary sinus, respectively. Palpation should then proceed to the preauricular and retromandibular regions. Is there a diffuse tender swelling as in parotitis, or a discrete nodule as in a parotid tumor? A deep lobe parotid tumor may be palpated with a gloved finger lateral to the retromolar trigone intraorally. The other major salivary glands in the head and neck region are the submandibular gland and the sublingual gland. The submandibular gland can be palpated in the digastric triangle. Each submandibular gland secretes via its duct through an orifice just lateral to the frenulum of the tongue in the anterior floor of the mouth. Frequently an obstructing stone can be palpated and removed from the duct orifice. Stensen's duct, which drains the parotid gland, is adjacent to the second upper molar on the buccal mucosa. Palpation and milking of an infected parotid gland may produce purulent discharge from the orifice of Stensen's duct.

Of the primary salivary gland tumors, 85% occur in the parotid gland and two thirds of these are benign mixed tumors. Submandibular gland tumors are malignant in about 50% of the cases. Tumors of the minor salivary glands, which are located in the mucosal lining in the oral cavity, are rare, but when they occur they are usually malignant. A parotid tumor associated with severe pain and facial weakness may imply a malignancy. Besides mixed tumor of the parotid glands (which constitute the predominant number) and the malignant tumors, Warthins's cysts are common in males between the ages of 40 and 60 and can be bilateral.

Plain film radiography can identify a calcified stone in the salivary gland regions. The use of sialograms has been advocated for many decades; however, their usefulness is somewhat limited today. Sialography will illustrate dilated ducts, implying a long-standing chronic inflammation. The sialogram may similarly outline a tumor mass. However, the decision of whether to surgically remove an infected gland or not should not be based on sialography but rather based on the clinical findings and history of the patient. A patient with an abnormal sialogram but with minimum clinical findings should not undergo surgical intervention; similarly a patient with multiple severe episodes of infection should be treated surgically irregardless of the sialogram findings. In rare cases where the clinical history is borderline sialogram perhaps may shed some light and help plan a course of treatment.

The student should be aware of the lymphatic drainage pattern in the head and neck area (Figure 11.4). As mentioned previously, the student should be aware of the different triangles of the neck as they relate to the normal anatomic structures, particularly the internal jugular vein. When palpating a neck mass, it is important to describe its size, firmness, and consistency, as well as whether it is mobile or fixed. A firm, hard mass that is fixed is more suspicious of malignancy whereas a more "doughy" and mobile mass is more suggestive of a benign lesion, such as a dermoid cyst. Auscultation of neck masses is also important. Masses associated with bruit may suggest a vascular tumor. A carotid body tumor is located at the bifurcation of the carotid arteries. Arteriography will illustrate a very characteristic "eggshell" appearance that is pathognomonic of carotid body tumors. Branchial cleft cysts are congenital cystic masses usually found in the anterior triangle of the head. They may give rise to a sinus tract into the tonsillar fossa or in the region of the pyriform sinus. A first branchial cleft sinus cyst or tract may be present as a draining sinus in the cartilaginous external auditory canal. This will give rise to recurrent external otitis of unexplained etiology. Hence, when treating patients with recurrent external otitis, particularly children,

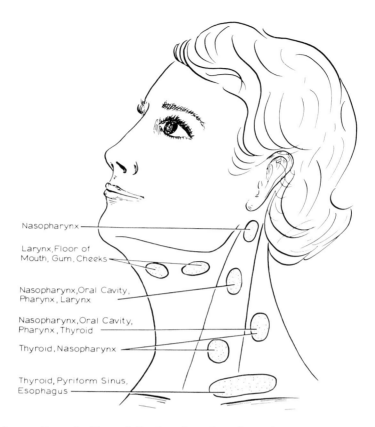

Nasopharynx

Larynx,Floor of
Mouth, Gum, Cheeks

Nasopharynx,Oral Cavity,
Pharynx, Larynx

Nasopharynx,Oral Cavity,
Pharynx, Thyroid

Thyroid, Nasopharynx

Thyroid, Pyriform Sinus,
Esophagus

FIGURE 11.4   Lymphatics of the head and neck region.

one should rule out the presence of a first branchial cleft sinus tract. The first branchial cleft sinus tract may have a cartilaginous core around it and may intertwine with the facial nerve. A first branchial cleft sinus cyst or tract is to be differentiated from the more common preauricular sinus tracts that occur as a draining site just anterosuperior to the tragus. The preauricular sinus tracts are usually shallow and do not intertwine with the facial nerve.

Thyroglossal duct cysts are generally in the midline of the submental area. The distinguishing feature of these cysts is that they move with the hyoid bone on swallowing. During the fourth week of gestation, a ventral (hyoid) diverticulum of endodermal origin can be identified between the first and second branchial arches on the floor of the pharynx. It is situated between the tuberculum impar and the copula. The tuberculum impar together with the lingual swellings develop into the anterior two thirds of the tongue whereas the copula is the precursor of the posterior one third of the tongue. The ventral diverticulum develops into the thyroid gland. As the embryo develops the thyroid diverticulum descends inferiorly and finally down to the adult position of the thyroid gland. At the sixth week of gestation this tract or pathway of descent should be obliterated and atrophied. Should it persist through the time of birth or thereafter, a thyroglossal duct cyst is present and may become infected. This tract is intertwined with the hyoid bone and may extend to the area of the foramen cecum. However, a submental mass may not necessarily mean a thyroglossal duct cyst. In children, reactive lymph adenopathy is a common finding. Also, lipomas or dermoid cysts may be present. Rarely, the submental mass may be the only thyroid gland that is present, and hence its excision may be detrimental to the patient's health. Therefore, prior to removal of these thyroglossal duct cysts it is essential to ascertain that the patient has a normal thyroid gland in the normal position. This can be accomplished by clinical examination or with the help of a thyroid scan. A lingual thyroid may be present at the junction between the posterior one third of the tongue and the anterior two thirds of the tongue. This too may be the only functioning thyroid gland in that particular patient.

Cystic hygromas, large fluid-filled lymph epithelial sacs, are common in the head and neck area in young children. These are cystic masses that transilluminate easily.

The isthmus of the thyroid gland can be palpated as a distinct band of tissue lying on the trachea just below the cricoid bone. The thyroid lobes lie deep to the sternohyoid and sternothyroid muscles, and in the absence of pathology the thyroid lobes may be difficult to palpate. Diffuse or multinodular enlargement of the gland, as well as discrete nodules, can be palpated by pressing and spreading the strap muscles laterally with the examining fingers. It is sometimes easier to palpate the thyroid gland by standing behind the patient.

In examining the neck, the examiner may be seated slightly to one side of the patient, facing the patient. Other examiners may prefer to palpate the neck from the back.

THE INTERNAL EXAMINATION

The internal head and neck examination is performed to investigate the mucosa-lined cavities of the head and neck through the natural orifices—the ears, nostrils, and mouth.

The Ear

The examination of the ear is most easily performed with an otoscope providing magnification and illumination. However, it is important to first examine the auricle itself as well as the external auditory meatus prior to picking up the otoscope. By proceeding with the otoscope too soon, a lesion on the external auditory meatus or auricle may be missed. Hence, it is a good habit to always examine the outer surface of the auricle carefully before using the otoscope.

The External Auditory Canal

The auricle is pulled slightly superoposteriorly to straighten the external auditory canal prior to introducing the otoscope. The largest possible otoscope speculum should be used. Care should be taken not to hurt the patient. The outer one third of the external auditory canal is cartilaginous and the medial two thirds of this canal is osseous. The ear canal is lined with squamous epithelium and is oftentimes afflicted with external otitis, which is a form of dermatitis of the skin lining of the external auditory canal. External otitis will give an appearance of weeping eruptions and severe tenderness. The external auditory canal diameter is compromised by this disease process. If it is possible to examine the tympanic membrane, it will be seen to be normal because it is uncomplicated in external otitis. In examining the external auditory canal one should pay attention to any eruptions or lesions that may signify an adenocarcinoma, squamous cell carcinoma, or basal cell carcinoma. Keratosis obturans is a disease process in which clumps of thick, hard, whitish plaques of squamous debris originate and accumulate in the external auditory canal, almost completely obliterating the area. This is to be differentiated from cholesteatoma, which usually originates from the middle ear. Although external otitis is a very painful process for the patient, it is rarely dangerous other than in patients with diabetes mellitus. Patients with diabetes mellitus may develop a fulminating external otitis, usually caused by *Pseudomonas aeruginosa*.

Exostosis of the external auditory canal is frequently seen in patients who swim habitually in cold water. Exostosis is a firm, rounded, bony mass similar to an osteoma. If small and not occluding the external auditory canal they need not be removed. However, when they become symptomatic in terms of producing either infection or a conductive hearing loss, they should be surgically removed. These whitish, bony, hard masses are not to be confused with any tumor or cholesteatoma.

The Tympanic Membrane

The tympanic membrane is visualized next. Figure 11.5 illustrates the otoscopic picture of a normal tympanic membrane. A portion of the membrane perpendicular to the light source will reflect light back to the examiner; this cone of light is known as the light reflex. A normal tympanic membrane will give rise to a clear light reflex whereas a diseased tympanic membrane may not give this light reflex. However, its significance is limited. The tympanic membrane should be examined for perforations, tympanosclerotic plaques, and drainage. Students should learn to appreciate the aeration of the middle ear cavity. Normal middle ear aeration allows the tympanic membrane to be suspended with an adequate lateral-medial distance (the distance between the tympanic membrane and the promontory). Normal tympanic membrane is made of four layers: a squamous layer laterally, two muscular layers, and a medial mucosal layer. A thin, retracted tympanic membrane may be made of the squamous layer alone. This thin layer may be draped over one of the ossicles, giving rise to some conductive hearing loss. Through a normal translucent tympanic membrane one can appreciate the air space behind the tympanic membrane. It is also possible to visualize bubbles of air pockets mixed with serous effusion in patients with serous otitis media. In patients with a great deal of serous otitis media of a long-standing nature, a dark greyish or even dark bluish tympanic membrane may be visualized with some bulging effect. The bluish tympanic membrane may also reflect a high exposed jugular bulb in the hypotympanum or a glomus tumor. In acute otitis media, an erythematous appearance with prominent capillaries may be visualized. A normal tympanic membrane should be mobile upon pneumomassage. This can be achieved with a Siegal otoscope. Patients with serous otitis media may have a less than mobile tympanic membrane.

Perforations of the tympanic membrane occurring in the anterior half are less worrisome than perforation that exists in the posterior half. A small, dry anterior perforation may be fairly innocuous, giving rise to minimum infection and minimal hearing loss. A perforation in the posterior aspect may give rise to recurrent infection leading to chronic otitis media and cholesteatoma formation. When there is a perforation it is essential that no water enters the external auditory canal because it may lead to ear infection.

Tympanosclerosis is a dry, hyalinized, fibrotic tissue that can be deposited on the tympanic membrane or in the middle ear. It is a reparative process after a perforation has occurred with recurrent infection. it is usually inactive and it is not to be confused with cholesteatoma, which is also a whitish clump of tissue. Cholesteatoma is usually friable, whitish, and moist secondary to chronic or acute infection.

Penetrating injury to the tympanic membrane may give rise to a perforation without any ossicular disruption. Traumatic perforation of this sort, when kept

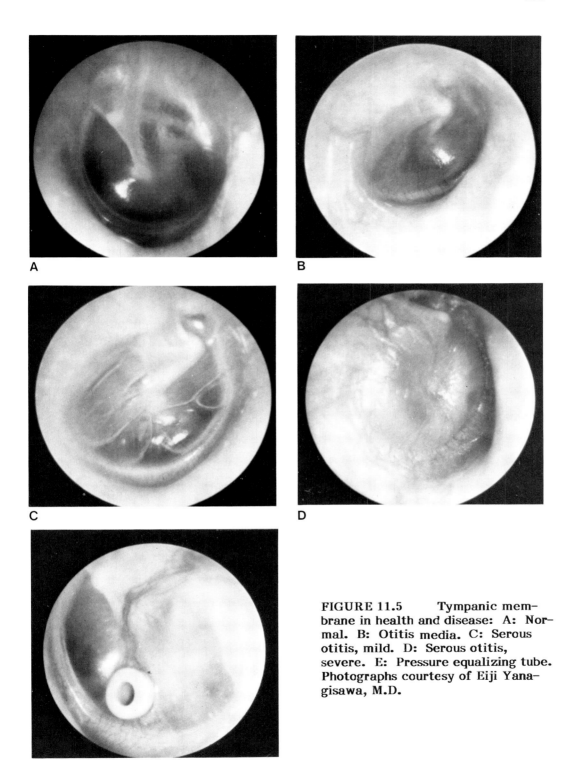

FIGURE 11.5   Tympanic membrane in health and disease: A: Normal. B: Otitis media. C: Serous otitis, mild. D: Serous otitis, severe. E: Pressure equalizing tube. Photographs courtesy of Eiji Yanagisawa, M.D.

uninfected, usually heals spontaneously. Dislocation of the malleus or incus at the time of injury will give rise to a conductive hearing loss that can be corrected subsequently. An injury to the tympanic membrane giving rise to vertiginous attacks accompanied by nausea, vomiting, ataxia, and the presence of nystagmus implies a labyrinthine fistula, most commonly due to a dislocated stapes. Once a labyrinthine fistula is identified it is important that it be repaired surgically within 24 to 48 hours to prevent a permanent sensorineural hearing loss. In the presence of a labyrinthine fistula, eardrops consisting of neomycin and polymyxin should not be used.

Testing Procedures

Hearing Tests. The use of the tuning fork can help to distinguish between a sensorineural hearing loss and a conductive hearing loss. Sensorineural hearing loss occurs when the end organ (the cochlea) or the neural elements are diseased. Presently there is no surgical or medical cure for sensorineural hearing loss. A properly prescribed hearing aid can be helpful. Conductive hearing loss occurs when the sound is not being conducted or transmitted to the end organ. This can arise from cerumen impaction in the external auditory canal, foreign body in the external auditory canal, a perforated tympanic membrane, otitis media, chronic otitis media with or without cholesteatoma, retracted tympanic membrane with poor ventilation of the middle ear space, ossicular disruption, otosclerosis, which is a hereditary fixation of the stapes. The 512-hertz tuning fork is the most useful in otologic examination. In Weber's test it is placed firmly on a midline structure such as the forehead, the dorsum of the nose, the anterior incisor, or the symphysis of the mandible. In a normal individual the sound is transmitted equally to both ears. In a patient with a conductive hearing loss in the right ear, sound is better transmitted to the right ear. In a patient with sensorineural hearing loss in the right ear, the sound is better transmitted to the left ear.

The Rinne test compares the loudness of the tuning fork when placed lateral to the external auditory meatus to the loudness when placed firmly against the mastoid. The tuning fork should be placed between 1 and 2 cm lateral to the external auditory meatus and then pressed firmly against the mastoid periosteum in the region of the antrum. A positive Rinne test is one in which the patient hears a louder sound when the tuning fork is placed lateral to the external meatus as compared to when it is placed on the mastoid periosteum. A positive Rinne test either is a normal sign or implies a sensorineural hearing loss. When the patient hears a louder sound when the tuning fork is placed on the mastoid cortex, this is a negative Rinne test and it implies conductive hearing loss on that tested ear.

When the hearing acuity between the two ears varies significantly it may be wise to mask the better hearing ear when testing the worse ear. This can be achieved by using a Barany masking noisemaker. A Barany noisemaker should be implanted firmly in the external auditory meatus of the nontested ear while the tuning fork tests are being done on the tested ear.

Nystagmus Testing. When the patient has dizziness it is essential to look for spontaneous nystagmus. Nystagmus is a rapid, jerky movement with a quick and a slow component. For nomenclature, the direction of the nystagmus is determined by its fast component. Hence, a nystagmus with a fast component going to the patient's right and a slow component going back to the left is called a right beating nystagmus. The test for nystagmus is to determine whether it is present in the straight gaze position, the right lateral gaze position, the left lateral gaze position, or in more than one direction. To observe for spontaneous nystagmus, first have the patient focus on your index finger in the straight gaze position. Presence or absence of nystagmus is recorded as well as the direction of the nystagmus. Subsequent to that, the index finger is brought toward the left at about a 45-degree angle from the midline. Do not have the patient look in an extreme lateral gaze on either side because it will lead to what is known as a fatigue nystagmus, which is a normal finding. After having determined the presence or absence of spontaneous nystagmus in the left lateral gaze, the patient is then checked for right lateral gaze spontaneous nystagmus.

The patient is said to have a first-degree spontaneous nystagmus when the nystagmus is present only when gazing in the direction of the fast component. Second-degree spontaneous nystagmus is when the nystagmus is present when gazing in the direction of the fast component as well as on straight gaze, and third-degree spontaneous nystagmus is when nystagmus is present in all three directions. It is not pathognomonic, but a first-degree spontaneous nystagmus implies a peripheral or labyrinthine-type lesion. A third-degree nystagmus implies a central nervous system disorder. Second-degree nystagmus may imply more of a central nervous system disorder but can also be due to a peripheral lesion.

Pendulum nystagmus, in which there is no fast or slow component, is usually due to a congenital benign nystagmus as seen in patients with albinism or in occular nystagmus. It has little clinical significance. Patients with disassociated nystagmus or with vertical or diagonal nystagmus usually have central nervous system disorder. Rotary nystagmus in the clockwise or counterclockwise direction is usually due to a labyrinthine disorder.

Vertigo Tests. Certain patients manifest positional vertigo, that is, vertigo that is present when the patient assumes a certain head or neck position. It is commonly seen when the patient rolls to one side while in bed. Positional testing is done in which the patient is brought swiftly from a sitting position on a stretcher to a recumbent position with the head hanging over the edge of the stretcher. First, quickly place the patient with his/her head hanging in the hyperextended position without turning the head to the left or the right. Next, bring the patient swiftly to the head-hanging position with the right ear down. The third component of the test is to bring the patient down swiftly with the left ear down. During all these maneuvers the patient is asked to keep his or her eyes open, and it is by observation of the eye movements that a diagnosis can be made. The patient with positional vertigo will usually experience violent vertigo with nausea and vomiting. Patients with positional vertigo of the benign paroxysmal type manifest what is known as a latency and a fatigue factor. There will be a latency of about 30 to 60 seconds between the assumption of the provocative position and the onset of the vertigo. When the patient is kept at the provocative position for more than 90 seconds, the vertiginous attack will subside (fatigue). With the violent vertiginous attack, the patient will manifest a rotary nystagmus, which will also have a latency component as well as fatigability. If the onset of the vertigo attack as well as the rotary nystagmus occurs immediately after assumption of the provocative position and is not fatigable, a central lesion is suspected. To further study the vestibular system, electronystagmography and other rotational tests can be performed. The discussion of these sophisticated tests is beyond the scope of this text.

Fistula Testing. When a patient is suspected of having a fistula of one of the labyrinthine canals or of the vestibule, a fistula test can be performed. In the fistula test a negative and a positive pressure are applied to the external auditory

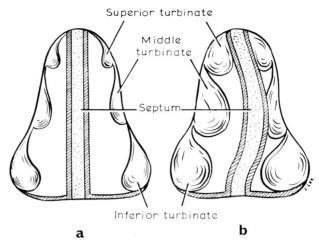

Superior turbinate

Middle turbinate

Septum

Inferior turbinate

a   b

FIGURE 11.6   **Cross-section of the internal nose. A: Normal septum. B: Deviated septum.**

canal and the middle ear space. A positive fistula test is said to occur when a negative and a positive application of pressure to the middle ear space elicit vertiginous attacks with nystagmus. A positive fistula test suggests that there is a fistula in the vestibular labyrinth. It is important to have a tight seal when doing the fistula test. It is also important to make sure that the positive and negative pressure are not applied too many times or it may produce a cooling effect. When the labyrinth is exposed to cool temperature the patient may feel dizzy and also manifest nystagmus. This is a normal caloric response and is not to be confused with a positive fistula test.

The Nose

Using a speculum and coaxial light source, the nasal vault is exposed through the nostril. Before inserting the nasal speculum it is wise to examine the nasal vestibule and the alae. Tenderness over the nasal vestibule can be due to vestibulitis; a common causative organism is *Staphyloccus aureus.* Dermoid cyst is a common finding over the nasal dorsum externally, with tracts leading internally spreading the nasal septum apart. After the insertion of the nasal speculum the nasal septum is inspected for deformities, curvatures, and bony spurs. These deformities may cause nasal obstruction. Superior, middle, and inferior turbinates protrude from the lateral wall of the nose (Figure 11.6). In normal state of health they are not obstructive and not edematous. In an infectious state they may be very hyperemic. In allergy states they may appear very "boggy," pale, and purplish in coloration. The nasal lacrimal duct opens anteriorly under the inferior turbinates. Nasal sinuses drain into the nasal cavity, mainly into the middle meati on both sides. Purulent discharge from the sinuses can be visualized through these meati. A nasal polyp is a rounded, greyish structure that is usually secondary to an allergic background. Most nasal polyps arise from the middle turbinates secondary to disease in the ethmoid sinuses. A choanal polyp is a large polyp in the posterior aspect of the nose or in the nasopharynx originating from the maxillary sinus. Choanal polyps usually have a stalk going into the middle meatus and through the maxillary osteum into the maxillary sinus. It is important to differentiate between a polyp or a mucocele and an encephalocele, particularly in infants. A staphylococcal infection of the nasal skin of the vestibule is to be treated aggressively. Because the lymphatic drainage of this midface triangle is directly into the cavernous sinus, severe staphylococcal infection of this region can lead to cavernous sinus thrombosis and hence give rise to a high mortality rate.

Epistaxis

Epistaxis is a very common afflication in the field of otolaryngology. so in an elementary differential diagnosis the student should be made aware of how to accurately diagnose epistaxis. Epistaxis is most commonly caused by dryness of the nasal mucosa causing the abundant capillaries in the nasal mucosa to rupture. The capillaries are particularly prominent over the nasal septum. Innocuous epistaxis arising from the nasal septum can be treated with digital pressure, lubricating ointments, or in severe cases cauterization and anterior nasal packing. When examining the nose for epistaxis it is important to identify the site of the bleeding. The second most common site of epistaxis is the lateral wall around the turbinates or within the turbinates. Another site of epistaxis is the superior aspect of the nasal septum in the region supplied by the ethmoid vessels. Treatment should be directed to the proper, particular site.

A particularly troublesome epistaxis is what is known as a posterior epistaxis, in which the bleeding site is posterior to the line of vision when examining the anterior nares. This can be posterior to the inferior turbinate or in the choanal region or even in the nasopharynx. Since this cannot be visualized anteriorly it is almost impossible to treat with cauterization or with an anterior nasal pack. Hence, a posterior nasal pack as well as an anterior nasal pack is essential. Severe epistaxis will also manifest as bilateral bleeding, although the original site of bleeding is unilateral. Hence, it is important for the examiner to accurately identify the location of the bleeding. It is important for the student or recent medical graduate to learn how to control epistaxis with an anterior nasal pack as well as with the posterior nasal pack.

The Sinuses

Diseases in the sinuses can be a frequent cause of headaches. **Allergic rhino-sinusitis** is a condition in which the mucosal lining of the sinuses is thickened or edematous, giving rise to a pressure-type headache. The patient may have other signs and symptoms of allergy such as sneezing, watery eyes, and congestion. These symptoms may be seasonal. However, one should be aware that a patient may be allergic to molds and dust, which can be perennial.

Sinusitis is not to be confused with allergic rhinosinusitis. A true bacterial sinusitis gives rise to all the signs and symptoms of an infection: temperature, pain, and erythema. Most commonly inflicted are the maxillary sinuses. They will manifest maxillary pain with purulent discharge in the nasal cavity. Percussion of the maxillary region will give rise to pain in that area. Fortunately, maxillary sinus infections seldom lead to severe complications. Transillumination of the maxillary sinus may reveal an air-fluid level or opacification. A sinus radiograph is of help in making or confirming the diagnosis.

Ethmoid sinusitis is characterized by tenderness in the medial canthal region adjacent to the nasal dorsum. Again purulent discharge can be visualized in the nasal cavity. Severe ethmoiditis can lead to exophthalmos with limitation of extraoccular eye motions as well as periorbital edema.

Frontal sinusitis gives rise to severe frontal headache as well as tenderness when the frontal sinus is percussed. A severe case may give rise to frontal "bossing," particularly if the periosteum is thickened and there is erosion of the frontal wall of the frontal sinus. "Pott's puffy tumor" is the term used to describe a severe frontal bossing with tenderness and accumulation of edema and perhaps an abscess formation. Frontal sinusitis is fraught with severe complication because any involvement of the posterior wall of the frontal sinus can lead to brain abscess or meningitis. Again, inspection of the nasal cavity may reveal purulent discharge from the frontal sinus duct. Mucocele of the frontal sinus giving rise to headache can be easily diagnosed by x-ray.

The sphenoid sinus is a deep-seated sinus. **Mucocele or infection of the sphenoid sinus** may give rise to a vertex headache. Mucocele of the sphenoid sinus can be well hidden, causing such patients to suffer for a protracted period of time without proper diagnosis. Hence, when examining a patient with severe vertex headache of unknown etiology it is well to rule out sphenoid sinus disease. This can be most easily achieved through a set of sinus radiographs, particularly the lateral sinus view and the submental-vertex view.

Dacryocystitis is an inflammation of the lacrimal sac, which is located in the inferior medial aspect of the orbit. The nasal lacrimal duct empties the lacrimal sac contents into the nasal cavity in the inferior meatus. Inflammation of the lacrimal sac gives rise to tenderness and erythema over the lacrimal sac as well as purulent discharge in the inferior meatus.

The Oral Cavity

Using coaxial illumination and gloves, the oral cavity is inspected and palpated, paying particular attention to the tongue and the floor of the mouth. Tumors of the tongue can escape visualization and hence palpation of the tongue is an essential component of intraoral examination. The region of the canine fossa, the upper gingiva, and the lower gingival sulcuses should be carefully examined visually and with palpation. The orifice of Stensen's duct can be seen on the buccal mucosa adjacent to the second upper molar. The hard palate should be examined for any bony erosion. A bony growth similar to an osteoma over the hard palate is called torus palatinus, which is a very common normal finding. This is not to be confused with a soft tumor mass, whose origin may arise from a minor salivary gland. As indicated previously, minor salivary gland tumors are usually malignant. The soft palate should be visualized for bifid uvula or a submucous cleft. Children with a bifid, stubby uvula and a short, soft palate should not undergo adenoidectomy because this can lead to severe velopharyngeal insufficiency speech.

The palatine tonsils should be examined for size, cryptic formation, lodged food particles, and any other sign of chronic or acute infection. Whitish clumps on the tonsillar crypts and pharyngeal mucosa may imply acute tonsillitis or acute pharyngitis. This is to be differentiated from food deposits in the tonsillar crypts. Unilateral swelling of a tonsil with severe pain may imply peritonsillar cellulitis or peritonsillar abscess. It is important to differentiate between these two. Patients with the former diagnosis have minimum or no trismus, whereas those with peritonsillar abscess have severe trismus and drooling. The reason it is important to differentiate the two is because peritonsillar cellulitis should be treated with high doses of antibiotics and not with incision and drainage, whereas the patient with peritonsillar abscess should be drained immediately. The posterior pharyngeal wall should be observed for any bulging suggestive of retropharyngeal mass or tumors. Fortunately, most tumors of the retropharyngeal or parapharyngeal area are benign in nature and are usually of a neurogenic origin. In infectious mononucleosis with tonsillar involvement symmetric tonsillar enlargement with whitish plaques and exudate is seen.

Ludwig's angina is a condition in which the anterior floor of the mouth is infected secondary to involved lymphatic spaces. Dental infection is a common etiology for Ludwig's angina. When Ludwig's angina is established airway obstruction should be avoided either with incision and drainage or a tracheotomy.

The oral mucosa should be examined for leukoplakia, which is a whitish discoloration of the mucosal lining in a streaklike fashion. These may be premalignant lesions and should be watched carefully or biopsied or removed. Lichen planus is a common affliction of the buccal mucosa; they too are whitish in a streaklike discoloration. These are benign lesions and perhaps are related to stress. It can be difficult to distinguish between lichen planus and leukoplakia. A biopsy may be necessary. Leukoplakia is known to be premalignant in some cases, whereas lichen planus is a benign process. Papilloma of the pharyngeal arches is not uncommon. These are wartlike growths on the tonsillar tissues or on the pharyngeal mucosa. They are of little significance but can be removed at the request of the patient. Intraoral cavity melanoma is rare and can be lethal, hence early detection is important. Squamous cell carcinoma of the tongue and oral cavity is common in elderly patients with heavy smoking and drinking histories.

The Larynx

The most challenging part of the head and neck examination is visualization of the larynx and the hypopharynx using a mirror-indirect examination. In most people preanesthesia is not necessary for indirect laryngoscopy with a laryngeal mirror. Occasionally spraying the hypopharyngeal and oral pharyngeal mucosa with Pontocaine spray or Xylocaine spray may be necessary. With the patient in the upright, forward sitting position, the patient's tongue is gently grasped with gauze and pulled anteriorly and inferiorly. A laryngeal mirror, previously warmed, is held up against the soft palate so that the examiner's light source is directed into the larynx through the reflection. It is important to first visualize the hypopharyngeal region, the base of the tongue, the vallecula, and the epiglottis. The lingual tonsil can be visualized at this stage. The pyriform sinuses are examined for any pooling of saliva suggesting esophageal obstruction. Any ulceration, unusual erythema, or growth on the mucosa should be identified. Subsequent to visualization of the lingual surface of the epiglottis, the laryngeal surface of the epiglottis should be examined. The aryepiglottic fold should be examined for any lesion. The arytenoid cartilages should be examined for any swelling or erythema. The arytenoids may be involved with rheumatoid arthritis as well as with any carcinomatous process.

The false vocal cord should be examined. Hoarseness can be secondary to the patient using the false vocal cord to phonate rather than the true vocal cord. This is usually due to laryngospasm or is of psychologic etiology. Subsequently the vocal cords should be visualized. The vocal cords appear as two whitish straps with sharp edges. In health there should be minimum erythema or capillaries. They should move well with phonation and respiration. A vocal cord nodule is a callous, hyperkeratotic lesion, usually seen at the junction of the anterior and the middle third of the vocal cord. It is usually of traumatic origin, such as secondary to smoking or voice abuse. A vocal polyp is a fluid-filled sac attached either pedunculated or sessile on the vocal cord edges. A pedunculated large polyp may not be visualized until the patient coughs or exhales strongly. Generalized hyperkeratosis of the vocal cord may be premalignant and should be watched carefully. Ulceration or an exophytic lesion usually implies a carcinoma of the vocal cord. Papilloma of the vocal cord is common in children. Mobility of the vocal cord should be visualized during phonation. If a vocal cord is paralyzed it should be noted whether it is paralyzed in the paramedian position or in the lateral position (see discussion of vagus nerve below).

Cranial Nerves

The cranial nerve examination is usually included as part of a general neurologic examination. However, it is important to recognize in the head and neck examination that certain cranial nerve disorders are often signs of diseases in the head and neck region.

The **first cranial nerve** can be tested by presenting the patient with several familiar odors to recognize and identify. The most common cause of decrease in olfaction is nasal obstruction either secondary to nasal polyps or due to a markedly impacted deviated nasal septum. In the absence of any nasal pathology, abnormality in olfaction could imply a neurologic disorder.

The **third, fourth, and sixth cranial nerves** should be examined carefully. The superior orbital fissure syndrome may imply an infectious process in that region or an entrapped piece of bone secondary to maxillofacial trauma.

The second division of the **fifth cranial nerve** exits through the foramen rotundum into the pterygomaxillary space and then crosses the roof of the maxillary antrum before finally exiting as the infraorbital nerve. If pain or numbness is attributed to this nerve, a search should be prompted for pathology along its course. Involvement of the third branch of the fifth cranial nerve may occur in the tongue, the mandible, or the infratemporal fossa.

The **seventh cranial nerve** shares the internal auditory canal with the eighth cranial nerve. It also travels through the temporal bone in the middle ear and mastoid, exiting from the stylomastoid foramen and dividing into its facial branches amid the parotid gland. A careful examination of the seventh cranial nerve is of vital importance. It is also important to separate a peripheral facial paralysis from a central facial paralysis. Peripheral facial paralysis involves the whole face, whereas a central facial paralysis will involve the lower two thirds of the face but not the frontalis muscle.

Examining the patient with facial paralysis, it is first important to determine whether it is a partial or a total paralysis. It is equally important to ascertain an etiology for the facial paralysis. An acoustic neurinoma or a facial nerve neurinoma should be excluded. Subsequent to that, any middle ear disease such as cholesteatoma, mastoiditis, or acute otitis media should be diagnosed or ruled out. Lesions in the external auditory canal or the parotid region should again be identified or ruled out. Facial nerve neurinoma usually gives rise to facial twitching followed by facial weakness and paralysis. It can be firmly diagnosed with polytomography of the facial nerve and computed axial tomography (CAT) scan. Acoustic neurinoma usually gives rise to a sensorineural hearing loss, loss of discrimination, and dizziness, followed by facial paralysis. This again can be identified with sophisticated audiologic evaluation, and by a CAT scan with air cisternogram. When a facial paralysis is diagnosed without any known etiology then the diagnosis of Bell's palsy is pronounced. It should be emphasized that a diagnosis of Bell's palsy should not be made until all known etiologies are ruled out. Bell's palsy implies a facial paralysis of an unknown etiology.

The next step in working up the patient with facial paralysis is to do what is known as topography mapping. The greater superficial petrosal nerve is a branch of the seventh nerve at the vicinity of the geniculate ganglion in the middle fossa. Hence, facial nerve paralysis and decreased tearing implies that the lesion is central to the geniculate ganglion region. A patient with facial paralysis who maintains normal tearing probably has a lesion distal to the geniculate ganglion. The stapedius reflex test can be performed by an audiologist to ascertain whether the lesion is proximal or distal to the stapedius nerve, which is a branch of the facial nerve in the vicinity of the stapes. The chorda tympani is the branch of the facial nerve just proximal to the stylomastoid foramen. Here the testing of taste sensation would help to topographically identify the site of lesion. The more serious student in this field should refer to the references listed for further information regarding Schirmer's test, the different electrical stimulation tests, and the salivary flow tests. It is important to mention in this basic text that the patient with facial nerve paralysis showing signs of degeneration should have the facial nerve decompressed before it is degenerated to get a better prognosis. Similarly, a patient with a traumatic facial nerve injury secondary to contusion or edema of the nerve can be followed with electrical stimulation. Should the electrical stimulation suggest imminent nerve degeneration then a facial nerve decompression is again warranted. However, if the tests do not imply imminent degeneration, careful follow-up may suffice. A patient with an immediate onset of facial nerve paralysis following trauma or surgery should have the nerve explored and resutured to get a better functional result. It is possible to do nerve grafting or a hypoglossal-facial nerve anastomosis for those patients with permanent facial nerve paralysis.

Recurrent laryngeal nerve paralysis can be identified through indirect laryngoscopy. Patients with thyroid tumors or thyroid surgery may manifest hoarseness secondary to recurrent laryngeal nerve paralysis. Patients with no head and neck diseases but who manifest hoarseness secondary to a left vocal cord paralysis should receive a pulmonary consultation and tomograms of the left upper lobe to rule out a left upper lobe or mediastinal lesion or a hypertrophied left ventricle.

Cranial nerves IX, X, and XI may be involved with a jugular foramen tumor such as glomus jugulare. The hypoglossal canal, which is adjacent to the jugular foramen, may be eroded, giving rise to hypoglossal nerve involvement. A glomus jugulare tumor usually presents at its early phase with a pulsatile bruit in the ear as well as a bluish hue or tinge to the tympanic membrane. As the disease progresses, cranial nerves IX through XII may be involved.

REFERENCES

1. Lee L, Lee KJ: A study of facial proportions and sketching of facial contours. *Ear, Nose, Throat* 1979;58:12-30.

2. Lee KJ: *Differential Diagnosis in Otolaryngology.* New York, Arco Publishing Company, 1978.

3. Lee KJ: *Essential Otolaryngology-Head and Neck Surgery,* ed 3. New York, Medical Examination Publishing Company, 1983.

4. Lee KJ: *Comprehensive Surgical Atlases and Text in Otolaryngology-Head and Neck Surgery.* New York, Grune & Stratton, 1983.

5. Paparella MM, Shumrick DA: *Textbook of Otolaryngology.* Philadelphia, WB Saunders, 1980.

12
The Urologic Examination

Ronald D. Lee, M.D.

INTRODUCTION

Males, as a rule, do not go for routine urologic examination. Some men may suddenly be filled with panic if a new little pimple appears, or they feel an unexplained pain. The given reason for consulting a physician may be far removed from the urogenital area. Instead, they may state that they are fatigued or are not feeling well, and finally comes the famous line, "Oh, by the way, I noticed I have an itch/ a discharge/a lump," or there is blood in the urine, or there is blood during ejaculation.

The rectal examination must be included in every physical examination. As one famous clinician once said, "If you don't put your finger in, you put your foot in your mouth later." Cancer of the prostate is increasing. There are approximately 60,000 new cases each year with 20,000 deaths. At the present time, cancer is detected in the early asymptomatic stage in only 10% of patients because doctors fail to examine the rectum. The symptom of hematuria must never be neglected. It should be followed up by the proper examinations, because tumors of the bladder account for 3% of all cancer deaths, especially in patients between 50 and 70 years of age. Seminomas of the testicles are also on the increase.

Dr. Lee has given us a simple outline on how to perform a thorough urologic examination, which is indispensable for proper diagnosis of problems with the male urogenital organs.

EXAMINATION OF THE KIDNEYS

The kidneys are paired organs that snugly lie in the retroperitoneal space between the T-12 and L-3 vertebrae, and are not readily accessible to the hands of the examiner (Figure 12.1). They are well protected by the rib cage and the surrounding muscle groups. Typical dimensions for an adult male kidney are a length of 13 cm and a width of 6 cm. Both kidneys are usually not visible through the skin, except in very thin persons, in whom they can be felt by bimanual palpation. When

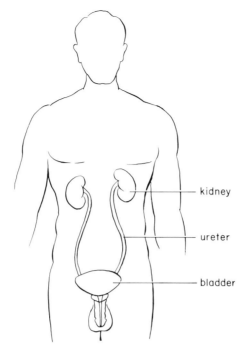

kidney

ureter

bladder

FIGURE 12.1   Location of kidney.

the kidney is enlarged due to a disease state, it becomes evident either as a flank mass or an anterior abdominal mass. The kidneys are best located by using a bi-manual approach (see Figure 12.2).

With the patient supine, one hand of the examiner is placed behind the patient in the costovertebral area. The opposite hand then is positioned under the corresponding costal margin. With anterior pressure being provided by the posterior hand of the examiner, and posterior pressure by the anterior hand, ask the patient to take a deep breath. As the kidney descends, its size, shape, and consistency may then be assessed using ballottement, which means bouncing the kidney gently between both hands like a basketball.

To elicit pain from the kidney area, light pressure by the examiner in the costovertebral angle, and not a punch, is sufficient. General palpation in the costovertebral angle that elicits pain may be caused by either renal distention or inflammation from renal or perirenal causes. Moving your hand through the flank area can sometimes cause crepitus sounds, as if there is something under the skin, which can represent perirenal abscess, fistula from pulmonary or gastrointestinal sources, or even recent penetrating traumas.

Auscultation of the renal area is performed by placing the stethoscope below the costal margin on the anterior abdominal wall lateral to the midline. The flank should also be auscultated. A bruit heard in the renal area may represent renal artery stenosis, aneurysmal dilatation, or arteriovenous fistula. This is another useful application of the stethoscope away from the heart.

The systemic manifestations of kidneys that do not function may vary from no symptoms through some generalized fatigue, weakness, pallor, and a distinct uremic odor to polyuria, polydipsia, bone pain, pruritis, congestive heart failure, severe

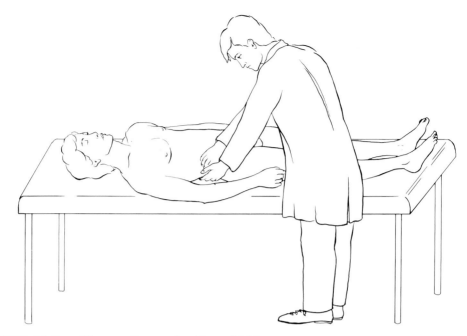

FIGURE 12.2   Bimanual examination of kidney.

electrolyte imbalances, electrocardiographic changes, radiographic changes (pseudo-fractures, osteoporosis, and osteomalacia), pigmentations of the skin, convulsions, seizures, and hiccoughs; this list is far from complete. The student will familiarize himself with the uremic syndrome, which is not the aim of this text.

The examiner will look for flank masses by the method described, estimating its size, its consistency, and its moveability. It is important to note if there are bilateral flank masses, as seen in polycystic kidneys. Often, there is a family history of visceral cysts with bilateral obstruction. Unilateral flank masses that arise in the kidney may occur from hypertrophic kidney or renal tumors, the most common type being renal cell carcinoma, usually associated with pain and hematuria, occurring in the sixth and seventh decades. The harder nephrotic kidney typically arises from obstruction, which may be unilateral or bilateral, or renal cysts, which are generally benign and sometimes can be transilluminated and differentiated from solid structures.

Flank masses may be found in trauma, or there may have been a history of bleeding diathesis. The presence of crepitations on the flank mass could represent an infection or even trauma. The finding of a left flank mass has to be differentiated from the spleen, which, at times, may be difficult.

Flank Pain

Pain in the costovertebral area is a very common complaint in clinical practice. Often, patients will say, "I have pain in my kidney area. There must be something wrong with my kidneys." As a rule, the pain does not result from kidney ailments but from a sprained back or a muscle injury. The pain may be present on a continual basis. It may arise from superficial cutaneous lesions, such as herpes zoster, and from trauma.

Flank pain that is accompanied with fever and chills should make the physician suspect pyelonephritis. If the urine has an increased white blood cell count the differential diagnosis of flank pain arising from the kidney area should consist of urolithiasis, infections, obstruction, tumors, perirenal abscess, vesicoureteral reflux (especially when given a history of recurrent upper urinary tract infections), and pain from ureteropelvic junction obstruction, which characteristically is pain that is worsened with increased fluid intake or diuresis. You will have to differentiate flank pain from pain that may arise from the gastrointestinal tract, as in a history of inflammatory bowel disease, blood or mucus in the stools, and gallbladder ailments, and from pain that arises from the pulmonary region, as seen in pneumonia or pleuritis.

EXAMINATION OF THE URETERS

The ureter is another structure not directly accessible to the examiner, who must, by a good history and appropriate testing, discover any illness of the ureters. Lying in the retroperitoneum, the ureter joins the renal collecting system at the ureteropelvic junction, then descends through the retroperitoneum into the bladder, where it terminates at the ureteral orifice. It is approximately 30 cm in length, and it is derived embryologically from the wolffian duct. As the ureter ascends to meet the metanephric cap in the developing fetus, it is not uncommon for it to err in its development, leading to the common partial or complete duplicated collecting system abnormalities one encounters. The wolffian duct not only gives rise to the ureters but continues cephalad, branching into the renal pelves, calyces, and finally the collecting ducts of the kidney.

Common Diagnostic Problems Associated with the Ureter

One of the most painful conditions in medicine is ureteral colic. As Sir Hutchinson, the great surgeon of the 19th century, stated, "Oh, Lord, take me not through my kidney." The characteristic pain of ureteral colic is an agonizing, deep, penetrating pain that makes the patient contort and twist his/her body in trying to get some relief. This is the kind of pain in which the patient does not lie still quietly for it to be relieved, but, instead, wanders around the room bent over, screeching in agony, as each spasm brings fear and despair. Often, it is associated with nausea, vomiting, diaphoresis, and feeling faint. As the stone passes down the ureter, the patient can actually trace the pain to where the stone finally stops, waiting to be extruded.

Ureteral colic may also be caused by a clot, tumor, or necrotic renal papilla, or even fungal material.

It is not possible to palpate a kidney stone. The examination of the abdomen may reveal an acute abdomen that is tense, with rebound tenderness. The examiner must go through an entire differential diagnosis on severe abdominal pain, which might include appendicitis, dissecting aneurysm, spermatic cord torsions, gastrointestinal illnesses such as perforation and duodenal ulcers, pelvic inflammatory disease in women, and pain from a variant origin.

The diagnosis of ureteral colic is made by the presence of blood in the urine and by a flat radiograph of the abdomen, which may demonstrate a radiopaque stone. If it is a uric acid stone, it may not be visualized. The aftermath of the presence of a kidney stone can be surmised by dilated ureters, and if obstruction resulted there may be hydronephrosis.

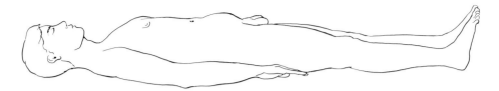

FIGURE 12.3   Distention of the bladder.

EXAMINATION OF THE BLADDER

The typical adult bladder is an intrapelvic organ. It acts as a reservoir for storage of urine, which is then periodically expelled through a coordinated contraction of the detrusor muscle and the urinary sphincters. Capacities of up to 400 ml may be considered normal. Embryologically the bladder is derived from both mesodern and endoderm. It is lined by transitional cell epithelium (urothelium) and is covered on the dome by the peritoneum, where the urachus or obliterated allantois may remain. The ureters enter the bladder posteroinferiorly and course lateral to medial through the bladder wall, then in a submucosal position to finally exit at the ureteral orifices, which mark the lateral borders of the trigone.

It is important to learn the examination of both the distended and the empty bladder. When the bladder is distended (Figure 12.3), the scaphoid abdomen will become asymmetrically shaped from the pubis cephalad, with lower abdominal swelling extending to or even above the umbilicus.

Palpation of the distended bladder will reveal a tense midline stricture that on pressing will cause the patient either pain or a desire to void. Bimanual palpation of the distended bladder will reveal a firm, fluid-filled, mobile midline mass. Bimanual palpation of the empty bladder should be performed with the index finger of one hand in the rectum or vagina and the opposite hand pressing on the lower abdominal wall. This should reveal a soft, midline, freely moveable structure. Occasionally one may palpate a poorly emptying diverticulum, or, in the case of vesical neoplasms, either paravesical masses or fixation of the bladder to the pelvic side walls. Percussion of a large midline lower abdominal mass, if it gives a fluid note, helps to make a diagnosis of bladder distention.

A lower abdominal mass rising out of the pelvis can be caused by a distended bladder. By having the patient void, or emptying the bladder with catheter drainage, the mass of the bladder will markedly diminish. Differential diagnosis of distention of the lower abdomen in the female includes pregnancy, uterine trauma, ovarian cyst, or plain obesity. Sometimes a bowel that is impacted with feces can cause distention or ascites.

EXAMINATION OF THE URETHRA

The urethra allows the egress of urine from the bladder. In men the urethra is approximately 23 cm in length, whereas in women it averages 4 cm. It is divided into anterior and posterior portions, and in men these are further subdivided into the glanular, penile, and bulbar portions of the anterior urethra and the membranous and prostatic portions of the posterior urethra. The lining of the urethra changes from squamous to stratified columnar to transitional cell as one travels from the meatus back toward the bladder. The meatus itself is lined by delicate pink mucosa and should be larger than a No. 18 French catheter in caliber. Narrowing of the meatus to less than this size in the adult is called stenosis.

TABLE 12.1   Differential Diagnosis of Urethral Meatal Masses

Diagnosis	Symptoms
Urethral prolapse	Protruding urethral mucosa that becomes more prominent with Valsalva's maneuver
Carbuncle	Abnormal fleshy growth of mucosa that does not change with Valsalva's maneuver
Condylomata acuminata	Typical epithelial-covered papillomas Often multiple lesions Usually spread through sexual contact
Urethral tumor	Usually firm on palpation Presents as hematuria, voiding dysfunction, or a mass May have associated inguinal adenopathy

Rupture of the urethra may be secondary to trauma, surgery, or tumor or may be iatrogenic, from urologic instrumentation including indwelling urinary catheters. When the rupture is located in the anterior urethra and confined within Buck's fascia, physical examination in the male will reveal a swollen, discolored penile shaft. With rupture in the bulbomembranous or membranoprostatic area, the extravasation may pass down into the scrotum and perineum ("butterfly hematoma"), as well as up to the abdominal wall toward the axillae.

A common manifestation of urethral illness is the urethral infection so common in females. It consists of burning on urination, sometimes blood in the urine, and/or a discharge, which may be venereal.

The meatal portion of the urethra should be examined for masses, the causes of which are given in Table 12.1.

EXAMINATION OF THE PENIS

The penis is an elongated, tube-shaped organ that serves a role in both excretory and reproductive functions. Embryologically, it is derived from the genital tubercle. In cross-section, the penis is composed of three erectile bodies (Figure 12.4). Two of these bodies, the paired corpora cavernosa, function to transform the flaccid penis into a turgid organ as their vascular channels fill with blood during erection. The third erectile body, the corpus spongiosum, also contributes to tumescence and, in addition, surrounds and accompanies the urethra.

The skin of the penile shaft is generally quite loose and elastic. On the under-surface, in the midline, a thin brown line, the **median raphe,** may often be seen. This represents the fusion of the urogenital folds and is continuous with a similar line on the scrotum. It is not uncommon to see dilated veins on the surface of the penile shaft.

The **urinary meatus** usually exits at the tip of the glans. More proximal locations of the meatus are described as hypospadias if located on the ventral aspect of the penis, or epispadias if located on the dorsal surface. Hypospadias is by far the more common of the two types of abnormal urethral placements encountered. Depending on the location of the meatus, hypospadias is classified into glanular, subcoronal, penile shaft, and penoscrotal positions.

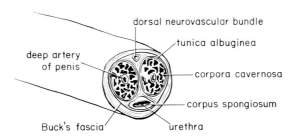

FIGURE 12.4   Cross-section of penis.

The **glans penis** is the enlarged distal end of the corpus spongiosum. Where it joins the penile shaft, the glans flares into a ring called the corona. On the under-surface of the glans, the frenulum, a loose fold of skin, joins the prepuce to the glans.

The **foreskin,** or prepuce, may be present depending on whether or not the man has been circumcised. If present, it should be retracted to thoroughly examine the glans and inner surface of the foreskin. If the examiner is unable to fully retract the foreskin, the patient has phimosis. This may be congenital, secondary to recurrent infections, or, if of sudden onset, suggestive of an underlying neo-plasm. When the foreskin is fully retracted and cannot be brought back down to cover the glans, the condition is called paraphimosis, and is a urologic emergency, since vascular compromise of the penis distal to the constriction of the retracted foreskin will ensue. This is why it is so important to pull the foreskin back down over the glans once the exam is completed. One may encounter a white, cheeselike substance under the foreskin. This is smegma and represents the secretions of the sebaceous glands in the area.

On the surface of the penis, various clinical abnormalities may be identified. Palpation of lesions is important not only to detect the presence or absence of pain but also to determine the extent of the lesion (see Table 12.2). One should always take care to use gloves when examining penile lesions.

With the penis in the erect state, several different observations may be made. Chordee, an abnormal bowing of the penis, usually in the ventral direction, may be seen. Most often it represents a congenital abnormality. Abnormal curvature of the penis may also be secondary to the presence of Peyronie's plaques. These are idiopathic thickenings of the tunica albuginea of the corpora cavernosa. Priapism is an abnormal prolonged erection unrelated to sexual stimulation and involving the corpora cavernosa and not the corpus spongiosum. Common etiologies include sickle cell disease, myeloproliferative diseases, medication, and idiopathic causes.

EXAMINATION OF THE SCROTUM AND CONTENTS

The scrotum is a saclike structure that serves not only to protect its contents but also to assist in thermoregulation of the testes. The wall of the scrotum con-tains the dartos muscle, which can contract in response to pain or cold and relax in response to heat. Embryologically, the scrotum is derived from ectoderm, with its homologue in the female being the labia majora. It typically has sparse hair growth with prominent folds or rugae, especially when the scrotum is exposed to cold. A dark brown line, the median raphe, may be seen running in the midline posterior to anterior and continuous with a similar line on the ventral aspect of the penis. The scrotum is quite elastic, allowing it to expand to a massive size when filled with hydrocele fluid or blood.

TABLE 12.2   Differential Diagnosis of Penile Lesions

Diagnosis	Symptoms
Gonorrhea	Short incubation period Purulent urethral discharge and dysuria
Syphilis	Ulcer with firm, nontender borders Serology often positive
Granuloma inguinale	Predominantly in the black population Often painless ulceration *Calymmatobacterium granulomatis* organism
Lymphogranuloma venereum	Painful ulceration Often bilateral painful inguinal adenopathy *Chlamydia trachomatis* organism
Chancroid	3–5 days' incubation Usually single vesicle changing to ulcerated lesions Painful but not indurated lesions "Soft chancre" Painful lymphadenopathy *Haemophilus ducreyi* organism
Herpes simplex	Prodromal symptoms Multiple vesicles followed by painful ulceration
Neoplasm	Often firm, painless exophytic lesions
Condylomata acuminata	Usually multiple small, pink, velvety projections May become massive at times
Condylomata lata	History of syphilis Flat lesions compared to condylomata accuminata
Candida	Usually present as balanitis or balanoposthitis
Molluscum contagiosum	Raised papules with central depression Whitish material may be squeezed from lesions DNA pox virus organism

Within the scrotum lie the normal scrotal contents, including the testes, epididymides, vasa deferentia, and spermatic cords surrounded by a small amount of fluid. Certain abnormal contents such as bowel, ovary, blood, or peritoneal fluid may, on occasion, be found in the scrotum (Figure 12.5).

Scrotal Contents

Testis

The normal adult testis is located in the dependent portion of the scrotum and measures greater than 20 ml in volume or 4 cm in its longest dimension. Serving both important hormonal and reproductive functions, the testes are an important

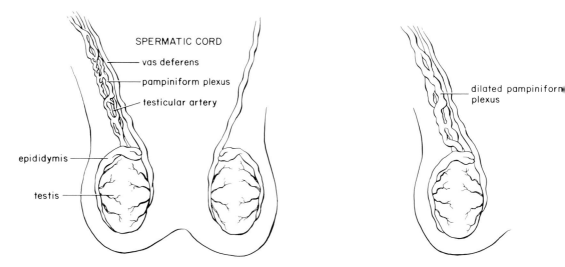

FIGURE 12.5   **Cross-section of scrotum, epididymis, testes, and spermatic cord.**

part of the genitourinary system. The incidence of undescended testes in adult males has been estimated to be approximately 0.7%, with monorchia, or congenital absence of one testis, occurring in 3% to 5% of boys undergoing surgery for cryptorchidism. In its superficial position, the testis is quite susceptible to trauma; however, the cremasteric muscles will often protect the testis by retracting it in a cephalad direction when exposed to noxious stimuli. Besides traumatic injuries, the testes may also be involved with neoplasm, infectious diseases, and ischemia secondary to spermatic cord torsion.

Epididymis

The epididymis not only serves in a storage capacity but also functions to transform testicular sperm, which are unable to fertilize ova, into sperm that can perform that function. Lying on the posterolateral surface of the testis, the epididymis is actually a single coiled tube of 3 to 4 m in length that connects the vasa efferentia of the testis to the convoluted portion of the vas deferens. Typically, the epididymis is soft and nontender. In cases of obstruction, it will be enlarged and thickened although usually not painful. Epididymitis, when acute, is recognized clinically as a tender swelling on the posterolateral aspect of the testis. Chronic epididymitis may also manifest as a painful swelling, although not quite as dramatic as in the acute form. The epididymis is divided into three parts: the head or caput, often called the globus major; the body or corpus; and the tail or cauda, often called the globus minor.

Vas Deferens

The vas deferens represents that portion of the excurrent duct system connecting the tail of the epididymis to the ampulla (Figure 12.6). Embryologically, the vas is derived from the wolffian duct. It is approximately 30 cm long in the adult and has the largest wall-to-lumen ratio of any hollow organ. Its luminal diameter is about 0.3 mm, but may be much larger in cases of obstruction. The

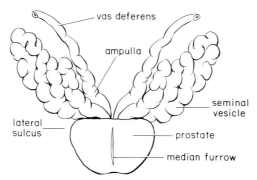

FIGURE 12.6   Cross-section showing vas deferens and prostate.

wall of the vas is composed of three muscular layers that, on contraction, help propel the sperm distalward.

At its proximal end, near the epididymis, the vas continues the curviform shape of the epididymis and is called the convoluted vas. As it progresses towards the ampulla, it gradually straightens and becomes the straight vas. Just before its entry into the urethra, the vas empties into the ampulla, which also drains the ipsilateral seminal vesicle. The ampulla then empties into the ejaculatory duct, which enters the prostatic urethra just lateral to the vera montanum.

Spermatic Cord

The spermatic cord is composed of blood and lymphatic vessels, nerves, various fascial layers and muscles, and the vas deferens. It passes through the inguinal canal into the scrotum. The normal cord is soft and pliable. In obese persons, a lipoma of the cord may be apparent as a soft mass that does not change with position or Valsalva's maneuver. The most common abnormality of the spermatic cord, seen in up to 15% of men, is the varicocele.

Varicocele

A varicocele represents a dilation of the pampiniform plexus secondary to reflux of blood through the gonadal veins. The pampiniform plexus forms a part of the spermatic cord and represents the major venous drainage of the testis and epididymis. The plexus is located on the spermatic cord just above the testis and extending cephalad.

Normally several valves in the gonadal vein prevent the reflux of blood into the pampiniform plexus. With a congenital absence of these valves or with wearing away from venous pressure, retrograde flow of blood may ensue, forming a varicocele. The pathophysiology of varicoceles is a subject of much discussion. Many theories, including increased peritesticular heat, toxic renal/adrenal metabolites, decreased oxygen tension, increased or decreased blood flow around the testis, and the like are invoked, but none can explain fully the deleterious effects of the varicocele.

Varicocele may be present in approximately 15% of males but seems to have a higher frequency of incidence in the subfertile male population. Usually, it is diagnosed during evaluation for testicular pain or atrophy, both of which may be related to the varicocele. It can also be seen as an asymptomatic finding on routine physical examination.

Varicoceles are classified into three sizes or grades:

III—Large enough to see through the scrotal wall

II—Easily felt upon examining the spermatic cords

I—Palpable with Valsalva's maneuver

The majority of varicoceles seen in men during work-up of male subfertility are of the Grade I variety.

The largest size varicoceles can be seen through the scrotum and appear as multiple dilated tortuous vessels. On occasion, there will be concomitant dilatation of the scrotal wall veins. This has been called a cirsocele, although, strictly speaking, this term applies to any varicocele, regardless of its location. Grade II, or intermediate, varicoceles are easily felt upon examining the scrotal contents. They have been classically described as feeling like a "bag of worms." Grade I varicoceles are the smallest and most difficult to diagnose.

Most often, varicoceles present on the left side. This has been thought to be due to the hemodynamics of the gonadal vein entering the renal vein at a 90-degree angle on the left side versus the much more acute angle of the entrance of the gonadal vein into the vena cava on the right. In addition, the "nutcracker" effect, that is, the compression of the left renal vein between the superior mesenteric artery and the aorta, may contribute to increased venous pressure.

The Physical Examination of the Scrotum

Inspection of the scrotum should reveal a nondistended, wrinkled sac. If one testis is congenitally absent, the ipsilateral scrotum may be poorly developed. Surface abnormalities may include sebaceous cysts; vascular anomalies, such as capillary hemangiomas; or exophytic lesions, including epithelial neoplasms. Dilated veins on the scrotal wall suggest an underlying varicocele. Very large varicoceles may sometimes be visualized through the scrotal wall. If the scrotum is distended, the examiner must differentiate between scrotal wall edema and fluid or a mass within the tunica vaginalis (Tables 12.3 and 12.4). Interstitial edema will make the wall of the scrotum thickened and dimpled, whereas fluid within the tunica vaginalis generally "thins out" the scrotal skin.

Next, the scrotal contents are examined, in both supine and standing positions. The examination begins with the testis, the consistency of which has been likened to a fluid-filled structure, that is, it should feel fluctuant. Palpation is best performed using both hands. The right testis may be gently stabilized near its upper pole using the left hand. The right hand is then used to gently palpate the whole of the testis. Any abnormalities in consistency either on or below the surface are noted. Occasionally tunica albuginea or mesothelial cysts are identified as small discrete lumps in the covering of the testis. They are benign in nature. The testicular and epididymal appendages, which may number up to five, are usually not palpable.

Of utmost consideration in the examination of the testis and related scrotal contents is gentleness, because this area may be exquisitely sensitive to palpation. Indeed, it is not uncommon to halt the exam before completion because of discomfort or light-headedness in the patient. The pain fibers of the testes are carried through the autonomic nervous system and, in fact, provide for a useful clinical test. Some diabetic patients with erectile dysfunction also have little or no discomfort on firm palpation of the testes, suggestive of an underlying peripheral neuropathy. Palpation of the epididymis is then performed proceeding from the

TABLE 12.3   Differential Diagnosis of Scrotal Swelling

Diagnosis	Symptoms
Interstitial scrotal wall edema	Usually from allergic reactions, insect bites Secondary reaction from intrascrotal pathology May be idiopathic
Intrascrotal fluid	
Hydrocele	Transilluminates May communicate with peritoneal cavity; if so, there will often be change in position Usually secondary to excessive fluid production/decreased fluid absorption of tunica vaginalis but may be seen as reaction to intrascrotal infection or neoplasms or as part of generalized edema, as in renal, hepatic, or congestive heart failure
Hematocele	Does not transilluminate History of trauma or recent intrascrotal surgery
Pneumatocele	May have associated crepitus in the scrotal wall Often a history of penetrating scrotal trauma or of pneumothorax Can be secondary to intrascrotal infection with gas-forming organisms

head to the tail. Thickening, induration, enlargement, and any areas of tenderness are noted.

Next, proceeding cephalad, each spermatic cord is palpated gently between the thumb and first two fingers of the examiner's hand, until the firm vas deferens is felt. The vas is then checked in both cephalad and caudad directions. Its consistency has been described as a "whip cord" or a large piece of uncooked spaghetti. Suffice to say, it is the firmest structure palpable in the normal spermatic cord. Two important abnormalities to search for in the examination are "beading" of the vas deferens and absence of the vas deferens. Beading may occur with many diseases, including tuberculosis, diabetes mellitus, and smallpox. On examination, one feels thickened, enlarged areas separated by variable lengths of more normal-feeling vas. Vasal aplasia occurs in approximately 2% of men presenting for evaluation of subfertility and is also a quite common finding in cystic fibrosis. The absent vas deferens is related to wolffian duct abnormalities in early embryonic life. In approximately 23% of cases of congenitally absent vasa deferentia, excretory urography reveals abnormalities ranging from renal agenesis to situs inversus.

The spermatic cord is next examined, paying careful attention for the presence of varicocele or any abnormal masses. Ideally the patient should be examined after standing for several minutes in a warm room. This will allow the scrotal wall to relax and the testes to descend on their spermatic cords. Even with this preparation,

TABLE 12.4   Differential Diagnosis of Intrascrotal Masses

Diagnosis	Symptoms
Testis	Irregular consistency noted secondary usually to neoplasm or infectious disease
Epididymitis	Tenderness along posterolateral surface of testis with swelling and induration also in this area Urine often infected
Spermatocele	Cystic structure usually a few centimeters in size Most often can be transilluminated Located anywhere along course of epididymis but commonly near globus major
Hydrocele of cord	Cystic swelling in region of spermatic cord Can transilluminate
Spermatic cord lipoma	Soft mass in cord region that does not change with position or Valsalva's maneuver
Paratesticular neoplasm	Usually a firm mass in the area of spermatic cord May have history of recent swelling in cord area
Spermatic cord torsion	Sudden onset May have history of previous episodes Testis often "high riding" and in transverse line Urine uninfected Uncommon after puberty
Intrascrotal appendage torsion	If early in course, will have localized pain and swelling in region of appendages, usually near globus major In Caucasians may be able to see ischemic appendage through skin ("blue dot" sign)
Hernia	Swelling present above testes and epididymis Bowel sounds may be present in scrotum Spermatic cord cannot be well delineated
Varicocele	Dilatation of the pampiniform plexus exaggerated by Valsalva's maneuver Thrombosis may present as a painful, swollen mass in the area of the cord

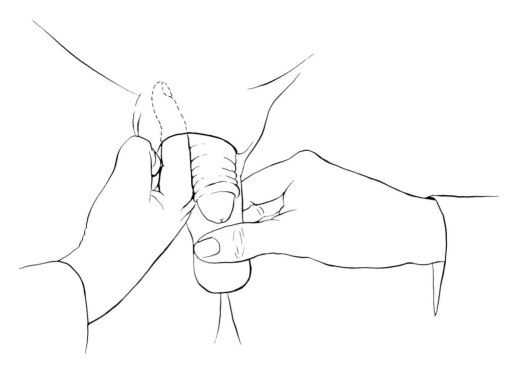

FIGURE 12.7   Deep palpation to check for inguinal hernia.

some obese men or men with small scrotums can be difficult to examine. A use-ful clinical maneuver to aid in testicular descent is to have the man stand close to a small lamp placed at scrotal height.

The spermatic cord on either side is grasped lightly between the thumb and first two fingers. A mental note is made of any disparity in cord size or consis-tency. Next the patient is instructed to inhale, hold his breath, and perform Valsalva's maneuver. Often, an "impulse" may be felt with the retrograde filling of blood down the gonadal vein. Sometimes, no impulse is felt but a thickening and increased consistency of the cord on the side of a varicocele may be appreci-ated. Examination of the scrotal contents is not complete without checking for inguinal hernias and inguinal adenopathy. The tip of the examiner's index finger is placed in the most dependent portion of the scrotum and the scrotum then inverted until the examining finger can palpate the external ring of the inguinal canal (Fig-ure 12.7). The patient is then asked to perform Valsalva's maneuver. Inguinal hernias may be felt as a bulge striking the tip of the finger. Palpation of the areas above and below the inguinal ligament is done to assess the presence, size, and consistency of any inguinal lymph nodes.

EXAMINATION OF THE PROSTATE

The normal prostate (Figure 12.6) is shaped like a chestnut and weighs approxi-mately 20 to 30 g. It is divided into several lobes, with the posterior lobe thought to be important in the development of prostatic neoplasm, and the periurethral glands, important in the development of benign prostatic hyperplasia. Prostatic

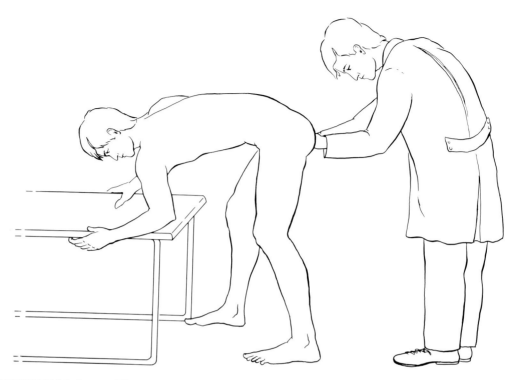

FIGURE 12.8   The rectal examination.

fluid contributes to seminal fluid content and is the largest source of zinc in the genitourinary system. Embryologically, the prostate is derived from endodermal buds in the urethra and it is an androgen–dependent organ.

The necessity of performing a gentle examination of this gland cannot be overemphasized. One of the major reasons that men refuse to go for a physical examination is because they fear the rectal and prostate exam. Hurt the patient once, and they will desist from any future examination, which would be a tragic loss to the early detection of cancer of the prostate and rectum.

Begin your examination with assuring words and place the patient at ease. It is important to describe in detail exactly what you are going to do. There are numerous positions in which the patient can be placed, either standing up, bent over a table, or with knees on top of a table with the right ear placed on the table and the arms crossed; for the elderly patient, lying on the side with the knees flexed toward the body is best (Figure 12.8). If possible, I prefer having the patient on the examining table with the right ear resting on a comfortable pillow and the buttocks in the air, because a full view of the rectal area can then be obtained.

The inspection is the initial part of the examination, with the gloved hand gently spreading the cheeks and making note of the presence of fissures, fistulas, hemorrhoids, lacerations, rashes, and the telltale signs of sexual contacts, such as condylomas. Some patients have a chronic rash from pruritis, which may occur on a psychoneurotic basis or be the result of parasitic infection or improper toilet habits.

With a gentle, well–lubricated finger of the nondominant hand, the tip of the finger is placed just at the anus. Do not insert the finger, but let it rest for a few

TABLE 12.5   Differential Diagnosis of Prostatic Nodules

Diagnosis	Symptoms
Neoplasm	Indistinct borders that blend into surrounding tissue
	If near lateral sulcus may involve pelvic side wall
	May have rapid onset of symptoms of urinary obstruction
Benign prostatic hyperplasia	Distinct border
	Resilient consistency
	May have history of slowly progressive urinary obstruction symptoms
Stone	Discrete raised lesion
	Pelvic radiograph may reveal prostatic calcifications
Granuloma	Often will have a history of prostatitis

seconds, and the anus will contract in anticipation. If the finger is kept neither moving forward or back, the sphincter will gradually relax, allowing further penetration by the examiner. By a series of slow movements, and a gentle voice of reassurance, detailing to the patient what you are doing, the finger is gradually inserted fully into the rectum. During advancement, an assessment of the sphincter and the presence of any anal masses is made. The prostate is next palpated, beginning at the apex in the midline and examining the median furrow. Next, each half of the prostate is examined from caudad to cephalad and from lateral sulcus to midline. Normal prostate consistency is soft and slightly resilient compared to the spongy. "boggy" feeling of an inflamed gland. The surface is smooth, with nodules (see Table 12.5). Some examiners have described the prostate as feeling like the contracted hand. Benign prostatic hyperplasia is approximated by opposing the thumb and little finger of the examiner's hand and feeling the thenar eminence. This feeling is firmer than normal prostate tissue, and often the prostate will have gently rounded lobes but with a smooth surface. Prostatic neoplasm has been likened to the feeling of the metacarpophalangeal joint of the thumb, again with thumb and little finger opposed. During this exam, one should also be sure to examine the pelvic side walls, coccyx, and the area of the seminal vesicles.

URINALYSIS

The urogenital examination should not be considered complete until a urine sample is taken. This is a simple, inexpensive office laboratory test that can give important information about a whole organ system.

Routine urinalysis utilizes a "clean catch midstream" sample of urine. In the circumcised male, no cleansing of the meatal area is needed. The patient begins voiding and, after approximately 1 ounce has been expelled, a sterile specimen container is introduced to collect several ounces of urine while the stream remains continuously flowing. In uncircumcised men, the foreskin must be fully retracted and kept this way until the specimen is obtained. In females, an antiseptic solution is used to clean the periurethral area, followed by rinsing of the solution with sterile water. A similar midstream method of collecting the urine sample is employed.

Twelve milliliters of urine are then placed into a sterile test tube and centrifuged for five minutes. While awaiting the centrifuged specimen, a dipstick analysis of the urine may be done testing simply for Ph, glucose, and protein or more extensively for blood, ketones, pyuria, and urobilinogen. The urine may also be examined grossly for color, turbidity, odor, and specific gravity. After five minutes, the centrifuged specimen is removed and the supernatant discarded except for a small amount of fluid over the sediment. The sediment is then resuspended in the fluid by hand agitation or by using a pipette. A drop of urine is then placed on a standard microscope slide and a coverslip placed. Examination of the urine is then performed looking for red and white blood cells, bacteria, casts, crystals, other infectious organisms, and debris. Culture of the urine may also be performed if infection is suspected.

More definitive localization of a urinary tract infection can be done using the three-glass urine test. Again, with a continuous stream of urine, the first half-ounce is collected into a container, a midstream portion is next collected in a second container, and the patient is told to continue voiding until one half ounce remains in the bladder. Prostate massage is then performed by gently stroking the prostate through the rectal wall. Prostatic massage should proceed on both sides of the median furrow using strokes in a cephalad-caudad direction and going from lateral to medial. On occasion a drop of prostatic fluid will be obtained from the meatus, and this should also be examined under the microscope. Following prostatic massage, the patient is instructed to empty the total content of his bladder into a third container. The three containers then represent respectively urethral, bladder and upper tracts, and prostatic origins, and appropriate culturing is performed. A similar test, using only two glasses, may be done in the female. Quantitative cultures of the different specimens will often help in localizing the site of urinary tract infection.

USEFUL TERMS

Anuria—Absence of urinary output.

Bacteriuria—The presence of bacteria in the urine. They may be present as contaminants or as true infection.

Dysuria—Painful urination; also used commonly to mean burning on urination. Usually seen in the presence of infection but may also be associated with obstruction, tumor, and inflammatory voiding; often synonymous with bedwetting but may be nocturnal or diurnal. Caused most often by neurologic problems or infection.

Frequency—An increase in the number of times per day a patient voids, the usual pattern being three to five hours between voids. May be due to infection, tumor, neurogenic causes, stones, inflammation, or obstructive uropathy.

Hematuria—Passage of blood in the urine either grossly or in microscopic form. Should be differentiated into initial stream hematuria, terminal stream hematuria, or total stream forms to aid in localization. Also should be separated into painless or painful hematuria. Multiple etiologies including neoplasm, infections, urolithiasis, trauma, and factitious. Must be differentiated from discoloration of the urine from other than blood cells, such as hemoglobinuria, myoglobinuria, certain foods or medications, porphyria.

Incontinence—Loss of urinary control, usually subdivided into four types:
  Stress—loss of urine with increased abdominal pressure, as in coughing or
      straining
  Overflow—loss of urine due to bladder overfilling, characterized by dribbling
      of urine when the intravesical pressure exceeds the intraurethral
      pressure
  Urge—loss of urine associated with a rapid and insistent sensation to void
  Total—continuous loss of urine, usually seen in injury to the urinary sphincter
      or congenital abnormalities

Nocturia—Voiding at night; seen often with obstructive uropathy, neurogenic
  bladder problems, inflammation, congestive heart failure.

Oliguria—Decreased amount of urinary output, especially in regard to fluid
  intake.

Pneumaturia—Etiologies include fistula, infection with gas-forming organisms,
  trauma, or recent urologic instrumentation.

Pollakiuria—Frequent small urinations, a prominent symptom of lower tract
  infection or inflammation.

Polyuria—Frequent voiding of large amounts of urine. May be seen in renal
  disease, diabetes mellitus, diabetes insipidus, or excessive fluid intake.

Pyuria—The presence of white blood cells in the urine, usually seen with infection or inflammation.

Ureteral colic—Sharp or dull pain that comes in waves from several seconds to
  minutes in duration. It may migrate from the flank down to the inguinal
  area and finally into the scrotal and penile area in men or the labia majora
  in women.

Urgency—An insistent sensation of needing to void, usually associated with
  infection or inflammation but also seen in neurogenic problems and tumors.

REFERENCES

1. Smith DR: *General Urology,* ed 9. Los Altos, CA, Lange Medical Publications,
    1978.

2. Felman YM, Nikitas JA: *Condylomata acuminata. NY State J Med*
    1979;79:1747.

3. Harrison JH, Gittes RF, Perlmutter AD, et al (eds): *Campbell's Urology,*
    ed 4. Philadelphia, WB Saunders, 1978.

4. U.S. Department of Health, Education and Welfare: *Syphilis. A Synopsis.*
    Washington, DC, US Government Printing Office, 1968.

5. Zimmerman LM, Anson BJ: *Anatomy and Surgery of Hernia,* ed 2. Baltimore,
    Williams & Wilkins, 1967.

13
The Dermatologic Examination

Ethan D. Nydorf, M.D.

INTRODUCTION

The examination of the skin is a fascinating part of physical diagnosis. The finger-prints of systemic disease can sometimes be revealed by a careful appreciation of the skin lesion. It is imperative that the examiner learn to describe the lesions thoroughly, as so elegantly outlined in this section. A good description is essential in arriving at a diagnosis. This is a thorough chapter on dermatology that is useful not only for the novice but for the person who wants to specialize in this discipline.

STRUCTURE AND FUNCTION OF THE SKIN

In order to examine the skin in an intelligent manner the function and structure of the skin must be understood. The skin serves protective and homeostatic func-tions. The skin prevents invasion of the body by pyogenic microorganisms and toxic chemicals. Its elasticity and durability allow motion without injury. The skin is relatively water impermeable and thus prevents dehydration.

The nervous structures in the skin allow the body to maintain awareness of touch, pain, temperature, and pressure. The pigment system of the skin prevents damage by ultraviolet light. The skin plays an immunologic role. Foreign antigens may incite an inflammatory response in the skin, making their presence known to the organism. Through sweating and vasodilation the skin serves as a temperature-regulating organ.

Epidermis

The three layers of the skin are the epidermis, dermis, and subcutaneous tissue (Figure 13.1). The epidermis is a thin layer of stratified squamous epithelium con-sisting of an outer dead cell layer, the stratum corneum, and an inner living cell layer. The living cell layer, called the **stratum malpighii,** consists of three zones. The zone closest to the dermis is the **basal cell layer.** The basal cells are young

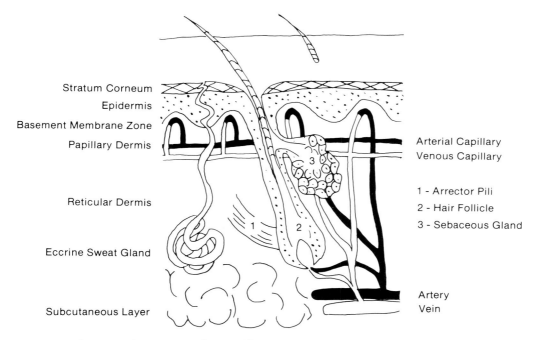

Stratum Corneum
Epidermis
Basement Membrane Zone
Papillary Dermis

Reticular Dermis

Eccrine Sweat Gland

Subcutaneous Layer

Arterial Capillary
Venous Capillary

1 - Arrector Pili
2 - Hair Follicle
3 - Sebaceous Gland

Artery
Vein

FIGURE 13.1   **Structure of the skin.**

keratinocytes that produce a structural protein called keratin. These cells divide every 19 days to produce two daughter cells, one of which migrates to the surface.

The next cell layer up is called the **squamous cell layer.** This is a 5- to 10-cell thick zone in which the cells are flattened. The uppermost level of the stratum malpighii is the **granular cell layer.** It is here that keratohyaline granules reach full development. These granules serve both to cement fibrils together and to form the inner lining of the dead stratum corneum cells. The dissolution of the nucleus and other cell organelles occurs in the granular cell layer.

The **stratum corneum,** or dead cell layer, represents the final differentiation product of the epidermis. These cells consist of keratin fibrils cemented together by an interfibrillary matrix and are enclosed by a marginal band and a cell membrane. The stratum corneum is thickest on the palms and soles. It is in these regions that a clear zone may be found under the stratum corneum. This clear zone, or **stratum lucidum,** contains phospholipids that prevent water evaporation from below.

The epidermis continually regenerates itself. Four to 6 weeks are required for a cell to move from the basal cell layer to the surface of the granular cell layer. It takes an additional 4 to 5 weeks for a cell to move through the stratum corneum.

Cells present in the epidermis, aside from keratinocytes, include melanocytes, Merkel cells, and Langerhans' cells. Melanocytes, located in the basal cell layer, produce pigment granules called melanin. Keratinocytes then take up the melanin. Merkel cells are sensory cells whose function is not entirely clear. Langerhans' cells serve to process foreign antigens and present them to lymphocytes. They are related to the monocyte-macrophage-histiocyte series.

Subepidermal Basement Membrane Zone

A subepidermal basement membrane zone serves to attach the epidermis to the underlying dermis. It is the site of pathologic alteration in several of the blistering disorders, such as bullous pemphigoid.

Dermis

The dermis provides the skin with structural support. The dermis is sparsely populated with cells, such as fibroblasts and mast cells. Fibroblasts produce the connective tissue of the dermis. Connective tissue consists of collagen, elastic fibers, and a mucopolysaccharide-rich ground substance. Collagen, the predominant fiber of the dermis, forms a finely woven meshwork in the upper or papillary dermis. In the deeper or reticular dermis, collagen fibers unite into thick bundles. Collagen resists breakage under mechanical stress. The fine elastic fibers give elasticity to the skin and thus allow it to return to its original position once stretched. Wrinkles occur in aged skin in which the elastic fibers degenerate.

Also present in the dermis are nerves, nerve end organs, blood vessels, lymphatics, and muscle. The skin is supplied with sensory nerves as well as autonomic nerves. The autonomic nerves, derived from the sympathetic nervous system, supply the blood vessels, the hair follicle muscles (arrector pili), and the eccrine and apocrine sweat glands. Specialized nerve receptors include the mucocutaneous end organ found in the papillary dermis of the mouth and genitalia. Meissner corpuscles, found in the dermal papillae of the palms and soles, mediate the sense of touch. Vater-Pacini corpuscles are large nerve end organs located in the subcutis that mediate the sense of pressure. The cutaneous blood vessels form a subcutaneous plexus of small arteries and veins. These vessels connect with a subpapillary plexus of arterioles and venules.

Subcutaneous Tissue

The fat layer, or subcutaneous tissue, serves to insulate the interior of the body from ambient temperature changes and mechanical shock. The fat also represents a stored form of energy. The subcutaneous layer is thinnest in the eyelids, penis, scrotum, nipple, areola, and area over the tibia.

Appendages

Hair, nails, sweat glands, and sebaceous glands are the appendages of the epidermis.

Hair

Hair, like the stratum corneum, is composed of keratinized epidermal cells. Hair is produced by hair follicles, which represent cylindrical ingrowths of epithelium. Hair follicles may be classified as vellus, terminal, and sebaceous. The **vellus follicles** are small and produce fine short hairs. **Terminal follicles** produce longer and thicker hairs, such as those found on the scalp, eyebrows, eyelashes, and axillary and pubic areas. **Sebaceous follicles,** present on the face and back, produce vellus hairs but have large sebaceous glands. It is in these hair follicles that acne occurs. Hairs are not present on the glabrous skin—the palms and soles.

Hair follicles cycle through a growing (anagen) stage to a regressing (catagen) phase and, finally, to a resting (telogen) stage. The length of time a follicle remains in a particular phase of its cycle depends on body location. For example, scalp hair spends most of its time in anagen, whereas eyelash hair divides its time equally between anagen and telogen.

Androgenic hormones affect hair growth differently in different locations. Thus, testosterone causes a reduction in hair growth rate on the scalp but increases hair growth rate in the beard area. The normal growth rate for scalp hair is 0.4 to 0.5 mm per day. About 100 of the 100,000 or so scalp hairs are shed daily.

Nails

The nail plate is composed of keratinized cells. These cells are produced by the nail matrix, which is located proximal to the proximal nail fold. The nail bed and proximal nail fold do not contribute to the nail plate.

Fingernails grow at about 0.1 mm per day and toenails grow at a rate of about 0.05 mm per day. Nail growth may be adversely affected by systemic disease and vascular insufficiency. Skin diseases that affect the epidermis can cause nail pathology as well. Thus, psoriasis, atopic dermatitis, and lichen planus can cause nail plate dystrophy.

Glands

The sebaceous (oil) glands and the apocrine and eccrine sweat glands originate from the epidermis. **Sebaceous glands** empty into hair follicles. They are most highly developed on the face, scalp, upper chest, and back. Rarely, they may empty directly to the surface of the oral mucosa or prepuce. Sebaceous glands are holocrine. This means that the cells themselves degenerate to form the secretion product, sebum. Sebum represents a mixture of lipids, epithelial cell remnants, and bacteria. Its production is androgen hormone dependent. Generally, patients with more severe acne have higher rates of sebum production.

Eccrine sweat glands are located throughout the body surface. They are found in greatest density on the palms, soles, and axillae. They are merocrine glands, meaning that their secretory cells simply excrete. Eccrine glands are made up of a dermal secretory portion, an intradermal duct, and a coiled intraepidermal duct. The temperature control center in the hypothalamus stimulates eccrine sweating. A dilute sodium chloride solution is produced that, on evaporating from the skin surface, results in cooling. Thus, the eccrine glands play a major role in the body's ability to regulate its temperature. Stress causes eccrine sweating from the forehead, axillae, palms, and soles. Abnormal sweating from these areas is called hyperhidrosis.

Apocrine sweat glands are located in the axillae, areolae, and periumbilical, perianal, and genital regions. These glands produce a secretion that, when acted upon by bacteria, becomes odoriferous.

APPROACH TO THE PATIENT WITH SKIN DISEASE

The diagnosis of skin disease requires four steps. The history includes the chief complaint, history of present illness, past medical history, review of systems, family history, social history, and list of medications and allergies. The second step consists of a careful examination of the skin, hair, nails, and mucous membranes. It is this step that will be discussed in depth in this chapter. Confirmatory laboratory tests are then carried out. Finally, a differential diagnosis and then a diagnosis is made.

History

The **chief complaint** in dermatology enables the examiner to focus his or her attention to a specific area of the body. One obtains the history of present illness through discussion of events surrounding the onset of the skin lesion and its evolution. For example, one may inquire when and under what circumstances the lesion

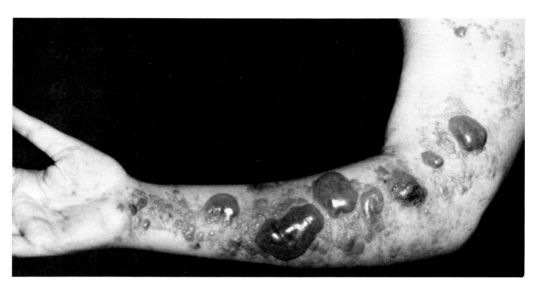

FIGURE 13.2   Herpes zoster with bullae.

developed, how long it had been present, and whether improvement or exacerbation had been noted.

Symptoms are then elicited. For example, itching may indicate local inflammation of the skin or underlying systemic illness. Skin diseases associated with itching include atopic dermatitis, contact dermatitis, seborrheic dermatitis, psoriasis, lichen planus, urticaria, xerotic eczema, dermatitis herpetiformis, drug eruptions, exfoliative dermatitis, insect bites, and scabies. Systemic diseases associated with pruritis include drug reactions, hepatobiliary dysfunction, thyroid disease, renal disease, polycythemia vera, carcinoma, and lymphoma.

Certain skin lesions may elicit pain or tenderness. Acute infections of the skin, such as cellulitis, are tender. Certain uncommon skin tumors produce pain spontaneously. Examples include glomus tumor, traumatic neuroma, angiolipoma, eccrine spiradenoma, and leiomyoma.

Finally, one must determine how the skin lesion was treated. The medication used may exacerbate the skin condition or produce a secondary reaction. For example, certain antifungal creams contain the potent sensitizer, ethylenediamine. Application of such a cream can result in an allergic contact dermatitis, which, to the patient, may dwarf the primary pathology in importance.

The **past medical history** should reveal the significant medical illnesses of the patient. For example, discovering that a patient has diabetes mellitus would aid in the diagnosis of a lesion of necrobiosis lipoidica diabeticorum.

A relevant and directed **review of systems** may be crucial in establishing a diagnosis. For example, in a patient presenting with grouped vesicles on an erythematous base in a unilateral distribution, the occurrence of preceding dermatomal pain may allow one to favor the diagnosis of herpes zoster over herpes simplex Figure 13.2).

A **family history** may aid in diagnosing hereditary conditions such as neurofibromatosis. Here about half of the patients have a positive family history for a symptom or sign of neurofibromatosis, such as café-au-lait spots, axillary freckling, acoustic neuromas, or neurofibromas (Figure 13.3).

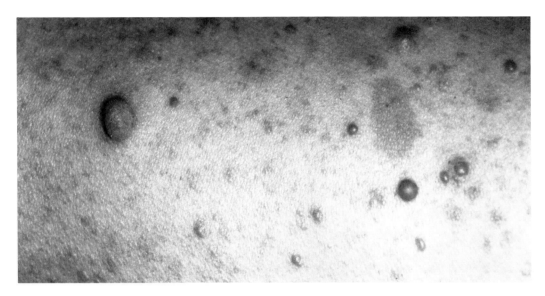

FIGURE 13.3   **Neurofibromatosis with café–au–lait spots and neurofibromas.**

The **social history** will reveal the subject's habits concerning tobacco and alcohol use, hobbies, and occupation. The latter becomes critical when the examiner must investigate the cause of an allergic contact dermatitis. In a patient with cutaneous signs of liver disease, such as spider angiomata, a history of alcohol intake could be important.

A **list of medications** taken and a **history of allergies** to drugs or other physical agents may be helpful. For example, a positive history of thiazide diuretic use combined with an intolerance to sunlight would be consistent with thiazide–induced photosensitivity.

Equipment and Laboratory Devices

Thorough examination of the skin necessitates adequate room lighting. A penlight will help to illuminate the scalp, mouth, and other areas not well visualized with room light alone. The Wood's lamp emits long-wave ultraviolet (black) light. It accentuates pigmentary changes and is useful in the diagnosis of vitiligo, freckling, and other diseases characterized by an increase or decrease in pigmentation. In addition, the Wood's lamp is useful in diagnosing certain skin infections. Black light turns skin a coral red color when superficially infected by corynebacterium in a condition of the groin and toewebs called erythrasma. Tinea capitis, or superficial fungal infection of the scalp, can, in some cases, turn the hair blue-green when illuminated by the Wood's lamp.

A tongue depressor will help in the inspection of the oral mucous membranes and tongue. A hand lens may be of use in detecting subtle surface characteristics of a lesion. A piece of clear plastic can be utilized to apply pressure to appropriate erythematous (red) lesions in an attempt to blanch them. This procedure is called diascopy and will be discussed later.

Certain laboratory equipment should be readily accessible. For example, a microscope is required in order to read a potassium hydroxide preparation, Gram's stain, Wright's stain, Tzanck preparation, scraping for scabies, and other insect

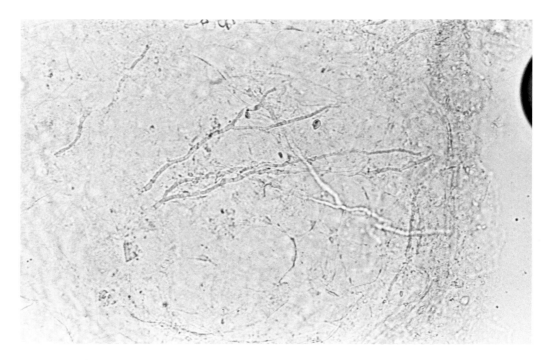

FIGURE 13.4   Branching hyphae from potassium hydroxide preparation.

specimens. The potassium hydroxide test involves lightly scraping the lesion suspected to contain a superficial fungus with a scalpel blade. The scale is collected
onto a glass slide and covered with a coverslip. A few drops of 10% potassium
hydroxide are applied to the edge of the coverslip, allowing the solution to coalesce
underneath the coverslip by means of capillary action. The slide is gently heated
with an alcohol lamp and is then examined at low power for hyphae (Figure 13.4).
The potassium hydroxide preparation enables one to diagnose superficial fungal
infections, tinea versicolor, and candidiasis of the skin while the patient waits.

Gram's stain serves to delineate superficial bacterial infections of the skin,
such as folliculitis. A pustule is opened using a number 11 blade and pus is smeared
on a microscope slide and stained. Wright's stain is useful for examining inflammatory and epidermal cells. In the common skin condition of the neonate, erythema
toxicum neonatorum, pustules loaded with eosinophils but without bacteria occur.
Simply scraping a representative pustule and staining its contents with Wright's
stain helps clinch the diagnosis.

When herpes simplex, varicella, or herpes zoster is suspected, a Tzanck smear
should be performed. Here, the roof of a vesicle is removed with a scalpel blade.
The base of the vesicle is lightly scraped and the scrapings are applied to a slide.
The slide is then stained with the Wright's stain and examined for multinucleated
giant cells.

A special darkfield microscope is required in order to visualize the living
spirochetes found in the exudate from a syphilitic chancre.

Culture media for certain viruses (herpes simplex and varicella-zoster), bacteria, and fungi should be available.

A skin biopsy may be required. The punch biopsy technique involves making
a circular cut in the skin using a 2- to 6-mm punch. The skin sample is removed

with forceps and the defect is either closed with sutures or packed with sterile material. Before packing, bleeding can be halted with Monsel's solution (iron subsulfate) or 20% aluminum chloride solution. Biopsies may be placed in a formalin fixative for routine hematoxylin and eosin staining or in specialized media for direct immunofluorescence or electron microscopy.

Patch test equipment should be available in order to elucidate the cause of a contact dermatitis. Suspect chemicals, diluted to safe concentrations, are placed onto absorbent pads and are applied to the skin for 48 hours. The production of vesicles under the applied patch represents a positive reaction.

Finally, blood testing may be required. Blood for VDRL, antinuclear antibody, and indirect immunofluorescence testing may be drawn to rule out syphilis, lupus erythematosus, and pemphigus, respectively.

EXAMINATION OF THE SKIN

One examines the skin in a logical sequence of eight steps. First, the type of primary lesion must be established. Second, the secondary changes are observed. Third, the layer of skin in which the pathology lies should be identified. Fourth, the texture of the lesion is noted. Fifth, its color must be determined. Sixth, the shape of the abnormality is seen. Seventh, its pattern is important. Eighth, the distribution about the body of the lesion helps in forming a diagnosis.

Types of Primary Lesions

The primary lesions of dermatology include the macule, patch, papule, plaque, nodule, tumor, vesicle, bulla, pustule, cyst, wheal, comedo, burrow, telangiectasis, petechia, purpura, and ecchymosis.

A **macule** is a flat area of skin with little or no surface change. It may vary from normal skin simply by a change in color. Examples include a hyperpigmented café-au-lait spot found in a patient with neurofibromatosis (Figure 13.3) or a hypopigmented "ash-leaf" spot seen in tuberous sclerosis.

A **patch** is a large macule. A large, flat capillary hemangioma (port-wine stain) represents such a patch. Another example is an area of vitiligo (Figure 13.5).

A **papule** is an elevated, palpable, solid lesion measuring less than 1 cm in diameter. A dermal nevocellular nevus (mole) is a papule.

A **plaque** is a plateau-shaped lesion that is raised or depressed with reference to the skin surface and is larger than 1 cm. An example is a plaque of psoriasis (Figure 13.6).

Nodules represent deeper lesions measuring less than 2 cm in diameter (Figure 13.7). They involve the reticular dermis or subcutaneous tissue. The border of a nodule is less well defined compared to that of a papule because of its depth. Erythema nodosum is an inflammatory nodule in the subcutaneous layer.

A **tumor** is a large lesion with a diameter greater than 2 cm. An example of such a lesion is a lipoma, which represents a benign proliferation of fatty tissue (Figure 13.8).

Vesicles are intraepidermal collections of fluid, measuring less than 0.5 mm in diameter. They appear like small bubbles in the skin. Vesicles occur in acute dermatitides, such as contact dermatitis.

Bullae are fluid-filled outpouches of the skin that measure more than 0.5 mm in diameter (Figure 13.2). The disease bullous pemphigoid results in bullae.

Pustules represent sterile or infected collections of pus. Folliculitis consists of multiple pustules about the openings of hair follicles.

A **cyst** is a compressible sac filled with material derived from the cells lining its cavity. For example, an epidermal inclusion cyst is filled with keratin. This cyst is commonly, although not accurately, known as a sebaceous cyst (Figure 13.9).

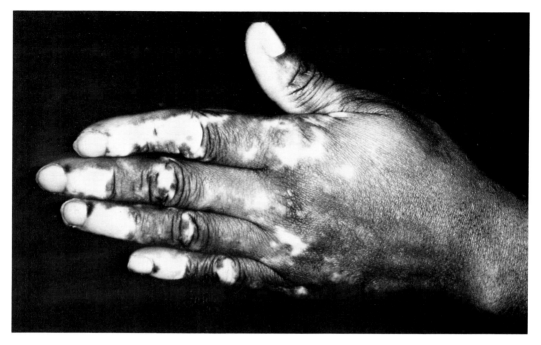

FIGURE 13.5   Vitiligo.

FIGURE 13.6   Plaque of psoriasis.

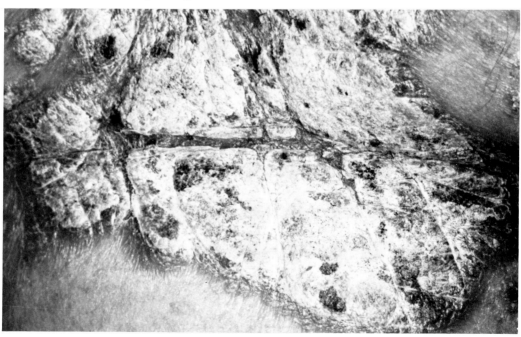

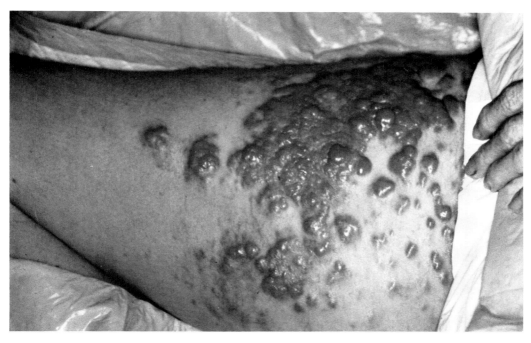

FIGURE 13.7   Metastatic nodules from ovarian carcinoma.

FIGURE 13.8   Lipoma.

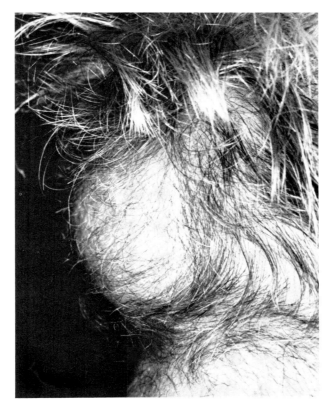

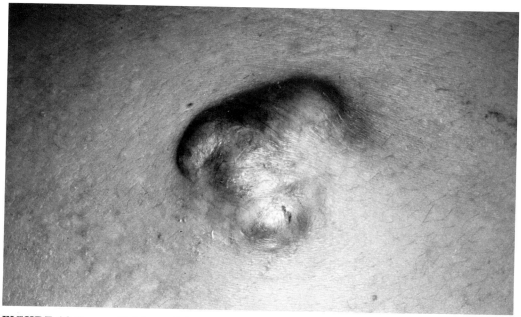

FIGURE 13.9   Epidermal inclusion cyst.

Wheals (hives) represent acute localized edema of the dermis due to a leakage of fluid from blood vessels in the skin (Figure 13.10).

The **comedo** is the primary lesion of acne vulgaris. Open comedones (blackheads) are dilated hair follicle orifices that often contain keratin and sebum. Closed comedones have more clinical significance in that they can develop into the inflammatory papules and pustules of acne. They also are formed from hair follicles expanded by keratinocyte and sebaceous gland debris, but have microscopically small pores.

Burrows represent tunnels in the skin created by parasites, such as the scabies mite or the larvae of roundworms.

Vascular lesions may present as **telangiectases,** which are widened superficial blood vessels, petechiae, purpura, or ecchymoses. **Petechiae** are pinpoint brown or red dots in the skin that do not blanch. Similarly, **purpura** are larger reddish spots that indicate that blood has leaked out of vessels and into the dermis. **Ecchymoses** are large bruised areas of skin in which bleeding has taken place.

Types of Secondary Lesions

Secondary lesions derive from primary lesions that have been altered either as a natural progression of the disease process or as a result of manipulation by the patient.

Once a vesicle, bulla, or pustule breaks, the serous exudate or pus dries to form a **crust.** When a crust is recognized, one must attempt to work backward to determine the nature of the primary lesion. Impetigo, caused by a staphylococcal infection of the skin, produces a vesicle in the epidermis. When the vesicle breaks, serum is released. On drying, the serum forms a honey-colored crust. Virally-induced vesicles can also crust. Examples include varicella (chicken pox), herpes zoster, and herpes simplex.

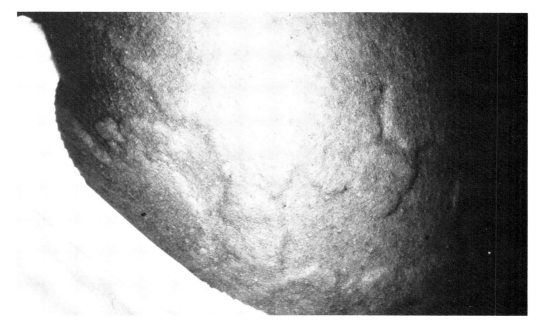

FIGURE 13.10   Urticaria.

Vesicular and other skin eruptions can become **impetiginized.** This refers to the secondary colonization of the skin with large numbers of bacteria, often *Staphylococcus aureus.* Itching dermatoses, such as atopic dermatitis, commonly become secondarily infected.

Erosions

Erosions occur when the epidermis is lost. Blistering diseases are associated with erosions. For example, in a lesion of bullous pemphigoid, the blister roof may be shed. The patient is then left with a circular erosion. In aphthous stomatitis (canker sores), intense localized inflammation results in focal loss of the mucosal surface of the mouth or lips. A small circular erosion results that appears as a white spot surrounded by an inflammatory red halo.

Naturally occurring linear erosions are called **fissures.** Hyperkeratotic (scaly) and xerotic (dry) skin is brittle and is susceptible to fracture (Figure 13.11). Cracks may be found on the hyperkeratotic palms and soles of patients with psoriasis or irritant dermatitis. In a condition called eczema cracquelé, xerotic skin of the shins becomes fissured.

Erosions caused by scratching are called **excoriations.** Certain pruritic diseases are associated with excoriation. Examples include insect bites, scabies, atopic dermatitis, and dermatitis herpetiformis.

Ulcers

Ulcers represent loss of the epidermis and part of the dermis. Ulcers heal with scarring. Natural disease processes associated with ulceration include pyoderma gangrenosum, certain tumors, stasis dermatitis, and vascular insufficiency.

Pyoderma gangrenosum (Figure 13.12) is a disease in which a small pustule rapidly ulcerates, leaving a dusky grayish-blue overhanging border and a moist base.

312

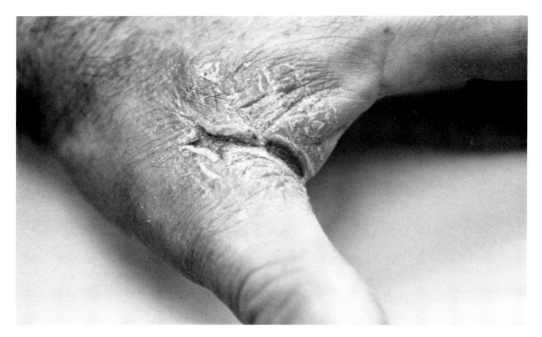

FIGURE 13.11   Fissure in patient with irritant hand dermatitis.

FIGURE 13.12   Pyoderma gangrenosum.

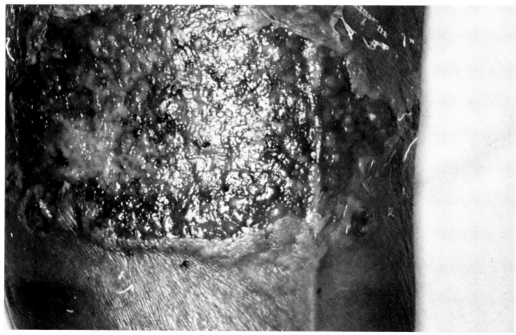

Most commonly, the lower extremities are involved. One often finds an associated systemic disease, such as ulcerative colitis. The lesions resolve spontaneously, with systemic corticosteroids, or after therapy of the underlying condition.

Skin tumors that ulcerate include basal cell carcinoma, squamous cell carcinoma, and lymphoma. Basal cell carcinoma, the most common skin malignancy, may present as a raised lesion of the face or scalp with a central, nonhealing ulcer (rodent ulcer). The borders are elevated and shiny and have telangiectases coursing along their surface. Basal cell carcinomas rarely metastasize but may expand locally, burrowing along tissue planes and through muscle into bone. Squamous cell carcinoma presents as an erythematous (red), crusted or scaly, ulcerated plaque on sun-exposed areas. The patient may note that the ulcer does not heal. Squamous cell carcinomas of the skin may eventually metastasize. Cutaneous T-cell lymphomas, such as mycosis fungoides, also ulcerate.

Stasis dermatitis of the lower legs tends to occur in the elderly or in patients with recurrent pedal edema due to venous disease. Normally, blood flows from the superficial veins of the legs through perforating veins with one-way valves to the deep venous system and then back to the heart. If the one-way valves are damaged, blood can back up in the superficial system, resulting in blood leakage and dermatitis. If tissue oxygenation is poor, chronic ulcers can develop after minor trauma.

Arterial insufficiency may also result in leg ulcers. Patients with sickle cell anemia can develop leg ulcers due to sickling of blood in arterioles.

Diabetics may present with ulcers on the soles or toes due to loss of sensory nervous function in the foot. This type of ulcer is called a neuropathic ulcer. Patients with lepromatous leprosy and neurosyphilis can also present with neuropathic ulcers.

Self-induced ulcers are called **factitial lesions.** They often take linear or geometrical shapes, depending upon the method of skin injury.

Scars

Scars form after injury to the dermis. Scars normally occur after surgical incision of the skin as part of the wound healing process. Diseases that scar are characterized by significant dermal inflammation and injury. Examples include lupus erythematosus and pyoderma gangrenosum. Scars may present as firm white lesions or as depressed areas of the skin.

Hypertrophic scars are tender, red scars, which often improve symptomatically with time. **Keloids** represent scars that outgrow the margins of the initial skin injury (Figure 13.13). Keloids are permanent.

Location of the Lesion within the Skin

In order to diagnose a skin disorder, one must answer the question: Which layer(s) of the skin is(are) involved?

Epidermal Disease

The epidermis is made up of the dead stratum corneum and the living stratum malpighii. **Scaling** (hyperkeratosis) represents excess stratum corneum. Hyperkeratosis can be seen in disorders of the epidermis, such as ichthyosis, or in diseases involving both the epidermis and dermis, such as psoriasis (Figures 13.6 and 13.28).

Many processes affect mainly the epidermis. Epidermal disease includes a variety of dermatitides, pigmentary alterations, tumors, and infections.

Dermatitis is defined as inflammation of the epidermis. Inflammatory cells leave blood vessels in the upper dermis and invade the epidermis. Fluid accompanies the migrating cells and, in many instances, forms vesicles. Included under the

314

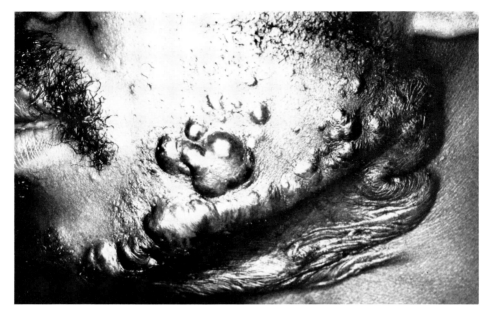

FIGURE 13.13   Keloid.

FIGURE 13.14   Lichenification.

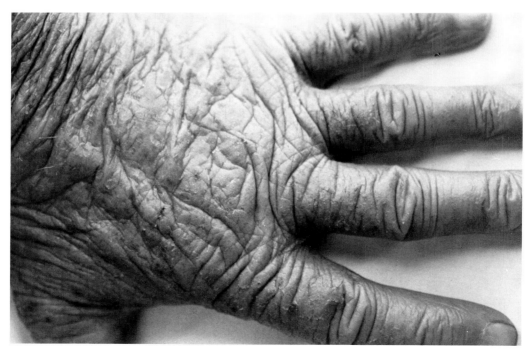

category of dermatitis are contact dermatitis, atopic dermatitis, nummular dermatitis, dyshidrotic dermatitis, stasis dermatitis, and lichen simplex chronicus.

Dermatitis can be acute, such as with contact dermatitis to rhus (poison ivy).
Here vesicles and bullae are seen. Subacute dermatitis presents as red scaling or
weeping areas. In nummular dermatitis, the subacute dermatitic plaques are well
defined and form coinlike shapes.

Atopic dermatitis may present in a subacute or chronic fashion. Erythematous,
weeping areas with poorly demarcated margins may be found. Scaling, fissures,
and lichenification indicate a long-standing process. Lichenification represents the
increased skin markings found in chronically rubbed skin (Figure 13.14).

Dyshidrotic dermatitis is a recurrent vesicular eruption of the palms and soles
of unknown etiology. Lichen simplex chronicus presents as an ill-defined, chronic
dermatitic plaque. It is caused by repeatedly scratching the skin.

Epidermal tumors are well-circumscribed, superficial lesions. Three examples
are benign seborrheic keratosis, benign actinic keratosis, and the premalignant
lesion of Bowen's disease.

Seborrheic keratoses are common hyperpigmented tumors of the epidermis
found predominantly on the face and trunk. Their surfaces are rough as a result
of increased folding of the epidermis. The lesions appear to be stuck onto the skin
and are often accidently peeled off by the patient (Figure 13.15).

Actinic keratoses are small, red, scaling spots that occur on the sun-exposed
areas of the face, ears, and hands of older people. An abnormality in cell proliferation presumably has been induced by ultraviolet light. A small number of actinic
keratoses can become invasive and evolve into squamous cell carcinomas.

Bowen's disease presents as a well-demarcated erythematous plaque with an
eroded and often moist surface. The lesion is caused by full-thickness disorganization of the epidermis. It is a precursor for squamous cell carcinoma. Bowen's
disease of the penis is called erythroplasia of Queyrat. Ingestion of inorganic ar-
senic can lead to Bowen's disease after a several-year latent period.

A common **viral infection** of the epidermis is a wart. Warts are discrete lesions
with hyperkeratotic papillated surfaces (Figure 13.16). The wart virus (human
papilloma virus) causes elongation of the dermal papillae and their capillaries along

FIGURE 13.15   Seborrheic keratosis.

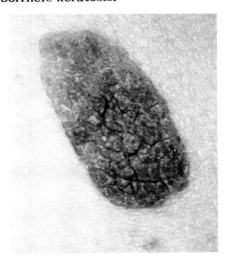

316

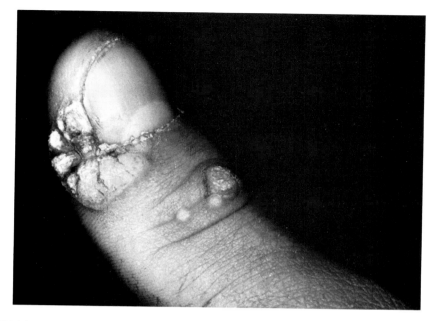

FIGURE 13.16   Verruca vulgaris (common wart).

FIGURE 13.17   Condylomata acuminata.

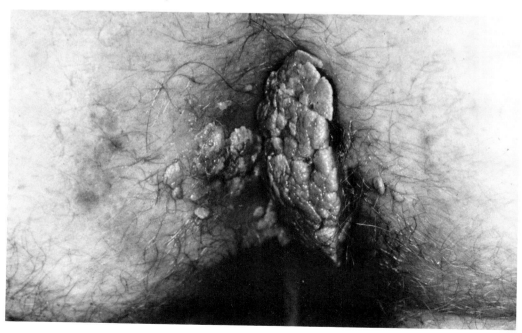

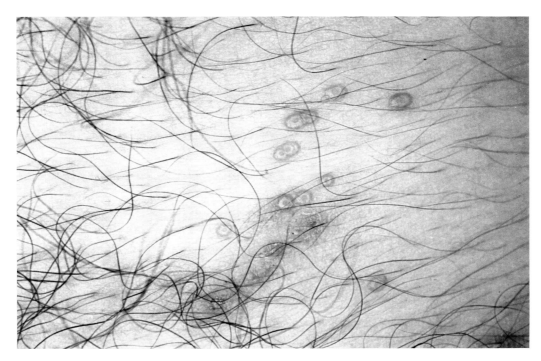

FIGURE 13.18   Molluscum contagiosum.

with proliferation of the epidermis. When a wart is shaved multiple small bleeding points are noted. These bleeding spots represent enlarged capillaries that have been cut. Warts occurring in the anogenital region are called condylomata acuminata (Figure 13.17).

Molluscum contagiosum also represents a viral infection of the epidermis. Here, multiple umbilicated papules are found (Figure 13.18). Herpes simplex and herpes zoster primarily involve the epidermis as well.

Bacterial infections limited to the epidermis include impetigo and erythrasma. Superficial fungal infections of the skin include diseases caused by dermatophytes, *Candida,* and pityrosporum ovale. Dermatophytes cause tinea capitis (scalp and hair), manuum (hand), cruris (groin), pedis (foot), and corporis (body). *Candida* contributes to infections of the mouth (thrush), groin (diaper dermatitis), and body folds (intertrigo). Tinea versicolor, caused by pityrosporum ovale, causes hypo- or hyperpigmented macules with fine scale on the trunk and shoulders.

The scabies mite creates short linear **burrows** in the epidermis (Figure 13.19). The mite may appear as a small black dot at the distal end of a burrow.

Diseases of the Dermal–Epidermal Junction
Many bullous conditions are caused by disruption of the dermal–epidermal junction. **Bullous pemphigoid** consists of multiple tense bullae on erythematous or urticarial bases, often in intertriginous areas. The disease is more common in the elderly. The primary pathology lies within the basement membrane zone in an area just beneath the basal cell layer of the epidermis. Here autoantibodies attack a normal attachment antigen, the bullous pemphigoid antigen. Inflammation and blistering results.

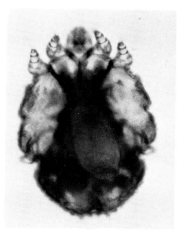

FIGURE 13.19   Scabies mite.

Pemphigus, on the other hand, occurs in a slightly younger age group. It is characterized by more flaccid bullae occurring on noninflamed skin. Blisters are commonly found in the mouth. Pemphigus is potentially a more serious illness as compared to bullous pemphigoid and must be treated promptly. Autoantibodies destroy the attachment of keratinocytes to one another in the lower portion of the epidermis.

Dermatitis herpetiformis is characterized by multiple grouped vesicles occurring symmetrically on the dorsal surfaces of the scalp, neck, buttocks, and extremities. The eruption is intensely pruritic and is often accompanied by excoriations.

Toxic epidermal necrolysis represents a severe disruption of lower epidermal cells often caused by an inflammatory reaction to a drug. The epidermis is shed in sheets, leaving large denuded areas that are prone to secondary infection by bacteria. Fluid loss from the dermis can become significant. In contrast, **staphylococcal scalded skin syndrome** is caused by an exotoxin excreted by the bacterial organism. The exotoxin creates a split higher in the epidermis. Although sheets of skin peel off the body, healing occurs within ten to 14 days. This disease, which tends to affect young children, has a much more favorable prognosis compared to toxic epidermal necrolysis.

Dermal Disease

Dermal lesions are often firm and discrete. Disorders primarily located in the dermis include erythemas, vascular lesions, granulomas, tumors, infections, and inflammatory and infiltrative conditions. Scars and ulcers also involve the dermis.

Erythemas are characterized by red lesions in which blood is confined to dilated blood vessels in the dermis. Blanching is noted when pressure is applied to the skin (diascopy). The most common type of erythema is urticaria (Figure 13.10). Wheals may be caused by an allergic reaction to drugs, foods, radiocontrast media, or undefined antigens. In the classic immunoglobulin E (IgE)-mediated type of urticaria, antigen links together IgE molecules on the surface of a mast cell to cause histamine release. Histamine and other mast cell mediators increase the water permeability of blood vessels. Fluid then leaks from the vessels into the dermis, causing transient elevation of the skin. Some antigens can stimulate mast cell release of histamine directly without IgE.

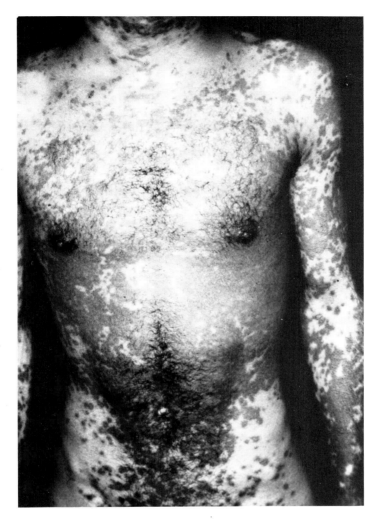

FIGURE 13.20   **Generalized drug eruption.**

Dermographism (skin writing) occurs in about 5% of the population. In this case, fluid leaks out of vessels after the skin is stroked with a blunt object.

Other erythemas include the common "maculopapular" drug reactions and viral exanthems (Figure 13.20).   Less common erythemas include erythema marginatum, a sign of acute rheumatic fever, and erythema chronicum migrans, an indication of Lyme disease. Erythema marginatum represents an evanescent, faint, rapidly migrating red lesion of the trunk. Erythema chronicum migrans starts as a small circular, raised area that spreads in a centrifugal fashion to form a ring. The lesion and its associated arthritic disorder is caused by a spirochete inoculated into the skin by a tick.

Erythema annulare centrifugum is a more slowly expanding, ringlike lesion with a peculiar central scale (Figure 13.21). This condition may occur in response to an underlying process, such as a fungal infection or tumor.

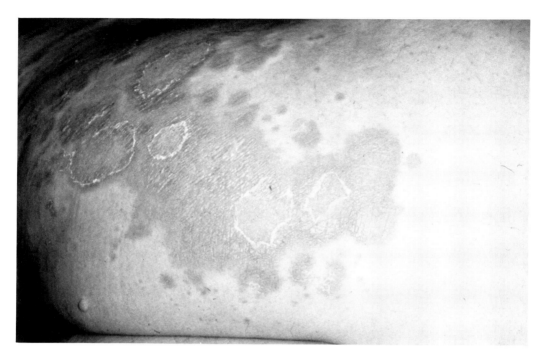

FIGURE 13.21   Erythema annulare centrifugum.

Vascular lesions appear red, purple, or brown. A telangiectasis is a dilated superficial blood vessel. Rectangular-shaped (mat) telangiectases can be found on the tongue, lips, fingers, and face in patients with scleroderma. Telangiectases in the cuticles of the proximal nail fold are seen in lupus erythematosus, dermatomyositis, and scleroderma—the collagen-vascular diseases.

Spider telangiectases appear as central, often pulsating, puncta with radiating legs. They may occur in normal adolescents, pregnant women, and patients with liver disease.

Telangiectases of the tongue, lips, nasal mucous membranes, and hands associated with gastrointestinal bleeding may indicate hereditary hemorrhagic telangiectasia (Rendu-Osler-Weber disease).

Blood that cannot be expressed from the skin by pressure represents purpura. Here, red blood cells have leaked out of blood vessels into the dermis. Small areas of blood leakage are called petechiae. Larger areas are denoted as ecchymoses.

Flat purpuric lesions can be caused by platelet disorders, such as thrombocytopenia, or by clotting diseases, such as hemophilia. Other etiologies include the capillary abnormalities found in scurvy or amyloidosis. The elderly often develop purpuric or ecchymotic spots on their extremities as a result of minor trauma and more fragile capillaries.

Raised, or palpable, purpura is indicative of vessel inflammation together with leakge of red cells. Examples include immune complex-mediated leukocytoclastic vasculitis and infectious vasculitis. Leukocytoclastic vasculitis is an acute inflammation of blood vessel walls. It is theorized that immune complexes, trapped in small vessel walls, lead to the activation of complement. Polymorphonuclear leukocytes are then attracted to the vessel walls, where they may be seen as whole or fragmented cells. Leukocyte enzymes may injure the vessels, leading to more disruption and inflammation.

An example of small vessel vasculitis is Henoch–Schoenlein purpura. This disorder, more common in the young, presents as palpable purpura of the lower extremities after an upper respiratory illness. Fever, renal disease, gastrointestinal bleeding, and pulmonary disease may accompany the cutaneous signs. Drugs, collagen–vascular diseases, and hepatitis can also cause leukocytoclastic vasculitis.

Infectious vasculitis occurs when bacterial, rickettsial, or other organisms with or without antibody attack vessel walls. Examples include the vasculitis of subacute or acute bacterial endocarditis, gonococcemia, meningococcemia, and Rocky Mountain spotted fever.

Granulomas represent collections of histiocytes in the skin. Lesions consist of papules that on diascopy leave a brownish "apple jelly" color. Granulomas may be caused by sarcoidosis, granuloma annulare, necrobiosis lipoidica diabeticorum, foreign bodies lodged in the dermis, and certain chronic infections.

Sarcoidosis is a multisystem disease primarily affecting the lungs and the skin. If a dyspneic patient with chest radiograph findings of hilar adenopathy and/or pulmonary fibrosis presents with brownish papules on the face, a diagnosis of sarcoidosis must be entertained. Skin lesions of sarcoid can appear in any location on the body and often present as papules or plaques.

Granuloma annulare, most commonly seen on the dorsal surface of the hand, represents a ringlike collection of papules. Although this disease can disseminate about the skin, systemic consequences do not occur. Occasionally diabetes mellitus may be noted.

A more consistent sign of diabetes is necrobiosis lipoidica diabeticorum. Here, yellowish plaques accompanied by thinning (atrophy) of the dermis are found on the shins. Because of the atrophy, blood vessels are more apparent in the lesions.

Foreign body granulomas occur when certain materials, such as silica, talc, thorns, or insect parts, enter the dermis and incite a chronic inflammatory reaction. A small nodule may result.

Infectious granulomas are chronic skin reactions caused by a variety of mycobacteria, certain fungal organisms, and leishmania. When mycobacterium tuberculosis is introduced into the skin of an already exposed, immune–competent host, a granulomatous lesion, called lupus vulgaris, results. The atypical mycobacterium *Mycobacterium marinum* causes granulomas of the hands in fishermen and fish tank caretakers who infect themselves through a scratch.

Chronic granulomas occur in hosts whose immunity to the infecting organism is high. The hypopigmented, hypesthetic granulomatous plaques of tuberculoid leprosy occur in patients with good immunity to *Mycobacterium leprae*. Few organisms can be found in these lesions. However, in the lesions of lepromatous leprosy, many bacteria are seen. Here, the host has little resistance. Similarly, the protozoan *Leishmania* causes granulomatous lesions in patients with high resistance.

Sporotrichosis presents as red nodules spreading up an extremity along the course of lymphatics. Here, a rose bush thorn may inoculate the fungus *Sporothrix schenckii* into a gardener's finger. A series of granulomas in a linear pattern may result.

Tumors of the dermis may result from overgrowth of one of the cell types normally found there. Examples of cells of dermal origin and their tumors include: fibroblasts (dermatofibroma), muscle cells (leiomyoma), nerve cells (neurofibroma), blood vessel cells (hemangioma), and mast cells (urticaria pigmentosa). However, tumor cells metastatic to the dermis may also occur. Malignancies that metastasize to the skin include breast, lung, kidney, and ovarian carcinomas as well as

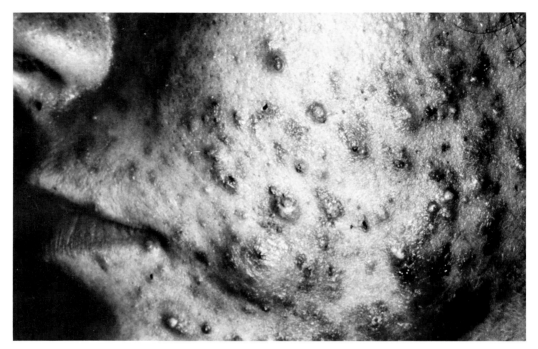

FIGURE 13.22   **Acne vulgaris.**

melanoma and lymphoma (Figure 13.7). Primary skin cancers that invade the dermis include basal cell carcinoma, squamous cell carcinoma, and melanoma.

Erysipelas is an **infection of the dermis** caused by streptococcus bacteria. Sharply demarcated erythema without a significantly raised border is noted. Folliculitis represents infection of a hair follicle either by the seriously pathogenic *Staphylococcus aureus* or by the more benign *Staphylococcus epidermidis*. A furuncle is an infection of a single hair follicle. A carbuncle represents a group of infected follicles that coalesce to form a tender nodule. Ecthyma is an erosive condition of the skin caused by *S. aureus* and group A *Streptococcus pyogenes*. Ecthyma gangrenosum represents a serious ulcerating infection of the dermis usually caused by Gram-negative bacteria, such as *Pseudomonas*.

A host of deep fungi can infect the dermis. North American blastomycosis, cryptococcosis, coccidioidomycosis, and paracoccidioidomycosis are diseases caused by such fungi. *Aspergillus* and *Nocardia* represent advanced bacteria that can invade the dermis.

Acne is an **inflammatory condition of the dermis.** A variety of lesions are found in acne. These include open and closed comedones, pustules, inflammatory papules, pustules, nodules, and cysts (Figure 13.22). Acne does not involve a true infection of the dermis. The closed comedo, the primary lesion of acne, forms when keratin is retained in the hair follicle wall. The follicle develops into an inflammatory papule after neutrophils are attracted to the hair follicle by soluble bacterial products. The plugged follicle may rupture as a result of the action of neutrophil-produced enzymes. If hair, sebum, or keratin escapes from the follicle and enters the dermis, a brisk inflammatory reaction results. Finally a nodule may form. Acne nodules may heal with pitted scars or sinus tracts.

Cells or cell products may infiltrate the dermis. **Infiltrative disorders** caused by lymphocytes are called lymphomas if malignant and pseudolymphomas if be-

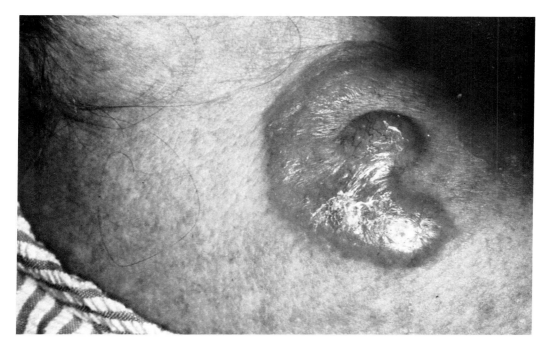

FIGURE 13.23   Mycosis fungoides tumor.

nign. Mycosis fungoides is a T-cell lymphoma of the skin that has three phases.
In the patch stage, dermatiticlike scaly areas are noted. The lesions become more
raised and firm in the plaque stage. The tumor stage represents advanced disease
and may be accompanied by lymph node and visceral involvement (Figure 13.23).
The tumors often ulcerate.

Pseudolymphomas appear as red plaques, often on the face. Nodules due to
persistent insect bite reactions may show dense infiltration of lymphocytes and
other inflammatory cells on biopsy.

Hyaluronic acid in excess can cause diffuse infiltration of the dermis of the
lower legs in pretibial myxedema. This sign of hyperthyroidism presents as an
orange peel-like (*peau d'orange*) thickening of the skin of the shins. The dimpling
seen in *peau d'orange* skin is due to tethering of the skin by the hair follicles.
Edema fluid may infiltrate the skin of the trunk after an infection or as a result of
diabetes in the condition known as scleredema. Uric acid deposits may be found in
the skin in tophi found over joints and in the ear lobes of patients with gout.

Combined Epidermal and Dermal Disease

Both the epidermis and dermis are involved in the papulosquamous diseases,
certain inflammatory conditions, and tumors. **Papulosquamous** diseases are characterized by scaling, well-demarcated papules and plaques. Psoriasis, pityriasis
rosea, lichen planus, and certain infections are included in this group.

Psoriasis presents as chronic erythematous plaques with micalike (micaceous)
scale (Figure 13.6). Areas of predilection include the scalp, ears, elbows, knees,
and intergluteal cleft. Here, mild dermal inflammation and dilatation of capillaries
are accompanied by epidermal hyperplasia and hyperkeratosis. The Auspitz sign
is evoked by peeling the scale off of a plaque. Small bleeding points are then revealed. Psoriasis may be associated with large or small joint arthritis.

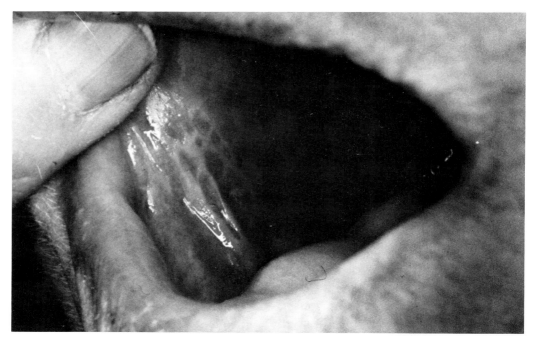

FIGURE 13.24   **Lichen planus of the buccal mucosa.**

Pityriasis rosea often begins as a single lesion, the herald patch. Subsequently, multiple small, oval erythematous to tan plaques erupt in a Christmas tree-like distribution on the trunk. A collarette of scale may be seen surrounding each lesion.

Lichen planus is a pruritic papulosquamous disorder of the oral mucous membranes, wrists, lower legs, genitalia, and fingernails. The classic lesion found on the skin is a violaceous (bright purple), flat-topped papule with fine white lines called Wickham's striae. The buccal mucosa reveals reticulated, or lacelike, white lines (Figure 13.24). These lines must be differentiated from the more banal linear bite lines. In lichen planus inflammatory cells collect just beneath the epidermis.

Tinea corporis (ringworm) can present as scaling papules that form ringlike arrays (Figure 13.25). It is the active, inflammatory border that, when scraped for a potassium hydroxide preparation, will reveal hyphae (Figure 13.4).

Secondary syphilis may mimic more classic papulosquamous diseases, such as psoriasis and pityriasis rosea. Patients with secondary lues often present with widespread papular or plaquelike lesions. Characteristically, the palms and soles are involved with copper- or ham-colored scaling oval plaques (Figure 13.26). The disease may be accompanied by an uneven (moth-eaten) alopecia, lesions of the oral mucous membranes and tongue, and moist papules of the angle of the mouth (split papules) or in the perirectal area (condylomata lata). Lymphadenopathy may also appear.

Inflammatory disease of the dermis along with epidermal alteration occurs in lupus erythematosus. The classic discoid lupus lesion is an atrophic, scaling, erythematous plaque with telangiectasia. The epidermal atrophy presents as a loss of skin markings and hair (Figure 13.27). Hair follicle plugging with scale is also characteristic of this disease. These plugs may be noted on the undersurface of scale that is lifted off from a discoid lesion (thumbtack scale). Such lesions tend to

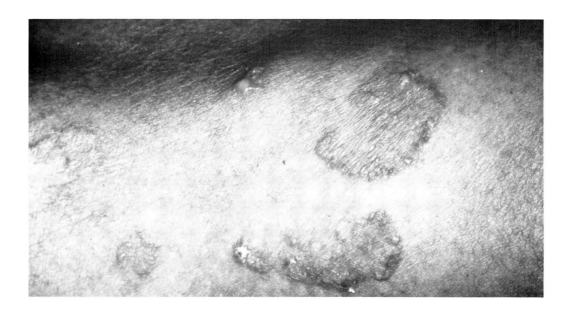

FIGURE 13.25   Tinea corporis.

FIGURE 13.26   Secondary syphilis.

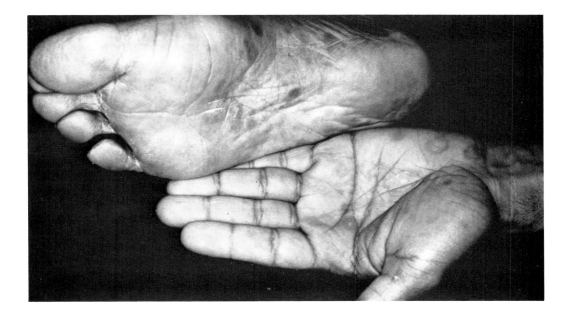

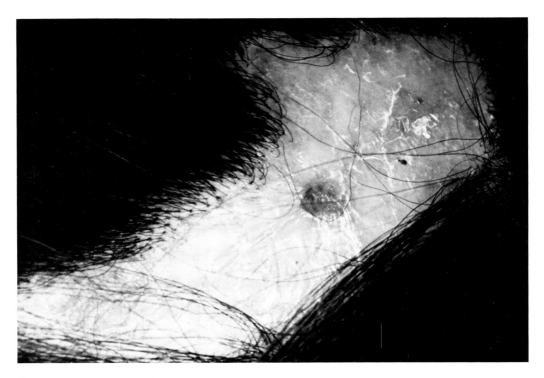

FIGURE 13.27   Discoid lupus erythematosus.

occur on sun-exposed areas of the body, such as the scalp, face, ears, neck, and anterior chest. Discoid lupus lesions may be present in patients with systemic disease.

Tumors of the skin that involve both the epidermis and dermis include basal cell carcinoma, squamous cell carcinoma, melanoma, and keratoacanthoma. The latter is a cup-shaped lesion with a central accumulation of scale. Keratoacanthomas may grow rapidly and then spontaneously regress. It may be difficult to distinguish a keratoacanthoma from a squamous cell carcinoma histologically, so that full excision may be required.

Diseases of the Fat

Inflammatory conditions and tumors may be confined to the fat. Erythema nodosum is an inflammatory reaction in the subcutaneous tissue. Here, lesions are not well demarcated because of their depth. Tender purplish-red nodules are noted, usually on the shins, in reaction to a systemic infection or drug. Tumors of the fat include the common lipoma, which represents a well-circumscribed overgrowth of fatty tissue (Figure 13.8).

Texture of the Lesion

The fourth step in the physical examination of the skin requires the determination of a lesion's texture. The texture of a lesion gives the examiner a clue as to where the pathologic alteration has occurred in the skin. Texture is discovered by palpation.

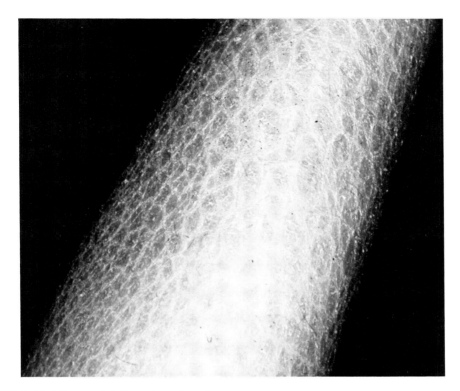

FIGURE 13.28   Ichthyosis vulgaris.

Epidermal Lesions

Epidermal change is indicated by a change in skin surface characteristics. For example, a thickened or less adhesive stratum corneum results in scale. Scale may also signify inflammation of the dermis with resultant edema or spongiosis of the epidermis. Scale may be loosely adherent, as in psoriasis, or branny, as with tinea versicolor. Ichthyotic (fishlike) scale represents scale that is large and often rhomboid shaped. Ichthyosis vulgaris is a common autosomal dominant condition in which large scales are found on the legs (Figure 13.28). Less usual types of ichthyosis include an acquired form found in association with Hodgkin's disease or sarcoidosis and rare congenital forms.

The term "hyperkeratotic" is used to describe a thickened stratum corneum. Chronic psoriasis or dermatitis of the palms and soles often presents with thick scale in these areas. Keratoderma refers to a uniform and often diffuse thickening of the stratum corneum of the palms and soles. Here, the scale is tightly adherent. Keratodermas can be acquired or inherited and can represent a local reaction to a more widespread skin disorder, such as exfoliative erythroderma or the rare condition pityriasis rubra pilaris.

Scale can be macerated, that is, saturated with water in moist intertriginous areas. Thus, one may find whitish, moist scale between the toes in patients who produce excess sweat or beneath pendulous body folds in the obese.

A verrucous (warty) lesion is one with many rough papillations. Such a lesion combines hyperkeratosis with an increase in folding of the epidermis (Figure 13.16). A skin disorder that demonstrates increased epidermal folds but does not

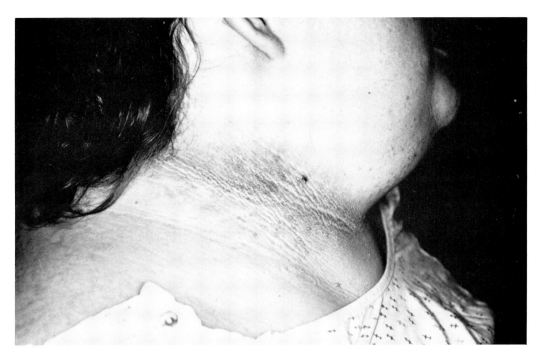

FIGURE 13.29   Acanthosis nigricans.

have excess scale is acanthosis nigricans. This velvety abnormality is found on the neck, axillae, and dorsal surfaces of the fingers in obese patients and in patients with underlying endocrinologic or malignant disease. The lesions appear hyperpigmented despite the lack of an increase in epidermal melanin (Figure 13.29).

Loss of normal skin lines and fine, cigarette paper-like wrinkling indicate epidermal atrophy. Such atrophy is found in aged skin, in early lesions of mycosis fungoides and in a condition of the genitalia called lichen sclerosus et atrophicus (Figure 13.30). The prominent skin markings found in lichenified skin represent a thickened epidermis (Figure 13.14).

Dermal Lesions

Dermal lesions have a feeling of substance rather than of surface change. Edematous lesions, such as hives, are raised but not unduly firm. Most benign tumors of the dermis that are not calcified feel solid, but not rock hard. Strictly dermal lesions are not fixed to the subcutaneous tissue and thus allow free mobility of the skin.

A dermatofibroma is a common, slightly hyperpigmented dermal papule often found on the lower legs. The lesion dimples upon application of lateral pressure (Fitzpatrick sign). The tumor is composed of proliferations of fibroblasts along with a vascular component.

A rock-hard lesion may indicate metastatic carcinoma, such as from carcinoma of the breast. Benign inflammatory cysts may become calcified or ossified and, thus, develop a stony consistency.

The term "infiltrative" refers to an excess number of cells or quantity of noncellular material in the dermis.

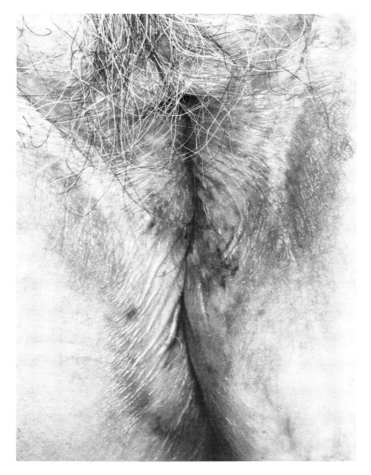

FIGURE 13.30   Lichen sclerosus et atrophicus.

Atrophy of the dermis can result in thinning of the skin. When dermal substance is lost the underlying blood vessels become more obvious. Dermal atrophy occurs in aged skin, topical corticosteroid abuse, and striae. As the skin ages both epidermal and dermal thinning occur. Such changes are commonly noted on the forearms. Telangiectases may be noted in skin thinned by overuse of potent corticosteroid creams. Striae occur on the abdomen, buttocks, thighs, breasts, and inguinal region when the adrenal glands produce an excess amount of glucocorticoids. Such is the case in adolescence, pregnancy, obesity, and Cushing's disease.

Subcutaneous Lesions

Induration indicates diffuse subcutaneous pathology. Here, the overlying skin is not freely mobile. For example, morphea presents with bound-down plaques with hypopigmented centers and lilac-colored or hyperpigmented borders. Similarly, scleroderma lesions are fixed and have lost their epidermal appendages and surface skin markings.

Atrophy of the fat creates a depression in the skin. Two examples are lipo-atrophy from insulin injections and lupus panniculitis. Insulin injections can produce gently sloping depressions on the upper arms and thighs. Lupus erythematosus can cause significant inflammation of the fat with resultant sharply punched-out lesions.

The compressibility of a lesion may be determined on palpation. Vascular lesions are often compressible since they contain blood-filled spaces. For example, a cavernous hemangioma represents a deep dermal or subcutaneous collection of enlarged vessels. These usually occur in the head and neck. Venous lakes are dilated venous channels that commonly occur on the lips. Compressibility is also a feature of most cysts. An epidermal inclusion cyst is an example (Figure 13.9).

Color of the Lesion

The fifth characteristic of a skin lesion is its color. Color change can be caused by an excess of natural pigments, such as hemoglobin, carotene, and melanin, or by foreign pigments, as with a tatoo.

Vascular Process Coloration

Inflammation leads to blood vessel dilatation, increased blood flow and, hence, a greater number of red blood cells circulating in superficial capillaries. Thus, inflamed skin lesions appear red or erythematous. With diascopy, blood can be expressed from inflamed lesions and from the dilated vessels seen in a variety of telangiectases. Petechial, purpuric, ecchymotic, and hemorrhagic lesions cannot be blanched because blood has leaked out of the vessels.

When red blood cells in tissue are destroyed, hemoglobin is converted to hemosiderin, leaving a brownish-yellow tinge. Small brownish spots evident on the lower legs in patients with stasis dermatitis and capillaritis represent the remnant of extravasated blood cells.

Cyanosis occurs when deoxygenated hemoglobin reaches a critical concentration (5 mg/dL). Diffuse cyanosis may be noted in patients with right-to-left shunts through the heart and in patients with shock, lung disease, and certain blood disorders. Acral cyanosis occurs when vessels in the hands and feet constrict, causing slower flow of venous blood and accumulation of deoxygenated hemoglobin. Examples include Raynaud's phenomenon and chilblains. The three colors found in Raynaud's phenomenon include white (vasospasm), blue (reduced venous flow), and red (reactive hyperemia). Chilblains represents chronic vascular inflammation and injury due to cold exposure. Bluish discoloration or nodules can be seen on the toes, shins, or earlobes.

Inflammatory Process Coloration

Erythroderma refers to diffuse erythema of the skin due to inflammation. Widespread scaling (exfoliation) often accompanies an erythroderm. Causes include primary skin disease, such as psoriasis or atopic dermatitis; drug reaction; and response to a systemic process, such as lymphoma.

Reddish-brown lesions that, on diascopy, leave an apple jelly brown-yellow color are indicative of granulomas.

Intense inflammation of the dermis produces the violaceous (purple) color seen in lichen planus and lupus erythematosus. Dusky and black colors signify varying degrees of skin necrosis. Erythema multiforme represents a reactive skin condition in which target-shaped skin lesions develop central dusky vesicles. The central color change is due to dermal inflammation and necrosis of the lower layers of the epidermis. Erythema multiforme most commonly occurs with herpes simplex or mycoplasma infection or in reaction to a drug. Meningococcemia and gonococcemia cause papules, pustules, or plaques with irregular gray centers. Here, intense vascular inflammation results in epidermal and dermal necrosis. Gangrene, representing ischemia and full-thickness skin necrosis, appears black.

Yellowing Processes
Excessive intake of carotene leads to a yellowish discoloration of the skin, but not of the sclerae. Jaundice, characterized by a yellow color of the skin and sclerae, indicates hyperbilirubinemia.

Melanin Coloration
The normal brown pigment of the skin, melanin, is found within the epidermis. The diffuse hyperpigmentation found in Addison's disease is due to increased melanin principally in the epidermis. Here, increased pigmentation is most prominent in sun-exposed sites, skin creases, sites of friction, and mucous membranes. Metastatic melanoma may present as widespread hyperpigmentation of the skin due to melanin production in the dermis. In hemochromatosis a bronze color is created by excess epidermal melanin and abnormal deposits of iron in the dermis.

The six types of **nevocellular nevi** (moles) are classified according to their morphology and quality of pigment. Nevi represent collections of nevocytes, or pigment cell precursors, in the dermis. Junctional nevi, common in young people, are small, macular, uniformly brown lesions that are benign. Their brown color is due to the presence of melanin near the dermal-epidermal junction.

Compound nevi are elevated moles with a uniform brown pigmentation. Here, there is nevus cell growth both at the dermal-epidermal junction and more deeply in the dermis. Dermal nevi are common flesh-colored papules in which the nevus cells are located in the dermis without involvement of the dermal-epidermal interface.

Blue nevi are small nodules that are made up of nevus cells that produce melanin deep in the dermis. Because of the Tyndall effect, deep brown pigment in a lesion gives it a blue appearance on the surface.

Congenital nevi are brown, often hairy, moles that are present at birth. Nevus cells often involve the dermal-epidermal junction, dermis, and subcutaneous tissue. A large congenital nevus, called a bathing trunk nevus, has the potential for developing into a malignant melanoma.

More atypical-appearing nevi, occasionally occurring in large numbers and in families, are called dysplastic nevi. These nevi may be flat or slightly elevated, but tend to have irregular borders or irregular pigmentation. Often a reddish hue is noted on their perimeter. At present it is unknown how often dysplastic nevi evolve into melanomas.

Melanoma represents a highly malignant tumor of nevus cells. The most common variety is the superficial spreading type. This type is only slightly raised and has very irregular borders (Figure 13.31). A number of colors may be noted, including brown, black, blue, gray, red, and white. A nodular melanoma is a melanoma with more vertical than lateral extension. Melanomas that occur on the digits are called acral lentiginous melanomas.

A **lentigo maligna** is a large flat lesion with irregular borders and various shades of brown that occurs in the elderly on sun-exposed areas. The lesion is caused by proliferation of atypical melanocytes in the epidermis. When the dermis becomes involved the lesion is called a lentigo maligna melanoma.

Benign, macular brown lesions include the common lentigo (liver spot) and ephelide (freckle) and the less common café-au-lait spot. The **lentigo** is a small tan area found on sun-exposed areas such as the face and dorsal surfaces of the forearms and hands. It represents an increased number of melanocytes in the

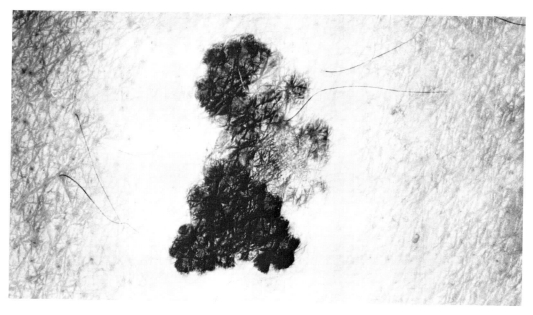

FIGURE 13.31   Superficial spreading melanoma.

epidermis. **Ephelides,** however, only show an increase in epidermal melanin rather than an increase in melanocyte number. The **café–au–lait spot** is a tan macule that, if numbering greater than five, may indicate the presence of neurofibromatosis (Figure 13.3).

Macular hyperpigmentation can result from the overstimulation of melano-cytes seen in melasma (mask of pregnancy). Here, the hormone alteration found in pregnant women or in women taking oral contraceptives is thought to play a role.

Inflammation in the skin of dark-skinned individuals can leave a hyperpigmented residue. The postinflammatory hyperpigmentation of acne occurs when epidermal cells laden with melanin are disrupted with release of pigment into the dermis. This pigment may remain in the dermis for several months. Inflammation of the skin can also produce the opposite effect: hypopigmentation. For example, in pityriasis alba, mild facial dermatitis prevents the normal incorporation of melanin into the epidermal cells. The result is a flat, slightly scaly hypopigmented patch on the face. Vitiligo, on the other hand, represents pigment cell destruction with total depigmentation of certain areas of the skin (Figure 13.5).

Shape of the Lesion

The sixth step in an examination of a skin abnormality is the determination of the lesion's shape. Several adjectives are employed to clarify the circular configuration of a lesion.

Circular Lesions

Annular lesions are ringlike areas, often with elevated borders. Dermatophyte infections of the skin may present as annular lesions with scaly, elevated rims and central clearing. Granuloma annulare consists of a circular array of granulomatous papules. Erythema annulare centrifugum forms erythematous rings with a central, trailing scale (Figure 13.21).

Arcuate lesions form an arc rather than a complete circle. Examples include urticaria and mycosis fungoides. The latter develops horseshoe-shaped lesions (Figure 13.23). Annular and arcuate shapes may fuse into polycylic forms.

Erythema multiforme forms targetoid or iris lesions in which centrifugal rings, similar to those of a dart board or arrow target, develop.

Umbilicated lesions are circular lesions with central depressions. An example is molluscum contagiosum (Figure 13.18). Herpes simplex, varicella-zoster, and variola viruses also produce umbilicated papules or vesicles.

Dermatitis occurring in coin-shaped plaques is called nummular eczema. This condition is caused by scratching and thus is found on the accessible areas of skin, especially the extremities.

Guttate lesions, as in acute guttate psoriasis, are small round papules usually large in number. Balanitis circinata refers to the scaly erythematous plaques that form a ring around the penis in patients with Reiter's syndrome.

Lesions of Other Shapes

Cutaneous pathology may present in a variety of shapes other than circular. Urticaria may form gyrate, or irregular, shapes (Figure 13.10). Roundworm larvae may invade the dermis and cause cutaneous larva migrans. The resultant lesion is described as serpiginous, or snakelike.

The term "reticulated" refers to a netlike or lacelike pattern. Patients with lichen planus develop reticulated white lines in the buccal mucosa (Figure 13.24). Livedo reticularis represents a temporary netlike, bluish discoloration of the legs due to vasospasm. Erythema ab igne results in brown reticulated lines on skin that has been exposed to excessive heat.

Geographic means widely variable and maplike. For example, in geographic tongue, irregular white and red areas appear where normal papillae have been lost.

A description of a lesion's three dimensional shape can aid in its diagnosis. Raised lesions may have broad bases, such as with compound nevi and seborrheic keratoses. Alternatively, lesions such as the common skin tag (acrochordon) may be pedunculated.

Pattern of the Lesion

The seventh step in the examination of the skin involves recognition of a lesion's pattern. Pattern refers to the arrangement of primary lesions.

Grouped vesicles on an erythematous base alerts the observer to consider herpes simplex or zoster. Vesicles arranged along the distribution of a sensory nerve in a unilateral, dermatomal pattern strongly suggest a diagnosis of herpes zoster (Figure 13.2).

Follicular lesions involve hair follicles. Examples include bacterial folliculitis and acne. Miliaria, on the other hand, represents inflammation of eccrine sweat glands. Here, multiple 1- to 2-mm erythematous papules or vesicles are located in a regular pattern between hair follicles.

A linear pattern often suggests trauma, such as from a scratch. Factitial pathology often presents in linear or regular geometric patterns (Figure 13.32). Contact with allergenic substances, such as rhus oil, often results in a linear arrangement of vesicles. Certain skin lesions may occur in a linear array in response to trauma. This occurrence is called the Koebner phenomenon. Diseases that show this pattern include psoriasis, lichen planus, and warts.

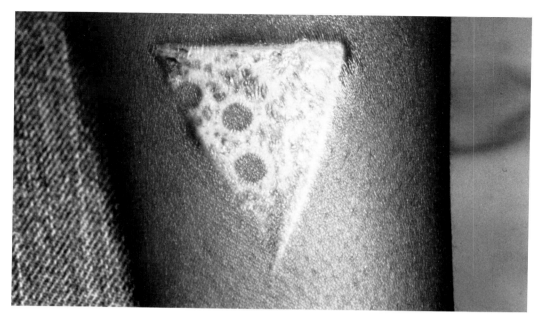

FIGURE 13.32   Factitial scar.

Male-patterned alopecia is a stereotypic arrangement of hair loss induced by testosterone. Typically, hair loss from the temples is followed by frontal hairline recession and occipital thinning (Figure 13.33). The term "patchy" indicates a spotty or irregular pathologic pattern. Patchy, or moth-eaten, hair loss from the scalp is seen in secondary syphilis.

Lesions may be classified as localized or diffuse. Localized lesions are limited to certain areas of the body, whereas those that are diffuse occur in many areas of the skin. The term "universal" refers to a generalized process. For example, alopecia universalis represents loss of hair throughout the body. On the other hand, alopecia areata represents loss of hair in localized, circular areas, usually on the scalp (Figure 13.34).

Whether or not a lesion is unilateral, bilateral, or symmetrical may be important. Disorders, such as vitiligo, psoriasis, tinea versicolor, and pityriasis rosea tend to be symmetrical.

Exanthematous means widespread. Thus, the viral exanthem of rubeola (measles) involves the entire skin surface over a period of a few days. Drug reactions also may become exanthematous (Figure 13.20). The term "morbilliform" may be used to describe a widespread measleslike eruption characterized by blanching erythematous macules and papules. "Maculopapular" is essentially synonymous with "morbilliform."

Distribution of the Lesion

The eighth and final step in the inspection of the skin involves a determination of the distribution of skin pathology. Certain diseases affect specific areas of the body.

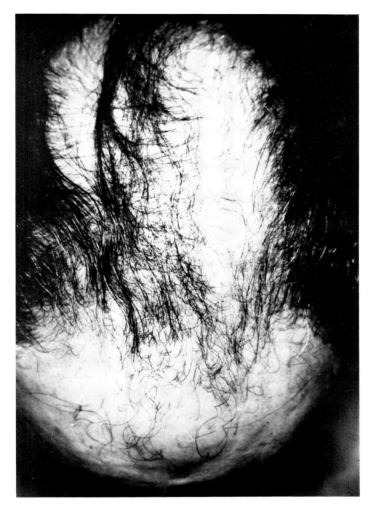

FIGURE 13.33   Male–patterned alopecia.

Area-specific Diseases

Seborrheic dermatitis produces erythema and loosely adherent, greasy scales on the scalp, eyebrows, nasolabial grooves, and chest. Psoriasis involves the scalp, ears, elbows, knees, intergluteal cleft, and nails. Lichen planus affects the buccal mucous membranes, wrists, ankles, and genitalia. Vitiligo tends to occur around body orifices and in areas exposed to friction, such as the dorsum of the hands.

Acne involves areas of the body that have large sebaceous glands. Such areas include the face, upper back, chest, and shoulders. Secondary syphilis may affect the trunk, mouth, perirectal area, palms, and soles. Herpes simplex causes vesicles on the lips, genitalia, buttocks, and fingers (herpetic whitlow). Scabies causes burrows and pruritic papules on the interdigital web spaces of the fingers, flexor surface of the wrists, axillae, belt line, buttocks, and genitalia.

Pemphigoid causes tense bullae on flexor surfaces of the extremities and anywhere on the trunk. Pemphigus often begins in the mouth. In neurofibromatosis, café–au–lait spots may occur in the axillae.

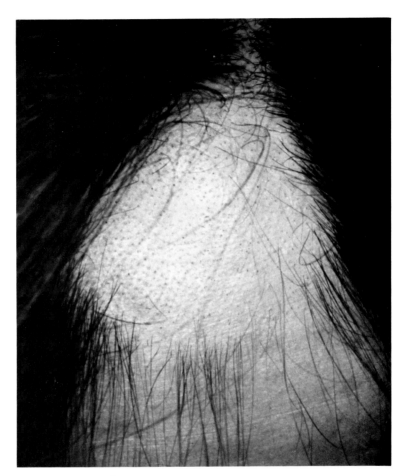

FIGURE 13.34   Alopecia areata.

Melanoma may occur anywhere on the skin surface or in the retina, but is more commonly seen on the back in males and on the legs in females. Lentigo maligna and lentigo melanoma occur on the face in the elderly.

Photosensitivity disorders present with erythematous plaques, hives, or vesicles on areas of the skin exposed to the sun. These regions include the forehead, cheeks, upper chest, and dorsal surfaces of the forearms and hands. Often the areas around the eyes, behind the ears, and under the nose and chin are spared.

Lupus erythematosus involves the scalp, ears, and face. Lesions include the nonspecific malar erythematous eruption seen in acute lupus or the specific, atrophic, chronic discoid lesion (Figure 13.27).

Scleroderma presents as induration and tightening of the skin, first of the face and hands. Characteristic matlike telangiectases are found on the lips, tongue, and fingers. Dermatomyositis causes proximal muscle weakness and a violaceous (heliotrope) eruption on sun-exposed areas. Papules over the knuckles (Gottron's papules) and telangiectases in the cuticles occur as well.

Diabetes mellitus may be associated with atrophic and granulomatous lesions of necrobiosis lipoidica diabeticorum on the shins; depressed, atrophic brownish spots (diabetic dermopathy) on the legs; and blisters (diabetic bullae) on the feet.

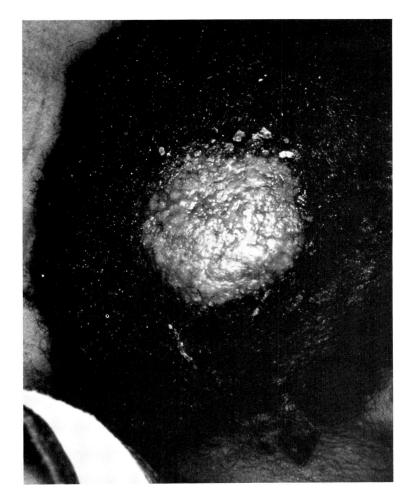

FIGURE 13.35   **Kerion.**

Regional Examination

One should examine specific regions of the body, keeping in mind a list of disorders that may affect that particular area. A scaling eruption of the **scalp** should bring to consideration seborrheic dermatitis, psoriasis, and tinea capitis. Seborrheic dermatitis (common dandruff) produces diffuse mild erythema with scale. Well-demarcated scaling plaques with thick micalike scale are found in psoriasis.

Tinea capitis often leads to an area of hair loss (alopecia). Broken-off hairs may be found. A kerion represents an inflammatory reaction to a fungal organism in the scalp and presents as a hairless, boggy tumor (Figure 13.35). Nonscarring alopecia can be caused by alopecia areata. Here, circular bald areas that often regrow spontaneously are seen (Figure 13.34). Scarring hair loss may be caused by lupus erythematosus (Figure 13.27) or more rarely by metastatic carcinoma or sarcoid.

The **face** is often the site of a photosensitivity eruption. An example is a photosensitivity induced by a drug, such as a thiazide diuretic. Malar erythema

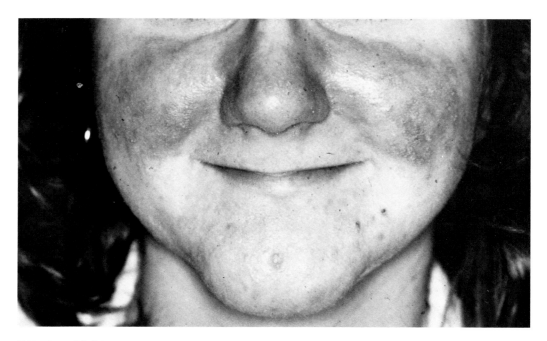

FIGURE 13.36   Acne rosacea.

may be caused by acne rosacea, seborrheic dermatitis, psoriasis, or lupus. Acne rosacea commonly affects middle-aged females and is characterized by malar erythema, papules, pustules, and telangiectasia. The central area of the face tends to be affected (Figure 13.36).

The **mouth** must be included in a thorough cutaneous examination. Here, one may find lesions of lichen planus, oral candidiasis, aphthous stomatitis, and blistering diseases, such as pemphigus or pemphigoid. Oral candidiasis (thrush) produces white patches on the tongue and mucous membranes. Pemphigoid, pemphigus, and lichen planus may cause severe erythema of the gums, called desquamative gingivitis. If the corners of the mouth are fissured as a result of excessive leakage of saliva, the term "angular cheilosis" (perlèche) is used.

The **palms and soles** may reveal the deep vesicles of dyshidrotic dermatitis, also known as pompholyx. Although dyshidrosis means abnormal sweating, sweat glands are not primarily involved in this chronic dermatitis. Pustular psoriasis of the palms and soles causes recurrent, culture-negative pustules. Dermatophytes can cause scaling on both soles of the feet but commonly on only one palm.

Systemic illnesses and diseases limited to the skin can affect the **nails.** Clubbing is a sign of chronic hypoxemia, characterized by a greater than 180-degree angle made by the nail plate with the proximal nail fold. The distal digit is somewhat bulbous in this disorder (Figure 13.37). Beau's lines are horizontal depressions in the nail plate caused by transient arrest of nail growth during an acute systemic illness (Figure 13.38). Splinter hemorrhages are linear dark red lines found in the nail beds as a result of trauma or bacterial endocarditis.

Cuticular erythema and telangiectasia is a sign of collagen-vascular diseases. Included in this group are lupus erythematosus, dermatomyositis, scleroderma, and mixed connective tissue disease.

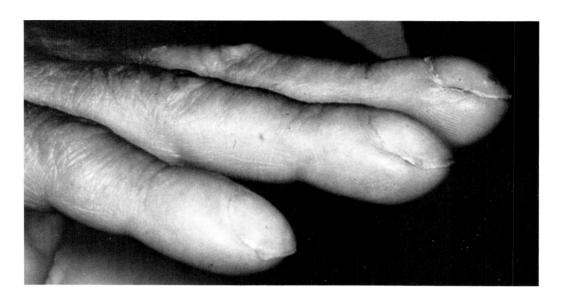

FIGURE 13.37   Clubbing.

FIGURE 13.38   Beau's lines.

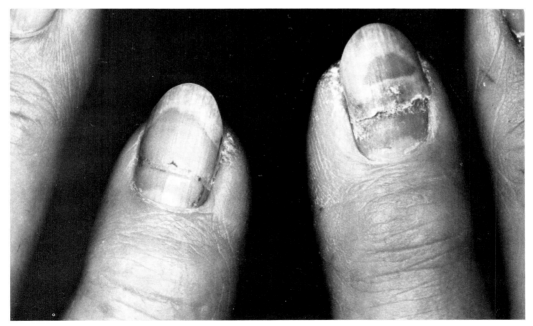

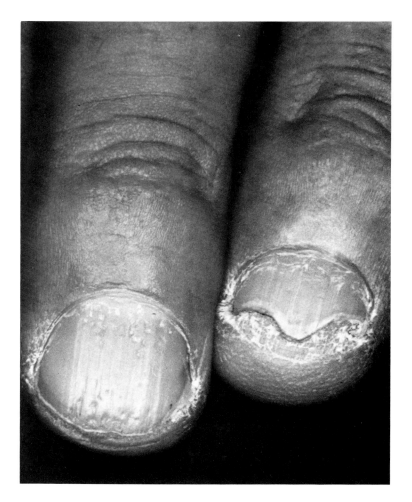

FIGURE 13.39   Pitted psoriatic fingernails.

Psoriasis of the nails produces characteristic pitting, lifting of the distal nail from the nail bed (onycholysis), and oil drop–like discoloration of the nail bed (Figure 13.39). Dermatophytes also produce onycholysis, but may, in addition, cause distortion of the nail and scaling about the nail bed.

A variety of infectious disorders affect the **groin.** Tinea cruris represents a dermatophyte infection of the inguinal creases. The scrotum is not usually affected. Candida infection of the groin may be confused with tinea cruris. However, candida causes erythema of the scrotum in men and satellite papules and pustules on the border of the lesion. Corynebacteria cause another type of inguinal erythema with a brownish hue called erythrasma.

Diaper dermatitis in infants is caused by irritation by urine and feces. The excess moisture encourages overgrowth of *Candida.* Thus, eczematous changes from irritant dermatitis as well as satellite pustules and papules due to *Candida* are noted.

Sexually transmitted diseases present with a variety of lesions of the **genitalia.** The primary chancre of syphilis is a single, nontender, punched-out ulcer with firm borders. Chancroid is a disease caused by *Haemophilus ducreyi,* a Gram-negative bacillus. The ulcers of chancroid are tender and often multiple and have shaggy margins. Gonorrhea and nongonococcal urethritis present with purulent urethral discharges.

Lichen sclerosus et atrophicus represents a white, atrophic noninfectious disease of the genitals (Figure 13.30). It tends to affect adolescent girls and middle-aged men and women. Perirectal involvement may occur as well as patchy involvement elsewhere on the skin surface.

Finally, the **lower extremities** develop particular dermatoses. Ichthyosis vulgaris or acquired ichthyosis especially affects the legs (Figure 13.28). Skin of the lower legs involved with stasis dermatitis becomes more susceptible to bacterial infection, contact dermatitis, and ulceration. Occasionally stasis dermatitis can be severe enough to induce widespread eczematous changes in the remainder of the skin. The production of a generalized eczematous change due to a local dermatitis is called an id or autosensitization reaction.

Small brown-yellow spots on the lower legs, representing the hemosiderin remnant of leaked red blood cells, can result from capillaritis. Capillary inflammation leads to increased vascular permeability and the subsequent extravasation of red cells. Leukocytoclastic vasculitis often presents with palpable purpura on the legs.

SUMMARY

A clear understanding of the normal anatomy of the skin is a prerequisite to the proper classification of skin disease. The patient with a skin disorder should be approached in the same logical manner required for all patients. Thus, a careful history and physical examination are performed. Use of appropriate equipment and laboratory tests will allow the examiner to confirm or contradict his/her hypotheses, often at the bedside. Finally, the examination of the skin must follow an orderly sequence. The examiner can then describe the lesion clearly, construct a differential diagnosis, and make a definitive diagnosis.

REFERENCES

1. Braverman IM: *Skin Signs of Systemic Disease,* ed 2. Philadelphia, WB Saunders Co., 1981.

2. Domonkos AN, Arnold HL, Odom RB: *Andrews' Diseases of the Skin,* ed 7. Philadelphia, WB Saunders Co., 1982.

3. Fitzpatrick TB, Eisen AZ, Wolff K, Freedberg IW, Austen KF: *Dermatology in General Medicine,* ed 2. New York, McGraw-Hill Book Co., 1986.

4. Lever WF, Schaumburg-Lever G: *Histopathology of the Skin,* ed 6. Philadelphia, JB Lippincott Co., 1983.

5. Moschella SL, Hurley HJ: *Dermatology*, ed 2. Philadelphia, WB Saunders Co., 1985.

6. Rook A, Wilkinson DS, Ebling FJG: *Textbook of Dermatology,* ed 3. Oxford, England, Blackwell Scientific Publications, 1979.

14
The Orthopedic Examination

John Shine, M.D.

HISTORY

The patient with a disorder affecting the muscoloskeletal system will ordinarily complain of pain, deformity, or limitation of motion and function in the spine or extremities. The history of a recent traumatic incident simplifies the diagnosis of fractures and sprains. The detailed history of the accident or fall describes the mechanism of injury and will aid in identifying the degree of injury to be expected and the precise anatomic structures that are damaged. For example, a swollen knee following a simple twisting while running represents a mild sprain without major ligament disruption. A similarly appearing swollen knee in a high-speed motor vehicle accident victim could actually be a spontaneously reduced knee dislocation with rupture of all the major knee ligaments and even injury to the popliteal vessels.

Conversely, a history of trauma can be misleading. Occasionally the swelling and pain of osteomyelitis or a bone tumor will be first noticed following a minor injury. This is especially true in young children, in whom the history of a fall may be rather vague.

Inflammatory arthritic joint symptoms are insidious in onset and initially only consist of morning stiffness and dull pain that is relieved somewhat with rest. These symptoms, or arthralgias, can spontaneously remit or recur intermittently while progressive joint deformity occurs.

Painless enlarging masses or complaints of significant night pain may be the first hints of either primary or metastatic tumors involving the muscoloskeletal system. A pathologic fracture is not infrequently the presenting problem of advanced metastatic disease.

History taking in musculoskeletal disorders will provide a major portion of our diagnostic acumen. The history combined with a physical examination should allow an accurate diagnosis in most orthopedic conditions. Supplemental laboratory and roentgenographic studies are often necessary to confirm the diagnosis before treatment is begun.

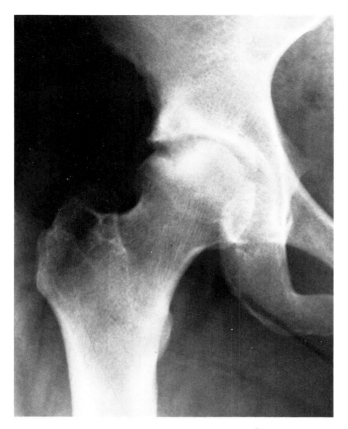

FIGURE 14.1   Osteonecrosis in sickle cell disease (hip radiograph).

INSPECTION

General Inspection

While the history is taken and during the early part of the physical examination, note the general appearance of the patient. Awareness of age-related problems will attune the examiner to the appropriate differential diagnoses. Hip dysplasia and sepsis are not unusual in the infant. During the adolescent growth spurt slipping of the proximal femoral epiphysis will produce a painful limp. Patients in their mid-twenties to mid-forties with hip pain are often suffering from muscle and disc disorders of the lumbosacral spine that refer pain to the buttock and lateral thigh. In the elderly, hip pain will usually arise from osteoarthritis of the hip or lower spine.

As the patient describes the pain, make sure that he/she points to the same anatomic site that he/she is describing. Some persons will complain of shoulder pain and yet point to the base of the neck or vertebral border of the scapula. Pain in these areas usually arises from the cervical spine rather than the shoulder joint. Frequently, a complaint of hip pain is really found on close questioning to be buttock or low back pain. True hip joint pain is usually felt in the groin and often radiates along the medial thigh and medial side of the knee. This referred pain is in the distribution of the obturator nerve that supplies a sensory branch to the hip joint.

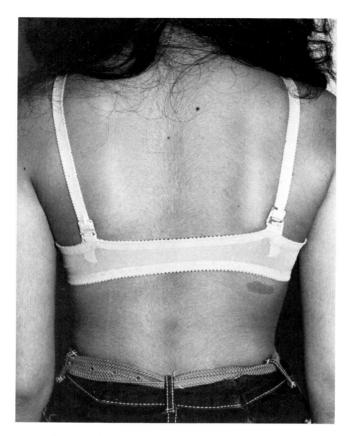

FIGURE 14.2   Café–au–lait spot.

Looking at the patient undressed and from a slight distance will make obvious any significant asymmetry of the trunk or extremities that might be caused by muscle atrophy, tumor, or congenital deformities. Malalignment of the lower limbs such as genu varum or genu valgum are also more easily appreciated this way. In bilateral varus knee deformity, or bowed knees, there is a space between the knees when standing with the feet together. In genu valgum, or knock-knee deformity, the knees touch but the feet are apart.

There are racial predispositions to certain musculoskeletal disorders. The osteonecrosis of sickle cell disease (Figure 14.1) and salmonella osteomyelitis occur in black persons, whereas these persons very infrequently incur a fracture of the hip. The offspring of American Indians and the people of Mediterranean countries have a high incidence of congenital dislocation of the hip.

A general inspection of the skin may disclose the café-au-lait spots (Figure 14.2) associated with neurofibromatosis of the spine. Hair loss and atrophic skin in the legs and feet can help explain buttock and leg pains that are due to peripheral vascular disease and not to degenerative disc disease. Skin abscesses, cellulitis, and draining sinuses may be sources or residuals of chronic osteomyelitis. After crushing injuries sympathetic dystrophy may result in an exaggerated diffuse pain with moist, reddened, atrophic skin. Avascular necrosis of the hip should be suspected in a patient complaining of hip pain whose skin is thin and easily bruised following long-term use of steroid medication.

In the Munchausen syndrome there are healed scars from multiple previous surgical procedures. Observe whether the patient's degree of complaint is consistent with their facial expression and body movements. Malingerers often show exaggerated and inappropriate grimacing and body movements. Hysterical patients tend to have an air of indifference to their complaint, even at times smiling as they explain how much pain is present.

By the time metastatic tumors have advanced to involve the musculoskeletal system, the patient looks thin and "grey." The day and especially more severe night pain seems to wear out the patient by its mere persistence. Early limited involvement by bony metastases can be rather subtle in their presentation and can be easily missed. A technetium bone scan is extremely important in the work-up of a patient suspected of having an occult metastic lesion to bone.

Posture and Gait

Posture

Posture is our static position when standing, sitting, or reclining. It requires balance and coordinated muscle activity. Normal posture is easily recognized by the relaxed, comfortable, unstrained appearance of the patient. Examining the patient in the standing position, the trunk and extremities should have an overall symmetrical appearance. There is a slight convexity or kyphosis of the thorax, and the cervical and lumbar spines are concave or lordotic. The shoulders and iliac crests are level and neither the abdomen nor buttocks are excessively protuberant.

The standing alignment of the lower limbs and feet gives a more dynamic view of any functional limb problems than does the supine view. The mechanical axis of weight bearing should pass through the center of the hip, knee, and ankle joint. The anterior-superior iliac spine is just anterior to the hip joint, so that a line drawn from that point to the midportion of the ankle will pass through the center of the patella. If the line passes medial to the patella there is genu varum, whereas if the line passes lateral to the patella there is genu valgum.

Abnormal posture may be caused by a variety of problems including pain, malunited fractures, ankylosed joints, and congenital skeletal deformities.

Observe the patient's posture during history taking. Is the neck held rigid because of painful cervical disc disease or tilted to one side, as in congenital muscular torticollis? Some persons tend to slouch or lean to one side purely from habit. On careful examination no skeletal deformity will be found.

Unequal height of the iliac crests when standing with both feet flat and knees straight indicates inequality of leg lengths. This inequality can be measured by comparing the distance between the anterior-superior iliac spine and the medial malleolus at the ankle on the right and left sides.

Scoliosis is a lateral curvature and rotation of the spine. Frequently there are double curves that may counterbalance one another so that there is no list or shift of the upper body from the midline. A single severe curve may cause the body to list to one side so that a plumb line from the palpable spinous process or T-1 falls wide to the midline of the gluteal crease. The relationship of each arm to the trunk will be noticeably different in such a case. The deformity of the spine and ribs in scoliosis is best seen with the patient bending forward from the waist and the examiner standing behind the patient looking up the spine (Figure 14.3). The unequal height of the paravertebral structures on one side is due to a rotation of the spine that accompanies the lateral curvature in scoliosis.

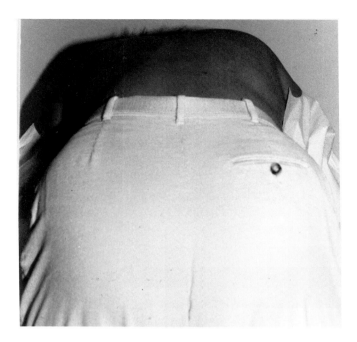

FIGURE 14.3   Right thoracic scoliosis.

Observing the patient from the side profile will show increased thoracic curvature in Scheuermann's juvenile kyphosis. The multiple spontaneous compression fractures in osteoporosis of the elderly will also cause an increased thoracic kyphosis. Pain in a ruptured lumbar disc syndrome may cause the patient to lean to one side, causing a "sciatic scoliosis." The curvature may be either away from or toward the affected side, depending upon the position of the ruptured disc in relationship to the affected nerve. This type of scoliosis is not a fixed deformity and usually resolves with cessation of the pain.

A curvature of the spine may appear with leg length inequality. To see if there is any true scoliosis with rotation of the spine, the patient should be examined bending forward in a sitting position to eliminate the leg length discrepancy. An alternative way would be to have the patient stand on a wooden block to level the pelvis prior to bending forward.

The normal weight-bearing foot shows a slight elevation or arch along the medial border, and the heel should be centered below the ankle or in, at most, 5 degrees of valgus. With flat foot deformity, or pes planus, the medial arch is lost and the heel appears to be tilted out into valgus (Figure 14.4). A very flexible flat foot may not show deformity in the non-weight-bearing position.

While standing and walking, the normal foot is turned slightly outward because of a 15-degree external rotation of the ankle relative to the knee. Developmental rotational deformities of the femur and tibia as well as malunited fractures may cause excessive internal or external rotation of the foot.

Observation of the patient's posture and attitude during the history taking gives important clues to making a diagnosis. There will be very little head and neck movement in a patient with an acute cervical sprain compared to the expressive motion seen during normal conversation. In acute tendinitis or bursitis of the shoulder, the affected extremity is held limply at the side. The patient may be

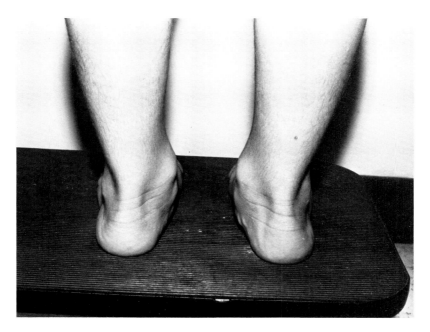

FIGURE 14.4   Heel valgus in pes planus.

lying supine with the hip and knee flexed in case of acute sciatica. This position relieves the tension on the lumbar nerve roots irritated by a herniated disc.

Gait

Normal walking requires a rather complex interaction of reflexes and coordinated muscular activity. Abnormal gait or limp is best understood by knowing the elements of normal gait.

Human locomotion is comprised of a series of gait cycles. Stance phase of the gait cycle begins with heel strike and continues through positions of foot flat, heel raise, and toe–off (Figure 14.5). Swing phase extends from toe–off to heel strike. Stance phase accounts for 60% and swing phase 40% of the gait cycle.

The body's center of gravity is located just anterior to the body of the second sacral vertebra. The goal of normal gait is to move the body's center of gravity through space with the most energy–efficient mechanism. During normal gait there is a double sinusoidal curve motion of the center of gravity through the rise and fall of stance and swing phase combined with the side–to–side motion of the alternating stance phase on either side. The vertical rise and fall of the center of gravity is about equal to the side–to–side horizontal displacement and measures approximately 4.4 cm. The rise and fall and side–to–side motions are kept to this minimal and energy efficient level by a combination of pelvic rotation, pelvic tilt, knee flexion and extension, and ankle motion.

There are many abnormal types of gait and each is less energy efficient than normal walking. When there is a leg length discrepancy of more than 2.5 cm there will be a lurch to the shorter side as the pelvis tilts down during stance phase. Accommodation for a shortened extremity can be made by walking on the forefoot and toes of the shortened extremity, flexing the knee of the long side, or wearing a shoe lift.

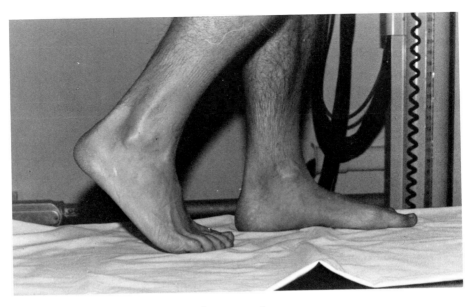

FIGURE 14.5   **Toe–off at end of stance phase.**

Weakness of the hip abductor muscles or bony instability of the hip joint will cause the pelvis to tilt down on the opposite side during the stance phase of the affected hip. In order to maintain balance the patient must lurch his upper body over the affected side to compensate for the tilting of the pelvis. This is called a gluteus medius gait. With painful conditions of the hip an antalgic lurch over the painful hip is often observed. By tilting the upper body over the affected hip, the center of gravity is brought directly over the hip, reducing the mechanical lever arm of the body weight and the opposing abductor lever arm. This results in a marked decrease in the joint forces and pain. An antalgic hip lurch can be reduced significantly by the use of a cane in the opposite hand. Observation of an antalgic hip lurch often helps to differentiate true hip pain from hip pain referred from the lower back.

A drop foot or steppage gait is due to paralysis of the dorsiflexors of the foot and ankle. In this type of gait the foot remains flexed so that during swing phase the leg has to be raised higher than normal to allow clearance of the toes and forefoot. An exaggerated steppage or placement of the foot occurs at the beginning of stance phase.

When there is paralysis of the quadriceps muscle, the knee is swung and locked into hyperextension in stance phase to prevent giving way of the knee. The patient may use his hand to help lock the knee into extension.

The most common gait abnormality in children is the intoeing gait due to torsional deformities in the lower extremities. In newborns, metatarsus adductus and internal tibial torsion are most common, whereas at 3 or 4 years of age femoral torsion is more likely to be the cause.

In patients with a stiff or arthrodesed hip, knee, or ankle, the gait is abnormal and less efficient than normal because of the exaggerated movements required to compensate for the stiff or fused joint.

The abnormal gait in neuromuscular diseases is often hard to describe since there may be varying combinations of ataxia, weakness, and spasticity. A gait analysis laboratory is most helpful in these difficult cases.

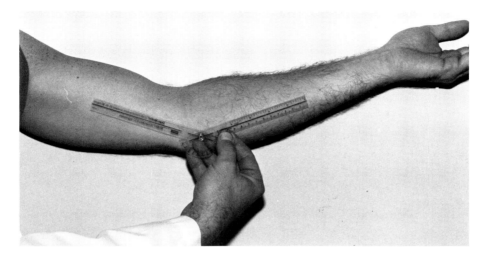

FIGURE 14.6   The goniometer for measuring joint motion.

Joint Motion

Joint motion varies from almost nil, as in the fibrous symphysis pubis, to true synovial joints such as the wrist, with a wide range of motion. Joint anatomy may be very congruous, as in the ball-and-socket configuration of the hip joint, or relatively unconstrained, as in the shoulder joint. The more constrained the bony architecture the less important are ligaments, and vice versa, in providing stability.

We are all aware of persons who are "double jointed," some of whom can perform tricks and position their joints in unusual positions. There is probably some genetic factor that determines an individual's degree of ligamentous laxity. Gymnasts depend on repetitive stretching and conditioning exercises to develop the suppleness and extra joint mobility they require. Pathologic hyperlaxity of joints is found in Ehlers-Danlos syndrome and Marfan's syndrome. Congenital absence of the cruciate ligaments will present with excessive mobility of knee at birth. Traumatic rupture of the posterior cruciate and posterior knee capsule will allow for excessive back knee motion. Children tend to be more lax than adults, and there is marked individual variation in persons of similar age.

Simple mechanical hinges merely flex and extend. Human joints move with a variety of complex kinematic interactions of the joint surfaces that may include flexion, extension, rolling, sliding, axial rotation, and variable axises and centers of rotation. During physical examination we can simplify this by just measuring the arc of motion in a single plane with the use of a goniometer (Figure 14.6).

By convention, the resting or zero position of our joints is the anatomic position, standing with arms at side as in the military position of attention.

Normal joint motion is painless, smooth, and silent. Painful joint motion can be due to problems within the joint, such as synovitis, or to abnormalities in periarticular structures, such as supraspinatus tendinitis of the shoulder. Severe pain accompanies the slightest joint motion and, in cases of septic arthritis where the joint is usually held in a position that allows maximum capacity, slight flexion. In tendinitis, active motion against resistance in the line of the affected tendon is quite painful and restricted whereas gentle passive motion is less restricted.

Obviously, the absence of active joint motion with normal passive motion after trauma may indicate a complete rupture of a tendon. Ruptures of the rotator cuff, quadriceps tendon, and patellar tendon will often show a discrepancy between active and passive motion. Rupture of the Achilles tendon can be masked by the ability of the long toe flexors to weakly flex the ankle joint. The brachialis muscle can likewise flex the elbow after rupture of the biceps tendon.

Limitation of active and passive motion can be caused by intra-articular and extra-articular fibrosis or loose bodies within the joint. A torn knee meniscus will act like a loose body if it is displaced and wedged between the articular surfaces of the femoral and tibial condyles. Exhuberant hypertrophied synovium or a large joint effusion may itself be a mechanical impediment to complete range of motion and may even cause subluxation.

Some joints will occasionally sublux during normal activity. This is most often seen in lateral subluxation of the patella or in anterior subluxation of the shoulder joint. The sudden, although minor, displacement can be very painful and cause a person to fall down or drop an object.

Lesser degrees of irregularity of joint motion that can be palpated are usually described as crepitation. This is associated with softening and irregularity of the normally smooth, glistening articular cartilage. Chondromalacia of the patella is a common condition that often demonstrates crepitation during the last 30 degrees of knee extension.

Other clicks and noises around joints can occur as tendons move over the joint margins. A fine crepitation from tendinitis may be best appreciated using a stethoscope over the affected tendon.

PHYSICAL EXAMINATION

Examination of the Cervical Spine

Cervical spine motion combines the movements in each of the seven cervical vertebrae and their associated joints. The ovoid atlanto-occipital joints contribute a major share of the "yes" nodding motion, and the atlantoaxial articulation provides a significant degree of lateral rotation. The latter is measured in degrees from neutral in a horizontal plane as if you were looking down on the head using the nose as one arm of a goniometer. Cervical extension is estimated in degrees of elevation of an imaginary line between the ear and eye. Flexion is measured in inches or finger breadths between the chin and sternum. Lateral bending of the head toward the shoulder is calculated in degrees of motion or distance from the ear lobe to the tip of the shoulder.

With acute cervical pain there is usually significant restriction of motion and a decrease in the normal cervical lordotic curve. The spinous processes of C-2 and T-1 are most prominent in the midline posteriorly. Deep palpation anterolaterally locates the carotid tubercle, the anterolateral mass of C-6, which is used as a surgical landmark.

Spurling's sign is positive when the head is gently rotated very slightly beyond the patient's active lateral motion and the shoulder or neck symptoms are reproduced (Figure 14.7). Pain arising in the cervical structures will be aggravated by careful manual downward pressure on the head and relieved by gentle upward traction. Adson's test, turning the head toward the abducted and elevated arm, reproduces the patient's radicular symptoms when it is due to compression of the lower cervical nerve roots between the scalenus anticus muscle and the first rib or a cervical rib (Figure 14.8).

351

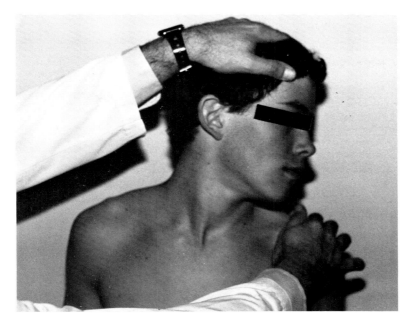

FIGURE 14.7   Spurling's sign.

FIGURE 14.8   Adson's test.

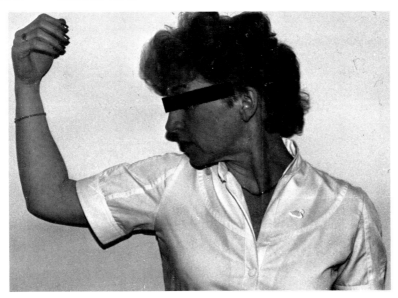

The first cervical root courses between the occiput and C-1. There are eight cervical nerve roots but only seven cervical vertebrae, so that below the cervical spine the nerve roots exit below the vertebrae of identical number. A herniated disc between C-5 and C-6 will compress the sixth root, causing pain, paresthesias, and numbness chiefly in the thumb and index finger; weakness of biceps contraction; and a diminished biceps reflex. The seventh cervical root will be affected by herniation of a disc between C-6 and C-7, resulting in weakness of the triceps muscle and a decreased triceps reflex.

Pain originating in the cervical spine may be referred to several areas, including the vertebral border of the scapula, the occipital area, and the shoulder, arm, and chest. Cervical spine pain that radiates to the shoulder will not be associated with significant shoulder stiffness or shoulder tenderness. Occasionally the extremes of shoulder motion may put traction on the cervical roots to the arm and thus reproduce the pain. Chronic neck pain that radiates to the shoulder and arm can give rise to "trigger points" in the shoulder and arm that reproduce the pain pattern on palpation but do not represent true sites of pathology. They may confuse the examiner trying to localize the origin of the symptoms.

Obviously in acute injuries of the spine the range of motion and tests of function are withheld until adequate x-ray studies have been performed to rule out fractures and dislocations.

Examination of the Back

The thoracic spine and the sacrum present a posterior convexity or kyphotic curve, whereas the lumbar spine is concave posteriorly or lordotic, as is the cervical spine. Abnormal increase of these curvatures can have various etiologies. Congenital failure of formation of the anterior portion of a thoracic vertebra will lead to localized kyphotic deformity, or gibbus, that is palpable and visible on inspection. Fractures, infection, or neoplasm may also lead to abnormal kyphosis by compression or destruction of one or more vertebral bodies.

Although kyphosis and lordosis describe curvatures in the sagittal plane when viewing the patient from the side, there is normally no curvature of the spine in the coronal plane when looking at the patient from the front or back. Any such lateral curvature of the spine is termed scoliosis. Accompanying the lateral bending of the spine is a rotation of the vertebrae and the paraspinal muscles that can be seen when the patient bends forward. The uneven height of the paraspinal soft tissues indicates the site and degree of scoliosis and is the earliest physical finding to look for. Most cases of scoliosis are idiopathic and occur during adolescence, progressing during periods of rapid growth. A smaller number of scoliosis cases occur with congenital vertebral anomalies, neuro-muscular disorders, or following radiation.

There are forms of scoliosis that are nonstructural and that do not show rotation. These can be found with poor posture, leg length discrepancy. and secondary to the pain of an acute herniated disc. Scoliosis in these cases can be corrected by improving posture, correcting the leg length discrepancy, or treating the acute disc problem.

When examining the back, indicate the motions of flexion, extension, and lateral bending. The angle at the waist between the upper torso and a vertical axis indicates the degrees of motion. Flexion of the back can also be measured by the distance in centimeters from the fingertips to the floor at full flexion or whether the patient can touch the knees, legs, or toes. It is easy to see that a patient with a very stiff back might still be able to bend over quite well by merely flexing at the hip joints. In ankylosing spondylitis there may be complete bony ankylosis of the

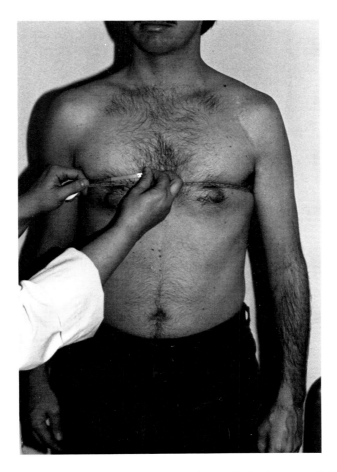

FIGURE 14.9   Measuring chest expansion for ankylosing spondylitis.

spine. By marking the back at the level of the first sacral spine and 10 cm above this and measuring that same interval with the patient fully flexed, the interval may be seen to increase to 15 cm in a normal spine but very little in the diseased spine.

Measure chest expansion just above the nipple line (Figure 14.9). It may be restricted to less than 2.5 cm because the costovertebral articulations are affected by ankylosing spondylitis. Ankylosing spondylitis primarily affects the sacroiliac joints. Patrick's test is painful. The hip and knee are abducted and the foot is placed just above the knee of the unaffected side. The thigh is pressed slightly out into more abduction, causing stress on the sacroiliac joint and pain if it is inflamed.

Palpate the spine for tenderness. Disease processes that primarily affect the vertebrae will show tenderness to palpation or percussion of the spinous processes. The paraspinal soft tissues will be more tender with musculoligamentous sprains or disc pathology. In severe trauma to the spine, palpate for soft tissue swelling and hematoma between the spinous processes. This finding indicates severe spinal injury and possible instability.

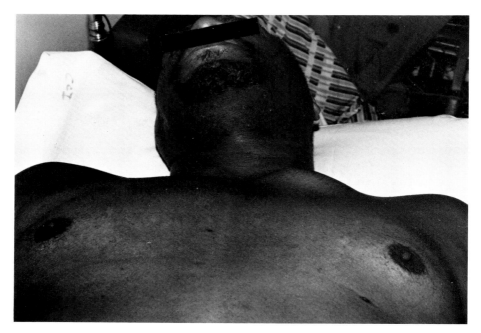

FIGURE 14.10   **Anterior sternoclavicular dislocation.**

Herniation of the intervertebral disc between the third and fourth lumbar vertebrae will cause weakness of the quadriceps and a depressed knee reflex due to pressure on the fourth lumbar root. Herniation between the fourth and fifth vertebrae will depress the posterior tibial reflex and cause weakness of great toe extension. The first sacral root is primarily affected by the L-5-S-1 disc herniation, showing a hypoactive ankle reflex and weakness of plantar flexion of the foot.

The acute nerve root pain in these syndromes is made worse by movements that put stretch on the sciatic nerve. In Lasègue's sign the leg is raised with the knee straight until the pain is reduplicated. It is lowered slightly and the foot is sharply dorsiflexed, again reproducing the pain pattern. The pain of pylonephritis, cholecystitis, pancreatitis, esophagitis, and posterior peptic ulcers all can be referred to the midback level. Cystitis and gynecologic pathology often refer pain to the lower lumbar spine and may be worse during menstruation.

Examination of the Shoulder

Observe the contours of the shoulder region both anteriorly and posteriorly. With the patient seated, inspect the shoulders from above and behind, comparing the affected side to the normal shoulder. In anterior dislocations of the glenohumeral joint, the normal rounded shape of the deltoid muscle is flattened. With dislocations of the sternoclavicular joint, the deformity at the medial end of the clavicle is best seen looking from below upward at the supine patient (Figure 14.10). In severe disruptions of the acromioclavicular joint there will be swelling of the joint and a drooping of the acromion in relation to the clavicle that can be masked by muscle spasm as well as the swelling. Standing radiographs of the acromioclavicular joint with the patient holding weights may be necessary to demonstrate the acute ac-romioclavicular separation.

The posterior aspect of the shoulder may show abnormalities in the contours of the trapezius, supraspinatus, and infraspinatus muscles. Congenital elevation of the scapula in Sprengel's deformity is due to failure of normal descent of the shoulder elements during fetal development. There is prominence of the trapezius muscle due to either scar tissue or an omovertebral bone connecting the scapula to the cervical vertebrae. The scapula is foreshortened and there is diminution of normal scapular rotation and abduction.

"Winging" of the scapula, or prominence of the vertebral border of the scapula, is associated with injury to the long thoracic nerve. Paralysis of the serratus anterior muscle, which it enervates, causes weakness of shoulder protraction. The winged scapula is seen best when the patient leans forward with his/her hands on the wall. Abnormal prominence of the scapula may also be caused by an osteo-chondroma (a benign tumor) located on the undersurface of the scapula.

Palpate the sternoclavicular and acromioclavicular joints in their subcutaneous position. The acromioclavicular joint is often the site of minor trauma that may lead to degenerative arthritis. The clavicle is entirely subcutaneous, and fractures of the clavicle can be easily identified by palpation. Tenderness in the supra-clavicular and infraclavicular fossae is associated with painful conditions of the brachial plexus. The tendon of the long head of the biceps can be rolled beneath the fingers deep to the interval between the deltoid and pectoralis muscle. The coracoid process is palpable approximately 3 cm medial to the acromioclavicular joint and 1 cm inferior to the clavicle. Tenderness just lateral to the coracoid process is found in the "impingement syndrome." In activities such as swimming, the coracoacromial ligament impinges on the rotator cuff as the arm is repeatedly elevated overhead. With chronic impingement, calcific nodules may occur within the rotator cuff that are the site of exquisite point tenderness and are often seen on x-ray.

Elevation of the arm combines the synchronous movement of four joints—the sternoclavicular, acromioclavicular, glenohumeral, and scapulothoracic joints. Raising the outstretched arm fully overhead 180 degrees includes 120 degrees of motion in the glenohumeral joint and 60 degrees of scapulothoracic rotation. If the scapula is restricted from moving, only 120 degrees of abduction can be ac-complished. During full shoulder abduction the clavicle tilts 30 degrees upward, half of which is provided by axial rotation of this crank-shaped bone.

For simplicity's sake, movements of the shoulder are described by the angular relationship of the arm to the trunk. A normal shoulder will usually allow 180 degrees of forward elevation and abduction. Tears of the rotator cuff cause a discrepancy in the active and passive range of forward elevation and side abduction. There may be only 70 degrees of active abduction while passively the arm can be fully elevated overhead. External rotation of the shoulder is measured with the arm by the side and elbow flexed 90 degrees. Zero degrees is the position with the hand pointing straight ahead, and progressive degrees of external rotation occur as the hand is moved laterally. Internal rotation is limited by movement of the hand against the trunk, so that the best description of internal rotation is the height to which the patient can place the thumb in the midline posteriorly (Figure 14.11). A condition of adhesive capsulitis or "frozen shoulder" causes severe restriction of internal rotation so that the patient may only be able to touch the gluteal crease.

Examination of the shoulder in the newborn infant includes observation for partial or complete absence of the clavicle, birth fractures of the clavicle, brachial plexus injury and partial absence of the pectoralis major. The newborn with a frac-ture of the clavicle or humerus will avoid moving the arm because of pain. This

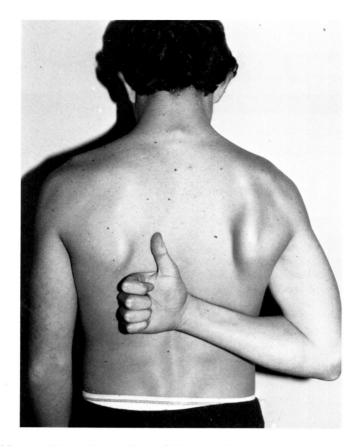

FIGURE 14.11   Internal rotation of the shoulder.

pseudoparalysis is only differentiated from a true brachial plexus injury by close observation, gentle physical examination, and roentgenographic study.

Congenital pseudoarthrosis of the clavicle is a developmental failure of union between the two clavicular growth centers. It is always found in the right clavicle and, unlike acute birth fractures, is not painful, so there is no associated pseudoparalysis of the arm.

Neuropathic joint disease is not uncommon in the shoulder. A patient with known diabetes or syringomyelia may present with a swollen, unstable, crepitant shoulder that is relatively pain free. Radiographs will show extensive destruction of the joint and soft tissue calcification.

Pain arising in the cervical spine often radiates to the shoulder. The distinguishing feature of shoulder pain is that it does not radiate up to the neck nor usually does it radiate below the elbow. Movement of the neck should not aggravate pain that arises from the shoulder. However certain movements of the shoulder may put stretch on the cervical nerve roots and exacerbate cervical root pain. Shoulder pain that radiates below the elbow with paresthesias extending into the fingers is more likely due to cervical radiculitis. Most shoulder conditions cause pain and tenderness in the anterior and lateral aspect of the shoulder, whereas cervical spine pain is frequently referred to the posterior aspect of the shoulder, especially along the vertebral border of the scapula.

Pain originating from the apical lung pleura will cause shoulder pain. Consider apical lung carcinoma in the older patient with shoulder pain and a history of smoking.

The diaphragm is supplied by the third, fourth, and fifth cervical nerve roots. Cholecystitis, pneumonia, or pulmonary infarction may irritate the diaphragmatic pleura and refer pain to the shoulder.

Examination of the Elbow

The range of motion in the normal elbow is from full extension to 135 degrees of flexion. In some loose-jointed individuals and children there is five to ten degrees of hyperextension. With the arm extended, there is normally a valgus inclination of 5 to 15 degrees at the elbow. This carrying angle is slightly greater in women. Pronation and supination involve rotation of the proximal and distal radius about the fixed ulna and are measured with the elbows at the side flexed 90 degrees. The zero or neutral position is with the palms facing medially and the thumbs up. Supination involves rotating the forearm and turning the palms up; in pronation the palms turn down. There is frequently 80 degrees of pronation and 80 degrees of supination.

Injuries involving the proximal or distal radioulnar joint will limit pronation and supination. If a young child is lifted suddenly by the arm, the annular ligament of the proximal radius may sublux partially over the head of the radius, causing the child to hold the arm slightly flexed and pronated. This "nursemaid's elbow" is often cured when the x-ray technician extends and supinates the elbow to obtain an x-ray film, resulting in repositioning of the annular ligament in normal position.

The bony landmarks of the flexed elbow form an equilateral triangle between the medial and lateral humeral epicondyles with the point of the olecranon. When the elbow is extended a straight line can be drawn through these points. A displaced supracondylar fracture of the distal humerus will not alter the relationship of these landmarks, whereas a dislocation of the elbow will significantly distort this equilateral triangle.

Ruptures of the biceps tendon will change the relationship of the biceps muscle contour to the elbow. If the disruption is through the distal biceps insertion, the muscle mass will appear displaced proximally. If the rupture is to the proximal origin of the biceps, the muscle mass will be displaced toward the elbow.

Normally a subcutaneous bursa allows the skin over the olecranon to be mobile. However, with trauma the bursa can fill with fluid and form a large, soft, tender swelling on the dorsum of the elbow.

Palpation behind the medial epicondyle will reveal the ulnar nerve. Tapping over the ulnar nerve will cause paresthesias in the ring and small fingers when there is entrapment of the nerve at the elbow. The radial head can be felt to rotate on the lateral side of the elbow just distal to the lateral epicondyle. In subtle nondisplaced fractures of the radial head there will be exquisite tenderness at this site, and there may be palpable fluid within the elbow joint noted as a fluctuant swelling just posterior to the radial head.

The origin of the forearm extensor group of muscles is the lateral humeral epicondyle. In tennis elbow, with the abnormal stress at this site, there is tenderness at the epicondyle or just distal to it over the radial head. If the patient attempts to maintain extension of the wrist against resistance, the pain is usually increased. With repetitive flexion of the wrist, a painful condition of the medial epicondyle can occur. Little League pitchers who attempt to throw curve balls with accentuated wrist action can develop this "Little Leaguer's elbow" or medial epicondylitis.

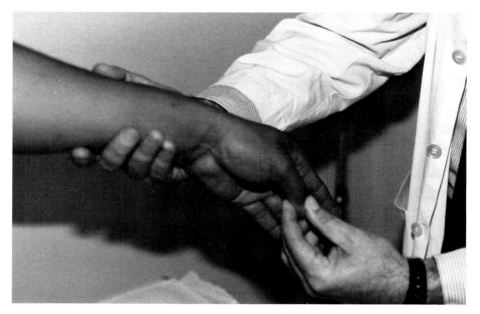

FIGURE 14.12   Testing for de Quervain's tendinitis.

Supracondylar fractures of the distal humerus are very common in children. There often is severe displacement with the injury. To reduce the fracture the normal carrying angle of the distal humerus must be achieved. If the fracture is allowed to heal with the distal fragment tilting medially, a so-called gunstock deformity, or cubitus varus, will occur. If the fracture is tilted laterally there will be abnormal cubitus valgus, or an increase in the normal carrying angle. It is possible for this to cause a delayed or tardy ulnar palsy as a result of stretch on the ulnar nerve.

Examination of the Hand and Wrist

The hand can be considered a complex biologic machine with which we can wield a hammer or play a fine instrument. It represents the main sensory organ of the musculoskeletal system. Blind persons "see with their hands." The hand may reveal information about the patient's general health, such as the pale color of the nailbed in anemia and the clubbing of the fingernails in chronic pulmonary disease.

From the neutral position the wrist can be flexed or extended almost 80 degrees. There is also radial and ulnar deviation, measuring the degrees of angulation along the second metacarpal. Circumduction or rotation of the hand is a combination of all of the above movements.

The major motor units of the hand come from the muscles of the forearm. The intrinsic muscles act to stabilize and refine the movements.

There are six dorsal compartments for the extensor tendons, whereas all of the flexor tendons except for the palmaris longus pass through the volar carpal canal with the median nerve.

Stenosis of the first dorsal compartment is found in de Quervain's disease, involving the abductor pollicis longus and the extensor pollicis brevis tendons. Passive flexion of the thumb causes increased pain in this condition (Figure 14.12). Compression of the median nerve in the volar compartment will cause pain and

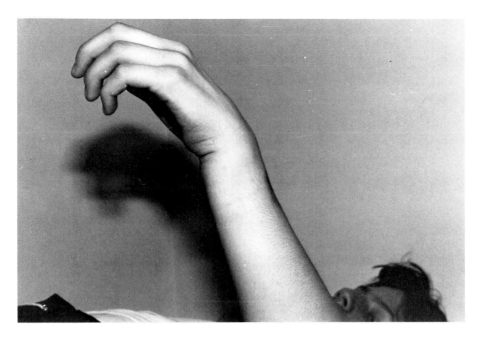

FIGURE 14.13   Silver fork deformity in a fracture of the distal radius.

paresthesia in the distribution of the median nerve from the thumb to the radial half of the ring finger. There may be atrophy of the thenar muscles supplied by the median nerve through its recurrent motor branch.

Wrist sprains are uncommon. Trauma to the wrist in elderly persons causes a fracture of the distal radius (Colles' fracture). The silver fork deformity is caused by dorsal angulation and displacement of the distal fragment of the radius (Figure 14.13). In younger persons a wrist injury may cause a fracture of the carpal scaphoid. There is tenderness in the anatomic snuff box on the radial side of the wrist between the extensor pollicis longus and the tendons of the first dorsal compartment. In growing children a fall on the wrist usually causes a fracture through the distal growth plate of the radius. If this is nondisplaced the radiograph will appear normal but the site of the growth plate will be tender.

Extensive movement of the thumb is necessary for opposition of the thumb to the individual fingers. The saddle-type joint at the base of the thumb metacarpal allows this wide range of motion—including rotation, flexion-extension, abduction, and adduction. Thumb movement in the plane of the palm is described as flexion and extension. Motion perpendicular to the plane of the palm is thumb abduction and adduction. Opposition is a combination of these maneuvers in bringing the thumb to oppose the individual fingers. Flexion and extension of the thumb interphalangeal joint is achieved solely by the long thumb flexor and extensor, whereas movement of the base of the thumb is through a combination of the forearm thumb muscles as well as the hypothenar muscles. In lesions of the ulnar nerve, which supplies the adductor pollicis brevis, thumb adduction is weakened so that when an attempt is made to grasp a piece of paper between the thumb and index finger, the thumb is acutely flexed at the interphalangeal joint (Froment's sign).

Laceration of the median and ulnar nerves in the distal forearm produces a claw hand deformity. There is denervation of the intrinsic hand muscles that normally

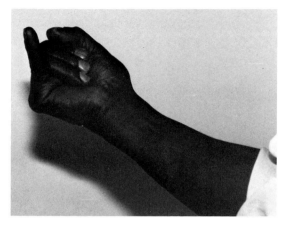

FIGURE 14.14   Old laceration of sublimus and profundus tendons to finger. Intrinsic muscles can flex the metacarpophalangeal joint.

flex the metacarpophalangeal joints and extend the interphalangeal joints. If only the ulnar nerve is affected there will be clawing of just the ring and small fingers, because the median nerve innervates the lumbrical intrinsic muscles to the index and long fingers.

Range of motion of the finger joints can be measured individually with a small goniometer. An easier and more functional assessment measures the distance between the fully flexed finger pulp and the distal palmar crease. Two flexor tendons supply each of the second through fifth fingers. The superficialis tendon flexes the proximal interphalangeal joint and the profundus tendon flexes the distal interphalangeal joint (Figure 14.14).

The integrity of the profundus tendon is noted by active flexion of the distal interphalangeal joint in each finger. By holding the fingers in extension the common profundus muscle belly of the ulnar three digits is blocked. Superficialis function can be examined by individually flexing each finger at the proximal joint.

The long extensor tendons of the index through small finger are joined by the intrinsic muscles to form an extensor hood. This divides into a central slip that extends the interphalangeal joint, and two lateral bands. The lateral bands combine to form a central tendon that extends the distal interphalangeal joint. Inability to fully extend either of these joints indicates injury of the extensor hood at the respective levels. Disruption of the extensor mechanism at the distal finger joint may occur with blunt injury to the fingertip. With this "mallet finger" there is a flexion deformity and inability to extend the distal joint. Alternately, a jammed finger can result in a boutonnière deformity if the central slip is avulsed at the proximal joint. There will be progressive flexion deformity and inability to extend the proximal interphalangeal joint.

Rupture of the ulnar collateral ligament of the thumb metacarpophalangeal joint occurs in skiing when the thumb is forcefully abducted by the ski pole and strap in a fall. In severe cases there is swelling over the ligament and instability of the joint in full extension with valgus stress. This is best demonstrated by comparison of a stress radiograph with one on the normal side.

The Allen test is performed to determine adequacy of the radial and ulnar arteries. The patient makes a tight fist and pressure is applied over both the radial and ulnar arteries at the wrist. The hand is opened and the skin appears very pale. Pressure over one artery is released and prompt refilling of the skin's capillaries is seen. The test is repeated by releasing pressure from the other artery. Failure of refilling may indicate thrombosis of one artery that might have occurred with previous trauma or arterial catheterization. A similar test can be performed in each finger to test for digital artery competence.

A trigger finger or snapping sensation as the finger is flexed and extended is due to a localized swelling in the flexor tendon where it enters the confined tendon sheath volar to the metacarpophalangeal joint. This can be an isolated entity or may be associated with rheumatoid arthritis.

A ganglion presents as a cystic nodule most commonly on the dorsal aspect of the wrist that varies in size and is quite mobile beneath the skin. It is filled with a gelatinous fluid and may or may not connect with the wrist joint itself. Similar but smaller cysts occur on the flexor sheath volar to the metacarpophalangeal joints, where they can be quite tender.

Dupuytren's contracture is a thickening and tightening of the palmar fascia with strands of fibrous tissue extending into the fingers, causing variable flexion deformities of the fingers. It predominantly affects the fourth and fifth fingers.

Examination of the Hip

Hip discomfort is usually located in the groin with radiation along the medial thigh to the knee. This referred pain is in the distribution of the obturator nerve, which sends a sensory branch to the hip. Tenderness of the hip capsule is found just lateral to the femoral pulse on a line between the anterior–superior iliac spine and the pubic symphysis. A painful bursitis can be located by palpation just lateral to the greater trochanter. Its location will move anterior and posterior with internal and external rotation of the femur, respectively. Pain elicited by palpation posterior to the hip joint is more likely to be related to an imflamed sciatic nerve as it exits the pelvis through the sciatic notch.

Hip motions include flexion, extension, adduction, abduction, and internal and external rotation. The pelvis should be steadied while determining hip motion; otherwise even an arthrodesed or fused hip will appear to be moveable. Flex both knees up toward the chest for the extent of hip flexion. Keep one knee on the chest while extending the opposite knee to test for a flexion contracture (this maneuver is known as Thomas' test [Figure 14.15]). Abduction, adduction, and internal and external rotation of the hip can be examined with the hip extended or flexed provided the pelvis is not allowed to move. An assistant can place his or her hands on the anterior iliac spines to steady the pelvis.

Examination of the hip is a vital element in the routine examination of every newborn. To examine a left hip, the examiner's left hand steadies the pelvis while the right thumb is placed on the inner side of the left thigh and the index and long fingers are placed over the greater trochanter. Keeping the knee flexed, the thigh is gently adducted and abducted. With hip instability the femoral head will sublux or dislocate posteriorly during the adduction maneuver. If the hip is fully dislocated a click or soft clunk will be sensed as the hip relocates on abduction. These physical findings are present in the first few days after birth, but as soon as the hip tissues tighten up the only sign may be limitation of abduction, which in the infant should be almost 80 or 85 degrees. If congenital hip dysplasia is diagnosed and treated early, most patients will develop a normal hip. If treatment is delayed, persistent subluxation or dislocation will lead to painful degenerative arthritis in early middle age.

Two other conditions in children that present with an antalgic hip lurch are Perthes disease, or avascular necrosis of the femoral head, and slipped capital

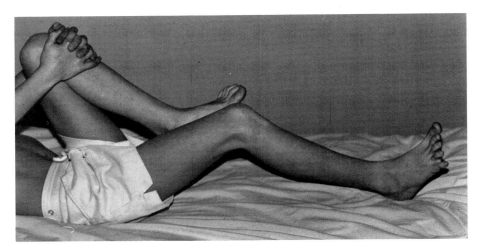

FIGURE 14.15   Thomas' test.

femoral epiphysis. The former is most common in boys between ages 4 and 8 following an episode of synovitis of the hip. Slipped epiphysis occurs most often in the rapidly growing adolescent due to weakness of the proximal epiphyseal growth plate. There is a posterior and varus tilting of the proximal epiphysis. The patient is either very tall and thin, indicating a very rapid growth spurt, or obese with undeveloped genitalia, indicating some hormone imbalance. The patient walks with an antalgic gait with the limb in external rotation. There is limitation of flexion and as the hip is flexed the thigh tends to go into external rotation.

Traumatic hip dislocation occurs in major high-speed motor vehicle accidents. With posterior dislocation the anterior capsule is intact, causing the hip to present in a position of flexion and adduction. With anterior dislocation the hip is abducted and externally rotated. A thorough examination of neuromuscular function is necessary because approximately 10% of hip dislocations are complicated by injury to the sciatic nerve.

Elderly individuals complaining of pain in the hip after a fall may have suffered either a fracture of one or both of the pubic rami or one of two types of hip fractures, a femoral neck fracture or an intertrochanteric hip fracture. Displaced hip fractures demonstrate shortening and external rotation deformity, best noted by comparing the position of the feet with the patient supine (Figure 14.16). External rotation of the extremity with a hip fracture is due to the effect of gravity and the psoas muscle acting as an external rotator of the hip after loss of continuity between the femoral head and the upper femur. The shortening associated with hip fractures is due to the upward migration of the femur and the varus tilting of the femoral neck.

In the normal femur there is 15 degrees of anterior tilt or anteversion of the femoral neck from the coronal plane of the distal femur. Increase of this femoral anteversion will tend to internally rotate the lower limb and is one cause for an intoeing gait in a child. Physical examination will show excessive internal rotation of the hip (Figure 14.17) in extension compared to external rotation (Figure 14.18). Usually in a child internal and external rotation are approximately equal.

Congenital partial or complete absence of the proximal femur is termed proximal femoral focal deficiency. The leg length discrepancy may be so severe that the foot of the affected extremity is at the level of the normal knee (Figure

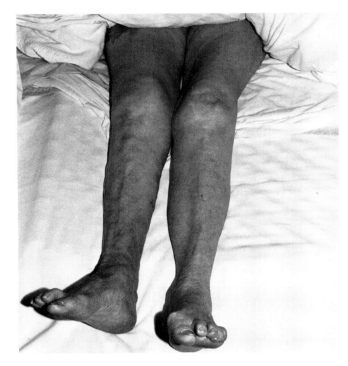

FIGURE 14.16   External rotation and shortening in a displaced femoral neck
fracture.

FIGURE 14.17   Increased internal rotation of the hip in femoral anteversion.

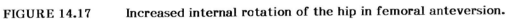

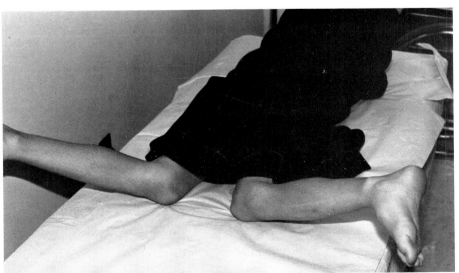

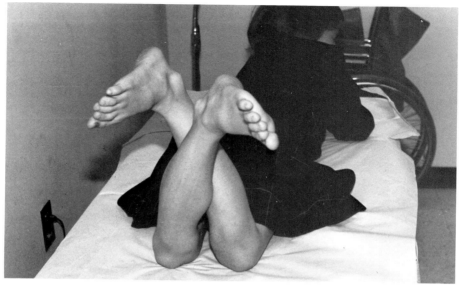

FIGURE 14.18   Decreased external rotation of hip in femoral anteversion.

14.19). Treatment often requires amputation of the foot and fitting of a prosthetic leg.

Examination of the Knee

The knee joint appears to flex as a simple hinged joint through a range of 135 degrees of flexion. However, there are many complex subtleties that occur during this motion, including 15 to 20 degrees of external rotation in the tibia during flexion and the converse in extension. There is both rolling and sliding motion of the femoral condyles on the tibial plateaus and menisci during this motion. The center of rotation is constantly changing.

The weight bearing or mechanical axis of the extremity passes through the center of the knee from the hip joint to the ankle. Since the femoral head is off-set from the shaft of the femur, there must be a physiologic valgus angle of approximately 7 degrees between the long axis of the femoral shaft and the tibia in the normal knee. When this physiologic angle is increased there is genu valgus, or knock-knee deformity. When there is decrease in the normal tibiofemoral angle there is genu varum, or bowlegged deformity. The degree of varus or valgus deformity can be measured with a goniometer along the anterior aspect of the extremity. A standing anteroposterior radiograph of the knee gives the most accurate assessment of knee alignment.

Blood, pus, or excessive synovial fluid in the knee joint will distend the synovial cavity, especially the suprapatellar pouch, which extends four finger breadths above the patella. This suprapatellar swelling is easily seen. If one hand is placed over the suprapatellar pouch, the fluid is forced into the retropatellar area. The patella then can be palpated and felt to ballotte against the anterior femoral condyles (Figure 14.20). Baker's cyst presents as a palpable swelling in the posterior aspect of the knee (Figure 14.21). It may be due to a distended bursa or may connect to the knee joint and be associated with a torn meniscus or chondromalacia of the patella. The size of the cyst may vary and when it is large it may cause

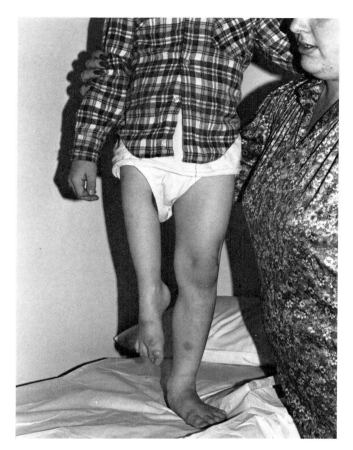

FIGURE 14.19   Proximal femoral focal deficiency.

limitation of flexion and extension because of its mechanical size. The cyst can be transilluminated, and aspiration produces gelatinous fluid. In older individuals an aneurysm of the popliteal artery may present as a mass in the posterior aspect of the knee. Giant synovial cysts in rheumatoid arthritis patients may rupture within the posterior calf musculature and give rise to symptoms and physical findings suggestive of deep vein thrombophlebitis.

A bursa located anterior to the patella allows for mobility of the overlying skin. In prepatellar bursitis it becomes distended with blood or synovial fluid, following repeated minor irritation or blunt knee trauma.

Cystic degeneration within the substance of the lateral meniscus will present as a mass on the anterolateral aspect of the knee joint at the level of the joint surface.

The patella is a sesamoid bone lying within the extensor mechanism and provides increased lever arm for the quadriceps muscle. Traumatic injuries of this extensor mechanism include lateral dislocation of the patella and rupture of the quadriceps tendon.

A blow to the medial side of the knee may cause partial or complete rupture of the lateral collateral ligament as the knee is opened on the lateral side. Conversely, and more often, there is a medially directed impact from the lateral side

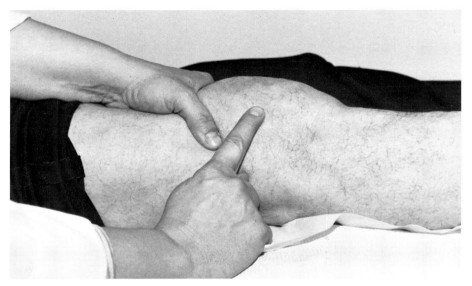

FIGURE 14.20   A knee effusion and ballottement of the patella.

or a valgus stress causing opening of the medial joint space. The medial capsule, medial collateral ligament, and even cruciate ligaments may be ruptured. With excessive anterior or posterior movements of the tibia in relationship to the femur the cruciate ligaments may be stretched or torn (Figure 14.22). The Lochmann test for cruciate stability is performed with the knee extended, one hand gripping the femur just above the knee, the other hand gripping the tibia just below the knee. Anterior and posterior movements of the tibia in relationship to the femur are evaluated and compared to the normal side. This test is especially helpful in an acute knee injury, in which it is difficult or impossible to flex the knee because of pain and swelling. The chronically injured knee can be flexed to 90 degrees and the anterior or posterior drawer sign is performed to test the anterior and posterior cruciate ligaments, respectively.

The medial collateral ligament and the lateral collateral ligament are tested by applying a valgus and varus stress to the knee while it is first in full extension and then in 30 degrees of flexion (Figure 14.23). The injured knee is compared to the normal knee. More extensive damage is indicated if the knee shows instability in full extension.

The pivot shift test is a dynamic test of anterior cruciate insufficiency and is performed with the patient rotated slightly to one side with a valgus stress on the knee. In a positive test, as the knee is flexed and extended there is a sudden displacement of the lateral tibial condyle that dramatically reproduces the patient's symptoms of instability.

A locked knee is one that will not fully extend because of interposition of a displaced fragment of meniscus or a loose body between the articular surfaces of the femoral and tibial condyles. MacMurray's sign is a clicking felt when the knee is fully flexed and then gradually extended as the tibia is rotated internally and externally. It is due to the movement of a displaced meniscus fragment between the articular surfaces. A loose body that is not causing locking may be positioned in the suprapatellar pouch, where it can be palpated.

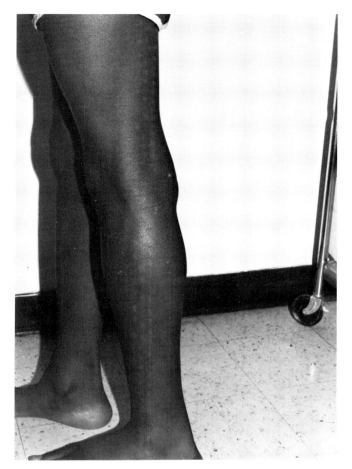

FIGURE 14.21   Baker's cyst.

The Q angle is the angle between a line drawn along the quadriceps tendon to the midpoint of the patella and a second line drawn from the midpoint of the patella to the tibial tubercle. When this angle is greater than 15 degrees there may be an excessive lateral bowstringing effect, causing recurrent lateral subluxation or dislocation of the patella. Malalignment syndromes of the patella in young persons may be a cause of chondromalacia or softening of the patellar articular cartilage. Physical examination reveals tenderness to the undersurfaces of the margins of the patella and palpable crepitations in the patellofemoral joint as the knee is fully extended. Physical diagnosis in the knee is often complemented by arthrography and arthroscopy.

Examination of the Ankle and Foot

Normally the ankle appears slightly externally rotated by 15 degrees compared with the knee axis of motion. The most common cause for intoeing deformity in infants is internal tibial torsion, so that the ankle axis is turned inward compared with the normal side. In the older child intoeing gait may be due to abnormal femoral anteversion (previously described).

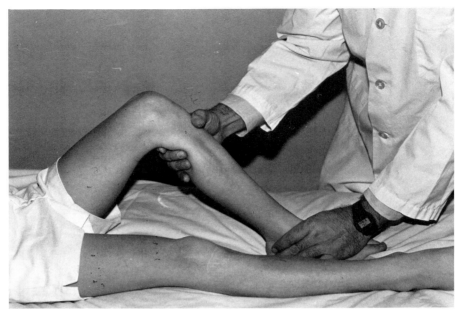

FIGURE 14.22   Testing for cruciate ligament injury.

FIGURE 14.23   Valgus stress test for medial collateral ligament injury.

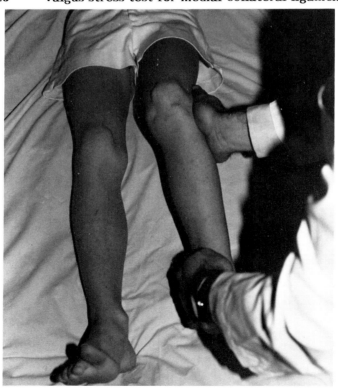

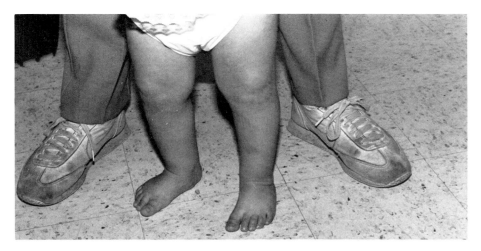

FIGURE 14.24   Metatarsus adductus and internal tibial torsion.

Ankle flexion and extension are measured in a single plane whereas pronation and supination of the foot occur through the subtalar joint and are more complex. The normal foot shows a straight medial border with a slight elevation of the medial arch. In the child a curvature of the inner border of the foot is found in metatarsus adductus. If this is associated with internal tibial torsion, the in-toeing gait is accentuated (Figure 14.24). Clubfoot deformity in a child combines inversion and adduction of the forefoot with inversion of the heel and equinus of the ankle. In untreated cases the patient eventually walks on the outer border of the foot and ankle, whereas in most treated cases there is some residual deformity with the foot appearing slightly smaller and the calf muscle slightly atrophied.

The physical examination of the acutely injured foot and ankle should include an understanding of the mechanism of injury and a general inspection as to the site of the significant swelling or deformity. An inversion type of injury while running or playing sports is most often a sprain of the anterior talofibular ligament. There will be tenderness and ecchymosis over the anterolateral aspect of the ankle. A similar injury may produce an avulsion fracture of the base of the fifth metatarsal, but the swelling and tenderness will be more inferior on the lateral border of the foot.

The characteristic history of a patient with a gastrocnemius muscle tear or ruptured heel cord is sudden severe pain in the lower leg following a forceful contraction of the gastrocnemius muscle as might occur on the tennis court reaching for a fast wide shot. The patient will often describe the feeling as one of being hit in the leg by an object. The ability to voluntarily flex the ankle and foot using the long toe flexors can mask a complete rupture of the Achilles tendon. In Thompson's test, the midportion of the posterior calf muscles is gently squeezed by the hand. If the ankle and foot flex, the Achilles tendon is intact. If they do not flex, the tendon is ruptured.

Heel spur pain occurs at the site of insertion of the plantar fascia on the bottom surface of the os calcis. The local area is tender to palpation and often there is associated pes planus, or flat foot, related to the excessive stress on the fascia. A flat foot deformity overstresses the peroneus longus tendon, causing pain and tenderness posterior to the lateral malleolus at the site where this tendon passes behind the fibula.

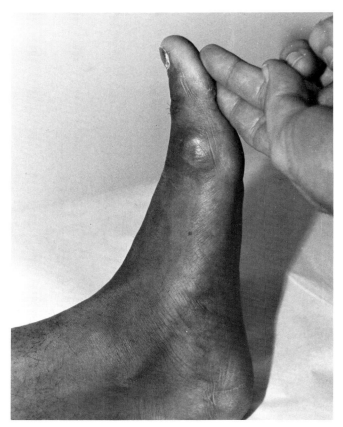

FIGURE 14.25   Hallux rigidus with restricted dorsiflexion of the great toe.

    A bunion is a valgus deformity of the great toe with prominence of the meta-
tarsal head medially. There is progressive swelling and inflammation of the overlying soft tissues, which become reddened and prominent. Lateral deviation of
the great toe causes crowding of the other toes and often overlapping of the second
toe. There will be transfer of weight bearing to the second and third metatarsal
heads and metatarsalgia. Foot pain that extends from the area of the metatarsal
heads out to between the fourth and fifth toes or the third and fourth toes can be
due to a Morton's neuroma or painful enlargement of the plantar digital nerve
between the metatarsal heads. Lateral compression of or direct pressure between
the metatarsal heads reproduces the pain. The patient will often remove his/her
shoes to obtain relief from the pain.
    Hallux rigidus is a painful stiffening of the great toe metatarsophalangeal
joint. In order to avoid stress on the joint, the patient walks on the lateral border
of the foot. There is excessive wear on the lateral aspect of the shoe. Examination
of the great toe shows increased motion at the distal interphalangeal joint, a callus
on the plantar aspect of the great toe, and very restricted dorsiflexion of the metatarsophalangeal joint that is painful (Figure 14.25). This condition is a sequelae
of sprains or fractures that involve the great toe metatarsophalangeal joint.
    Numerous foot deformities are associated with congenital or developmental
neuromuscular diseases. The actual deformity in any case depends on whether the

dorsiflexors, plantar flexors, inverters, or everters are primarily affected and whether the muscles are primarily spastic or weak. In cerebral palsy the most common deformity is equinus resulting from spasticity of the gastrocnemius and soleus muscles.

ARTHRITIS

Osteoarthritis

Osteoarthritis, also known as hypertrophic arthritis and degenerative arthritis, is the most common form of arthritis. The usual age of onset is during the fourth and fifth decade, and women are affected more often than men. Unlike inflammatory forms of joint disease, osteoarthritis is not a systemic disease but seems to affect primarily the joints of the spine and the major weight-bearing joints, especially the hip and the knee.

Osteoarthritis is usually divided into primary and secondary types. Secondary osteoarthritis can occur after any traumatic, inflammatory, circulatory, or metabolic condition that causes injury to a joint surface. If the damage is severe enough, there can be progressive wearing out and destruction of the articular surfaces. In primary osteoarthritis the etiology is unknown, but there are probably genetically determined predisposing factors.

Osteoarthritis of the cervical and lumbosacral spine is very common and often is asymptomatic. The patient may present after a minor twisting injury of the neck and show radiographic changes of a narrowed disc space, sclerosis of the joint margins, and hypertrophic spur formation. These hypertrophic spurs, by encroaching on the neural foramen, can cause arm pain with depressed reflexes and muscle weakness.

Osteoarthritis of the lumbosacral spine with narrowing of the disc spaces, erosion of the facet joints, and hypertrophic osteophytes will cause chronic or recurring back pain with episodes of sciatic-type pain. Narrowing of the spinal canal and neural foramen by hypertrophic spurs in osteoarthritis is known as spinal stenosis.

With osteoarthritic involvement of the cervical and lumbosacral spine there is diminution in the normal range of spinal motion. There are relatively painless quiescent phases, but during painful episodes or following minor trauma there will be restriction of motion and exacerbation of radicular symptoms.

Primary osteoarthritis of the hip or knee usually progresses slowly so that the patient has a gradually progressive feeling of stiffness and pain in the affected joint. The pain is exacerbated by overactivity and inclement weather. As the joint becomes more progressively involved, there is an increasing degree of rest and night pain. The course is unpredictable, with some cases plateauing and others progressing relentlessly.

In the hip joint, the progressive loss of joint space and the hypertrophic spurs cause restriction of motion with flexion and adduction deformity. In order for the patient with a severe adduction contraction to avoid crossing his legs while standing, he must elevate the affected hemipelvis. This causes an apparent shortening of the leg on the affected side. There will be a significant antalgic lurch as the patient tries to bring the center of body weight over the hip joint to reduce the joint forces during stance phase of the gait cycle. Use of a cane in the opposite hand significantly reduces the joint forces and the degree of lurch.

Osteoarthritis of the knee joint affects primarily the patellofemoral, the medial tibiofemoral, or the lateral tibiofemoral compartments. Osteoarthritis affecting the medial tibiofemoral compartment causes a progressive varus deformity and secondary stretching of the lateral ligaments, so that on weight bearing there

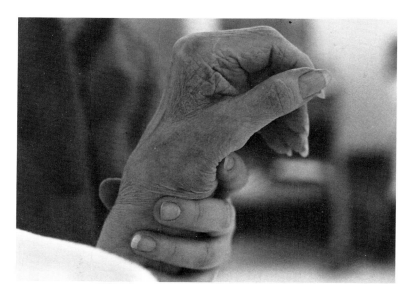

FIGURE 14.26   Swelling of the metacarpophalangeal joints in rheumatoid arthritis.

will be a lateral thrust of the knee. A valgus deformity will occur with primary involvement of the lateral tibiofemoral compartment. In any of the varied forms of osteoarthritis of the knee there are usually atrophy of the thigh muscles, hypertrophic spurs that are palpable, general enlargement of the joint, increased joint fluid, and decreased range of motion. There will be crepitation and even a grinding sound during range of motion as the exposed eburnated surface of one bone rubs on the opposing surface.

In secondary osteoarthritis following trauma or other pathologic conditions of joints, any joint can be affected, especially the ankle and wrist, which are so commonly affected by intra-articular fractures. Heberden's nodes are fusiform swellings of the distal interphalangeal joints of the fingers considered to be osteoarthritic in nature.

Rheumatoid Arthritis

Rheumatoid arthritis is the synovial joint manifestation of a chronic systemic immunologic disease. Women are affected three times more often than men, and the usual onset is in the fourth decade. The clinical course is variable. Often there is a gradual swelling and stiffness of the metacarpophalangeal and proximal interphalangeal joints of the fingers, especially the index and long fingers (Figure 14.26). Characteristically the patient complains of morning stiffness that eases up with activity but later in the day is aggravated by continuous activity. Many cases undergo a spontaneous remission after a brief period of illness leaving little or no residual joint deformity or disability. In a fewer number of cases there is a relentless progressive symmetrical involvement of the hips, knees, ankles, shoulders, elbows, wrists, hands, and feet.

There is fusiform swelling of each affected joint as a result of the profuse synovial inflammation and thickening. On palpation the joint feels warm and boggy; swelling is due to synovial thickening and effusion. In early cases limitation of motion is due to the acute pain and the increased synovial tissue and fluid within

the joint. In later cases limitation of motion is due to intra-articular fibrous adhesions and fixed contracture of the capsule and tendons. Synovial granulation
tissue (panis) migrates over the articular cartilage and erodes into the subchondral
bone. Lysosomal enzymes released from the inflamed synovium destroy the articular cartilage. The cumulative effect of loss of the joint cartilage space and the
stretching of ligaments from chronic inflammation eventually leads to instability
and malalignment. For example, a knee with valgus deformity will concentrate the
mechanical joint forces to the lateral joint compartment and cause further mechanical erosion of bone and further valgus deformity. Most chronically affected joints
will also show atrophy of the periarticular muscles and a fixed flexion deformity.

The rheumatoid hand often illustrates several pathognomonic deformities.
"Ulnar drift" is a slanting of the fingers at the metacarpophalangeal joints toward
the ulnar border of the hand. This deformity is due to a combination of the slight
ulnarward pull of the long extrinsic tendons and the effect of gravity on the
chronically swollen metacarpophalangeal joints. In swan neck deformity the proximal interphalangeal joint is hyperextended and the distal interphalangeal joint is
flexed. This is due to contracture of the intrinsic muscles. A boutonnière deformity occurs at the proximal interphalangeal joint when the extensor hood is stretched,
allowing the head of the proximal phalanx to protrude through like a button through
a hole. The lateral bands of the extensor mechanism are subluxed volarward and
lead to further flexion deformity with attempts to actively extend the interphalangeal joint. The tenosynovitis of the rheumatoid hand may lead to trigger finger
symptoms and spontaneously ruptured tendons. The swollen tenosynovium may
cause a median nerve neuropathy at the volar carpal canal.

Cervical spine involvement by rheumatoid arthritis may affect the articulation
of the first and second cervical vertebrae. Stretching of the alar and transverse
ligaments allows a forward slip of the atlas on the axis so that the odontoid
impinges on the spinal cord. Physical findings of a slowly impending quadriplegia
are masked by the patient's generalized arthritic symptoms. The key to diagnosis
of this complication is the finding of pathologic hyperactive reflexes in the extremities with a history of a recent degradation in the patient's ambulatory status. A
lateral radiograph of the cervical spine in flexion and extension will show more
than the usual 3-mm distance between the anterior odontoid and the posterior arch
of C-1.

The main features differentiating osteoarthritis from rheumatoid arthritis are
the following:

The proximal interphalangeal joints and the metacarpophalangeal joints are
more commonly involved in rheumatoid arthritis, whereas in osteoarthritis
the distal interphalangeal joints are swollen.

Periarticular osteoporosis and soft tissue atrophy are uncommon in osteoarthritis but common in rheumatoid arthritis.

Subcutaneous nodules are often found in rheumatoid arthritis along the extensor
surface of the forearm but are not seen in osteoarthritis.

Rheumatoid arthritis is a manifestation of a systemic illness, whereas osteoarthritis involves only one or a few major joints.

Weight-bearing joints are more often involved in osteoarthritis, whereas
rheumatoid arthritis involves the weight-bearing joints and the joints of
the upper extremity equally.

Rheumatoid arthritis, being an immunologic problem, is a panarthritis affecting the entire joint, whereas osteoarthritis, often mechanical in nature, may affect only the highly stressed areas of a joint.

REFERENCES

1. American Society for Surgery of the Hand: *The Hand, Examination and Diagnosis,* ed 2. New York, Churchill Livingstone, 1985.

2. American Academy of Orthopedic Surgeons: *Joint Motion Method of Measuring and Recording.* New York, Churchill Livingstone, 1984.

3. American Orthopedic Associates: *Manual of Orthopedic Surgery.* American Orthopedic Associates, 1984.

4. Dec JB, Saunders M, Inman VT, Eberhart HD: The major determinants in normal and pathological gait. *J Bone Joint Surg* 1953;35A:543-558.

5. Tachdjian, MO: *Pediatric Orthopedics.* Philadelphia, WB Saunders Co., 1972, chap I.

Index